NOTICE

Medicine is an ever-changing science. As new research and clinical experience broaden our knowledge, changes in treatment and drug therapy are required. The editor and the publisher of this work have checked with sources believed to be reliable in their efforts to provide information that is complete and generally in accord with the standards accepted at the time of publication. However, in view of the possibility of human error or changes in medical sciences, neither the editor nor the publisher nor any other party who has been involved in the preparation or publication of this work warrants that the information contained herein is in every respect accurate or complete, and they disclaim all responsibility for any errors or omissions or for the results obtained from use of the information contained in this work. Readers are encouraged to confirm the information contained herein with other sources. For example and in particular, readers are advised to check the product information sheet included in the package of each drug they plan to administer to be certain that the information contained in this work is accurate and that changes have not been made in the recommended dose or in the contraindications for administration. This recommendation is of particular importance in connection with new or infrequently used drugs.

OBESITY SURGERY

Edited by

Louis F. Martin, MD

Professor of Surgery and of Public Health and Preventative Medicine
Louisiana State University Health Sciences Center
New Orleans, Louisiana

McGRAW-HILL
Medical Publishing Division
New York / Chicago / San Francisco / Lisbon / London / Madrid / Mexico City / Milan
New Delhi / San Juan / Seoul / Singapore / Sydney / Toronto

The *McGraw·Hill* Companies

Obesity Surgery

234567890 DOCDOC 0987654

ISBN 0-07-140640-9

This book was set in Times Roman by Binghamton Valley Composition, Inc.
The editors were Marc Strauss, Kathleen McCullough, and Peter J. Boyle.
The production supervisor was Catherine Saggese.
Coughlin Indexing Services prepared the index.
R.R. Donnelley was printer and binder.

This book is printed on acid-free paper.

Library of Congress Cataloging-in-Publication Data

Obesity surgery / [edited by] Louis F. Martin.
    p. ; cm.
  Includes index.
  ISBN 0-07-140640-9
  1. Obesity—Surgery. I. Martin, Louis F., MD.
  [DNLM: 1. Obesity, Morbid—surgery. 2. Gastric Bypass—methods. 3. Gastroplasty—methods. 4. Postoperative Care—methods. 5. Peroperative Care—methods.
  WD 210 S9659 2004]
  RD540.S96 2004
  617.4'3—dc22
                                                              2003067157

Contents

CONTRIBUTORS

F. Merritt Ayad, PhD
Assistant Professor of Clinical Psychiatry
Department of Psychiatry, Section of Psychology
Louisiana State University School of Medicine
New Orleans, Louisiana
Chapter 4

Peter Benotti, MD
Valley Hospital
Ridgewood, New Jersey
Chapter 5

Simon Biron, MD
Department of Surgery
Laval University
Quebec, Canada
Chapter 12

Robert Brolin, MD
Director of Bariatric Surgery
St. Peter's University Hospital
New Brunswick, New Jersey
Adjunct Professor of Surgery
University of Pittsburgh Medical Center
Pittsburgh, Pennsylvania
Chapter 15

Merita Burney, BSN
Chief, Operating Office
Director of Nursing

St. Charles General Hospital
New Orleans, Louisiana
Chapter 8

Jiande Chen, MD
Associate Professor
Division of Gastroenterology
University of Texas Medical Center
Galveston, Texas
Chapter 13

Valerio Cigaina, MD
Unit of Digestive Surgical Electrophysiology
Umberto I Hospital
Venezia-Mestre, Italy
Chapter 13

George Cowan, Jr., MD
Emeritus Professor of Surgery
College of Medicine
University of Tennessee Health Science
  Center
Memphis, Tennessee
Chapter 16

Vonda Gaitor-Stampley, APRN, MSN
Nurse Practitioner
Weight Management Center
St. Charles General Hospital
New Orleans, Louisiana
Chapter 8

Frank L. Greenway, MD, PhD
Medical Director and Professor
Pennington Biomedical Research Center
Louisiana State University
Baton Rouge, Louisiana
Chapter 3

Scott E. Greenway, MD
Resident Surgeon
School of Medicine
University of California, Los Angeles
Los Angeles, California
Chapter 3

M. Lloyd Hiler, MD
Associate Professor of Surgery
College of Medicine
University of Tennessee Health Science Center
Memphis, Tennessee
Chapter 16

Frédéric-Simon Hould, MD
Department of Surgery
Laval University
Quebec, Canada
Chapter 12

Stéfane Lebel, MD
Department of Surgery
Laval University
Quebec, Canada
Chapter 12

Walter Lindstrom, Jr., Esq.
Obesity Law and Advocacy Center
San Diego, California
Chapter 6

Picard Marceau, MD, PhD
Department of Surgery
Laval University
Quebec, Canada
Chapter 12

Simon Marceau, MD
Department of Surgery
Laval University

Quebec, Canada
Chapter 12

Louis F. Martin, MD
Professor of Surgery and of Public Health and
  Preventative Medicine
Louisiana State University Health Sciences
  Center
New Orleans, Louisiana
Chapters 1, 2, 5, 8, 10, 14, 16, and 18

Barbara J. Moore, PhD
President and Chief Executive Officer
Shape Up America!
www.shapeup.org
Chapter 1

Ninh T. Nguyen, MD
Associate Professor of Surgery
Department of Surgery
Medical Center, University of California,
  Davis
Sacramento, California
Chapter 9

Tracy Martinez Owens, RN
Director of Program Development
Alvarado Center for Surgical Weight Control
San Diego, California
Chapter 6

Walter J. Pories, MD
Professor of Surgery and Biochemistry
Department of Surgery
Brody School of Medicine
East Carolina University
Greenville, North Carolina
Chapter 11

William J. Raum, MD, PhD
Medical Director
Weight Management Center
Associate Professor of Medicine and Surgery
Louisiana State University School of Medicine
New Orleans, Louisiana
Chapters 3, 7, 8, and 18

John Scott Roth, MD
Professor of Surgery and Biochemistry
Department of Surgery
Brody School of Medicine
East Carolina University
Greenville, North Carolina
Chapter 11

Scott A. Shikora, MD
Director, Center for Minimally Invasive Obesity
  Surgery
Tufts–New England Medical Center
Boston, Massachusetts
Chapter 13

Melinda S. Sothern, PhD
Pennington Biomedical Research Center
Louisiana State University
Baton Rouge, Louisiana
Chapter 17

John N. Udall, Jr., MD, PhD
Chief, Pediatric Gastroenterology
Department of Pediatrics
Louisiana State University Health Sciences Center
New Orleans, Louisiana
Chapter 17

Terry Wheeler, MBA
Chief, Executive Office
St. Charles General Hospital
New Orleans, Louisiana
Chapter 8

Bruce M. Wolfe, MD
Department of Surgery
Medical Center, University of California, Davis
Sacramento, California
Chapter 9

The most common question asked of bariatric surgeons is, "Why did you choose this field?" Bariatrics—the medical science for the prevention and control of obesity—is not glamorized in the press. Adolescents preparing for college or medical students preparing to choose a field for training and practice usually do not realize that it exists. Very little of our medical training, however, actually prepares us for establishing medical practices. During training we rotate among specialty services that typically last one or two months and have limited opportunity to follow patient outcomes. We usually find a field that allows us to enjoy our interaction with patients and to take pride in our work and accomplishments. Fortunately, as physicians we have as many variations in personality as there are variations in the types of practice we can establish. As a resident I enjoyed the challenge of treating trauma victims and the adrenaline rush of life and death scenarios in the operating room. In establishing a practice after residency, I found that most trauma victims have horrific memories of their experiences that inadvertently includes their treating physicians. Although the practice of treating trauma victims is very stimulating and challenging, the variability of the time requirements and the number of different operations performed make it difficult to maintain a schedule and push the envelope of your surgical skills in a direction of your choosing.

I used bariatric surgery initially as a means to develop my skills by completing challenging operations under difficult technical circumstances. However, as I followed patients after operations, I soon realized I enjoyed watching morbidly obese patients lose weight, while most of their medical problems evaporated. It was incredibly rewarding to see patients vastly improve their quality of life. Not everyone will like this type of practice. The surgical procedures do not work unless there is adequate psychological, dietary, behavioral, and exercise support so that patients can permanently change their eating and exercise habits. You must be the captain of this multidisciplinary team. The patients require long-term followup, not days to weeks but months to years. You must help them make these changes and prevent the development of complications that the procedures can create. The discrimination that society heaps on the morbidly obese will also be directed at you. Even some of your medical colleagues may hold illogical and antiscientific beliefs regarding obesity or be insensitive to people with this genetically and socially connected disease that affects over three percent of our population. Most physicians tell their patients all they have to do is "push away from the table." This level of discrimination and misunderstanding is especially embarrassing in medical and allied health professionals.

A bariatric surgical practice quickly teaches you that there is not an obese personality. Whether grouped by gender, race, or illness, obese people, like any other large group, exhibit a bell-shaped curve of characteristics. Over half of all Americans now meets criteria to be considered overweight, and one-third are obese. They need multiple treatments to choose from if they are all to be helped. If you provide these services, you can develop a very busy and rewarding practice. I am certainly happier treating my population of patients than I would be caring for people who present with headaches, backaches, hemorrhoids, or my former choice, trauma. But this is my choice, and I am glad that these other groups of patients find physicians who enjoy working with them.

The preoperative preparation and operative treatments are exciting and challenging. The recent expansion of our field to include procedures that can be accomplished laparoscopically have amplified these pleasures. I enjoy going to work—the ultimate reward if you need to work 50 to 60 hours each week to maintain your lifestyle.

This book will help you decide if you would enjoy practicing in this field. It can also help any physician or allied health worker better understand why the surgical treatment of morbid obesity is not only justified but cost-effective and the best treatment available. Chapters trace the evolution of the field to its current state and provide complete explanations of the major accepted procedures and some of the evolving therapies. The text outlines what is involved in setting up the outpatient office, the special needs of patients who are hospitalized for operations, and how to monitor and treat patients short- and long-term to minimize the complication rate. Data is presented to explain how obesity develops, the physiological and psychological changes that morbidly obese patients undergo after surgery, and how to treat complications or outcome failures.

Starting this type of practice is somewhat akin to starting an organ transplantation program. The treatment requires a multidisciplinary team of professionals and substantial costs for a hospital to purchase the extra equipment to treat patients who exceed the weight limits of most hospital equipment. (Patients over 300 pounds cannot use regular hospital beds, operating room tables, gowns, etc.) The surgeon needs the full support of the hospital administration and the full support of the hospital's medical staff and the allied health professionals who will work with these patients. This needs to be contracted in advance, not as you develop problems that require outside expertise. Programs that start without this support often are shut down after the first complications develop and surprised colleagues are asked to intervene in a situation where malpractice risk is already present.

It is difficult to run a part-time bariatric surgical practice while also having substantial involvement in other fields. This is especially important to note for recent residency graduates who want to develop expertise in several areas of laparoscopic surgery while bariatric procedures provide the base income. This can work as an established practice adds new members devoted at least part time to other specialties but who also cover their bariatric team members on-call and assist in the operating room. The field of bariatric surgery is relatively understaffed compared to the number of patients eligible for treatment. Once starting to perform bariatric surgery, a large volume of patients may quickly find you. Maintaining another area of expertise, unless you have other interested surgeons willing to help with the practice, becomes difficult.

It is also much more difficult to obtain medical insurance clearance to proceed with bariatric operations than it is for any other commonly performed general surgical procedure (except for the special clearances needed to perform organ transplantation). This is again because society allows the medical insurance industry to discriminate in a way that is not acceptable in most other diseases. Probably fewer than half the people who qualify as candidates for surgery using National Institutes of Health guidelines (established through multiple separate consensus conferences) have medical insurance that will cover these procedures. This is slowly changing as the insurance industry's ridiculous claim that obesity is a cosmetic condition rather than a medical disease is countered by documentation that obesity is the second leading cause of death in our society. It still requires considerable effort (one full-time employee equivalent in an office) to obtain insurance approval for a bariatric surgeon(s) to perform 4 to 30 cases per month. Most bariatric surgeons feel that competence is developed and maintained only if one is performing 20 to 50 cases per year.

This book attempts to outline the positive and the negative aspects of the surgical treatment of obesity. Bariatric operations cannot be performed with the limited pre- and postoperative evaluation and followup common in hernia repair, cholecystectomy, antireflux surgery, and other general surgical procedures. There are 50 years of research behind the results reported in this book. We have learned that few of the procedures we have tried work the way we thought they would. Most procedures now used are the results of 15 to 50 years of experimentation. Also, as previously mentioned, the procedures do not work without extensive allied support.

If the detailed instructions outlined in this book are not followed, a high rate of complications and poor long-term weight loss will result. In the bariatric practice of the 1970s and the early 1980s, which was not multidisciplinary, well over half the patients regained the majority of the weight they initially lost. Although extremely motivated patients may find mentors among prior patients or may learn success strategies from the Internet, this is certainly not the norm. Many patients come to bariatric practices expecting to receive an operation within a week, like other procedures. Surgeons who provide this type of treatment are not meeting the current standard of care. This book will help you understand what the standards of care are for the field in general and for each of the operations regularly used to treat obesity. Welcome to the field.

ACKNOWLEDGMENTS

One of the most important steps in rating a quality publication is to find the right publisher and medical editor to guide and promote the book through its journey to find its audience. I was led to our editor, Marc Strauss at McGraw-Hill, through a chain of knowledgeable, helpful friends and colleagues. First, our surgical department chair and acting dean at the Louisiana State University School of Medicine, Dr. J. Patrick O'Leary, a gentleman, unparalleled teacher, and bariatric surgeon, referred me to Ms. Wendy Husser, executive director of the Journal of the American College of Surgeons, whom he felt had the most extensive contact with medical publishers. She referred me to her colleague, Martin Wonsiewicz, the vice-president and publisher for clinical medicine at McGraw-Hill's New York office, who introduced me to Marc Strauss.

Bariatric surgery and all medical treatments of obesity struggle constantly to demonstrate their need, cost-effectiveness, relative value to our society against a backdrop of corrupt weight loss scams advertised on late night television, in print, and on the Internet. The portion of our population who can control their weight feel morally superior to those who cannot. More discrimination is openly practiced against the obese than any other segment of our society. Many dedicated physicians, either in spite of this or at times defiantly because of it, have worked for over half a century to document the mortality and morbidity associated with becoming massively (twice normal size or more) obese. I was just a baby when these early efforts were initiated, especially at the University of Minnesota, so I must defer to and acknowledge those who taught and influenced me and properly document the early history of the surgical efforts to treat this newly termed disease, "morbid" obesity.

Foremost in stature and the length of the shadow he cast in bariatric surgery is Edward Mason, professor emeritus at the University of Iowa, who trained at the University of Minnesota. He was chairman of the department of surgery at Iowa when I was in residency training, and I was lucky enough to visit his department several times, learning new skills each time. He is known as the "father of bariatric surgery" both for his creative scientific efforts and for nurturing the profession. In the late 1970s, it had become obvious that the small-bowel bypass operations used to treat morbid obesity from the 1950s were causing too many serious complications, in spite of the weight loss they produced. Negative media attention terminated not only the use of these procedures but almost the whole field. Dr. Mason's work in the 1960s and 1970s documented two bariatric procedures, gastric bypass and vertical-banded gastroplasty, that were safer, yet very effective. And, every June starting in 1980, he invited the entire community of bariatric surgeons to the University of Iowa campus and to his home to share their scientific observations and practical experiences. His support and the enthusiasm and defiance of these bariatric surgeons saved the field and encouraged my generation to establish bariatric practices. I never met a more honest, ethical, creative, and caring physician than Dr. Mason.

I initially learned the technical aspects of bariatric surgery at the University of Louisville under Lewis Flint. I met Dr. Flint because Dr. C. James Carrico realized that a medical intern at the University of Washington Hospitals in Seattle had made the wrong choice and should have entered a surgical training program. He helped me correct my initial mistake by convincing Dr. Flint, his former student, along with the other members of the surgery department at the University of Louisville to accept me into their training program.

My interest in a career in academic medicine and development of the skills to succeed in this field were stimulated and nurtured by Hiram C. Polk, Jr., chairman of the department of surgery at Louisville for the last quarter of a century. I consider him the second most important man in my development, holding only my father in higher esteem. Dr. Polk's protege, Dr. Donald Fry, supervised my initial clinical and basic science research and allowed me to initiate obesity research projects, even though it was not his primary field of interest. He convinced me that it was not hard to write scientific papers and I did not learn otherwise until I tried mentoring residents and medical students myself.

My first academic position at the Penn State College of Medicine in Hershey allowed me the freedom intellectually and financially to develop my own interests, which led me to a career in bariatric surgery. The chairman of surgery at Penn State, Dr. John Waldhausen, was recruited to Hershey as the medical school was evolving and dedicated over 30 years of his life to creating an ideal atmosphere and structure not only within his department but also within the school for it to grow into an academic and clinical powerhouse thanks to its artificial heart program run by his friend and colleague, Dr. Bill Pierce.

My colleague and friend at Penn State, Dr. Kathleen LaNove, tried her best to supervise my development in basic sciences, but clinical medicine proved more enjoyable. Dr. Ed Bixler, a scientist and biostatistician from the department of psychiatry at Penn State, set up the initial database for our bariatric program. He and Dr. Tjiauw-Ling Tan, a psychiatrist, convinced me how important it was to tend to the psychological and behavioral modification needs of the patients both pre- and postoperatively. I firmly believe that preoperative psychological preparation of patients decreases perioperative complications as much as medical treatment does, an opinion I would have strongly disagreed with before our association.

I also want to acknowledge the importance of the support of the pharmacology and medical device industries for the development of the bariatric medical field. Several companies have developed important new medications and procedures that have helped bring media attention to this field. There has been a more positive attitude in the press toward obesity treatments—in spite of the controversy over fenfluramine, which was removed from the pharmaceutical market when side effects were identified with its use. Nevertheless, the work of Dr. Michael Weintraub at the University of Rochester demonstrated that pharmacological treatment of obesity can provide effective long-term weight loss. Pharmaceutical companies like Knoll Pharmaceutical and American Home Products have helped demonstrate both the promise and the limitations of drug therapy, while ethically promoting the need for medical treatments of obesity.

INAMED Health (formerly BioEnterics), Transneuronix, Inc., and Johnson & Johnson have all initiated clinical trials of new medical devices to treat obesity in the last five years. Many members of these companies, especially Vernon Vincent of INAMED Health, have tirelessly worked to cross-fertilize this field by transporting new ideas between surgeons in the United States and the rest of the developed world. Now several Fortune 500 companies have begun manufacturing bariatric surgical instruments, demonstrating a significant increase in the acceptance of surgical therapy for morbid obesity. I would like to recognize the support of both Laura Moreno of Ethicon Endo-Surgery, a Johnson & Johnson subsidiary, and Tom Nolan of U.S. Surgical, a division of Tyco Healthcare, for organizing and promoting their companies' efforts to support educational activities for bariatric surgeons. The behind-the-scenes effort and creativity of the engineers, veterinarians, and numerous other employees of these companies have impressed me over the last several years.

Dr. J. Patrick O'Leary, our current dean and my friend, recruited me to New Orleans with the promise that I could develop the bariatric program of my dreams. Former dean Dr. Robert Marier helped support the program as it first developed. Dr. J. Turkowitz, the former medical director of what is now Tenet Healthcare Louisiana, recommended to his business colleagues that they support the development of a hospital-based, multidisciplinary clinic devoted to obesity treatment. Their vision and early support were crucial.

I thank my colleagues in bariatric surgery for their dedicated and underappreciated service to this formerly neglected area of medicine. The free sharing of ideas and techniques were essential to my early development as a bariatric surgeon and again when we initiated our laparoscopic program. Dr. Harvey Sugerman of Richmond, Virginia, was an early mentor, and his initial technical suggestions overcame some of the awkwardness I felt moving from the role of resident to responsible attending surgeon. Dr. Mickew Belechew of Belgium and later Drs. Allan Wittgrove and Wes Clark of San Diego supervised my laparoscopic bariatric training. More recently, Dr. Paul O'Brien of Australia and Dr. Henry Buchwald of Minneapolis have lent their senior advice, which has helped me to create this book.

Finally and most importantly, I would like to acknowledge my family. My wife of 26 years, Debbie, has supported me through all the trials and tribulations of an academic career, including the relocation of our family to Paris for a year. My parents, my wife, and my three sons have provided me with the love that has allowed me to make career choices without ever doubting that I would always have their support. I thank them all for their love.

OBESITY SURGERY

WHY SHOULD OBESITY BE TREATED?

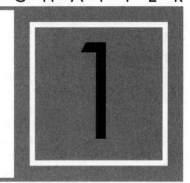

BARBARA J. MOORE /
LOUIS F. MARTIN

In December 2001, US Surgeon General David Satcher issued a *Call to Action to Prevent and Decrease Overweight and Obesity.*[1] With this report, the imprimatur of the Surgeon General's office was added to the efforts of former Surgeon General C. Everett Koop to raise awareness of the growing threat of obesity and its toll of expense and human suffering borne by the American people.[2] In 1994, Dr. Koop founded Shape Up America! to provide information on obesity and weight management. The organization launched its web site—www.shapeup.org—in 1996 and published a set of guidelines established by a consensus of experts to help family physicians treat their overweight and obese patients.[2]

The 2001 Surgeon General's report[1] and more recent data[2–4] document upsurges in obesity prevalence in all ages and ethnic groups, and reinforces the well-established but poorly understood connections between obesity and type 2 diabetes, hypertension, heart disease, stroke, respiratory problems such as sleep apnea, and certain cancers. In his report, Dr. Satcher attributes 300,000 deaths annually to obesity.[1] This same statistic was greeted with skepticism when Dr. Koop reported it soon after the launch of Shape Up America! in 1994.[5] A 1993 study published by McGinnis and Foege[6] was the first to blame 300,000 to 500,000 "preventable deaths" annually to "poor diet and inactivity," but not to obesity per se. Another report,[7] published by a large group of obesity experts led by Allison, in 1997, helped to validate the annual mortality figure associated specifically with obesity by outlining how it was produced. Today, the figure of 300,000 deaths a year attributable to obesity is widely accepted. The Centers for Disease Control and Prevention (CDC) recently established that morbid obesity, the disease associated with being more than 100% over ideal body weight, increases the prevalence of numerous chronic debilitating diseases when compared to those of normal weight, including type 2 diabetes (7.4 times higher prevalence rate), hypertension (6.4 times), arthritis (4.4 times), asthma (2.7 times), elevated cholesterol levels (1.9 times), and poor (or fair) overall health (4.2 times).[4]

In our view, the two most important new developments that have changed public attitudes toward obesity are the dramatic rise in obesity prevalence especially among children[1,4] (see Figure 1–1), including the connection between pediatric obesity and pediatric type 2 diabetes,[8] and the evidence-based consensus reports from Shape Up America![2] the National Institutes of Health (NIH),[9] and the World Health Organization (WHO),[10] which all reported the importance of the contribution of obesity to the morbidity of hypertension, diabetes, atherosclerosis, osteoarthritis, and other expensive diseases. In children, there is no governmentally sanctioned definition of "obesity" (*this term is considered politically incorrect by pediatricians concerned with the self-image of their patients*), but "overweight" is defined in terms of gender- and age-specific body mass index (BMI) percentiles (see Chapter 17). Thus, "overweight" is defined as a BMI at or above the 95th BMI percentile where BMI is defined as weight (in kg) divided by the square of height (in meters).[1] Using that definition, the prevalence of overweight has increased from approximately 4% in the 1960s[1] to 15% in both children and teens in 1998.[1,4,11] In Hispanic and African American children, however, the prevalence of overweight is strikingly higher— 22% for both ethnic groups (see Figure 1–1).[11] Overweight in the teenage years is not a benign condition. A study by Whitaker[12] shows that teenagers whose BMI is at the 95th percentile or above face an extremely high likelihood of remaining obese in young adulthood. These adolescents are set up for a lifelong struggle with the problem of obesity, the comorbid medical conditions listed in the consensus reports from Shape Up America!,[2] the NIH,[9] and the WHO,[10] and the social and financial discrimination that obese persons face.[13]

The consensus reports published by Shape Up America!,[2] the NIH,[9] and the WHO[10] point out the ridiculousness of the argument made by medical insurance companies that treatment for obesity should not be a covered medical benefit because it is only a cosmetic problem without medical consequences (refer to Walter Lindstrom's Web site www.obesitylaw.com). These reports also document that the success rates of medical treatment of obesity and the surgical treatment of morbid obesity is at least as successful, and often more successful, than many other treatments that medical insurance companies routinely cover.

OBESITY AND DIABETES

The presence of obesity increases the risk of type 2 diabetes in all age groups, including children and adolescents.[1,14] As a consequence, the growth in type 2 diabetes prevalence parallels the growth of obesity prevalence. By the early to mid-1990s, obesity prevalence in adults had escalated from less than 10% to greater than 15% in many midwestern states, from Michigan to Wisconsin and down the Mississippi River to Louisiana. Over the next 10 years, highest levels of obesity prevalence spread from the heartland to both the east and the west coasts. Today more than 20 states have a prevalence of obesity greater than 20%.[1]

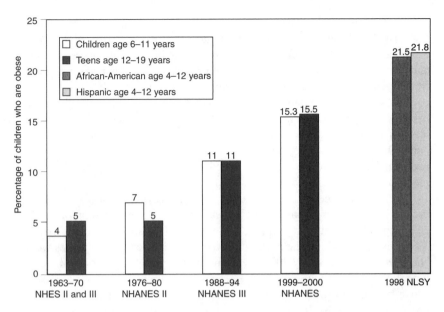

FIGURE 1–1   Prevalence of overweight among US children and adolescents. NHES, National Health Examination Survey; NHANES. National Health and Nutrition Examination Survey; NLSY, National Longitudinal Survey of Youth. (Data are a combination of that reported in the *Surgeon General's Call to Action*[1] and by Ogden et al.[2] and Strauss and Pollack.[11])

The spread of increased diabetes prevalence followed a roughly similar pattern to the spread of obesity, with the highest prevalence emerging first in the heartland and then moving eastward and westward. Prior to 1990, diabetes prevalence was under 4% of the US population, but by 2000, the vast majority of states had a prevalence of diabetes greater than 7%.[15] It is important to appreciate that although the diabetes prevalence data collected through the CDC's Behavioral Risk Factor Surveillance System includes both type 1 and type 2, 90% to 95% is type 2 diabetes,[15] and is therefore preventable. In 2001, the direct and indirect costs of diabetes were estimated to approach $100 billion dollars yearly.[15]

Type 2 diabetes can be prevented by weight reduction and lifestyle modification; weight management is central to the treatment of type 2 diabetes. The results of the Diabetes Prevention Program[16] demonstrate a remarkable 58% reduction in the onset of diabetes in high-risk overweight adult individuals. At the start of the study, the subjects were not diabetic but had impaired glucose tolerance and were thus at high risk for the disease, which most subjects successfully averted through a modest but sustained weight reduction effected by lifestyle change, including increased physical activity. Study participants in the lifestyle change group took off 7% of initial body weight and kept off 5% by the end of 3 years.[16] This landmark trial demonstrated that weight loss through lifestyle change is possible and is significantly more effective than pharmacotherapy in preventing diabetes in high risk overweight individuals.[16]

The morbidly obese patient with a BMI of 40 or higher is at extremely high risk for the development of type 2 diabetes.[17] Pories and his colleagues collected data on the benefits of bariatric surgery in morbidly obese patients and demonstrated its value in both preventing and resolving diabetes in this extremely vulnerable population.[18] Long-term (6 to 10 years) followup of these patients shows that the unoperated controls (usually patients unable to secure insurance coverage for the procedure) experience a greater use of diabetes medications and higher rate of mortality[19] than do their surgically treated counterparts. The surgically treated patients decrease their use of diabetes medications and their glucose levels and glycosylated hemoglobin invariably normalize or move in a positive direction (Figure 1–2).[19]

In the past, the vast majority of cases of pediatric diabetes was type 1, previously known as juvenile onset diabetes. Type 2 diabetes among the pediatric population is currently growing alarmingly. One study[8] reported that in 1990, fewer than 4% of the newly diagnosed pediatric cases of diabetes were classified as type 2. But by 2000, the proportion of pediatric cases classified as type 2 diabetes had increased by 500% or more.[8] These data may be conservative because, in many regions throughout the United States, anecdotal reports[8] suggest that half or more of all new cases of pediatric diabetes are now type 2 and that these afflicted children are invariably obese (Figure 1–3).[8]

Although obesity prevalence is increasing in all socioeconomic groups, it is noteworthy that the association between obesity and lower educational attainment and, consequently, lower socioeconomic status, remains a strong one.[20] Thus, millions of obese individuals, who will become ill prematurely as a consequence of their obesity, will be uninsured. American society will bear the expense of treating the comorbidities of obesity in the uninsured through Social Security disability pensions, lost tax revenue, missed days of work, and lower productivity rates. Additionally, the ethical ramifications of our current failure to cover the costs of treatment of the obese will be a challenge since it disproportionately afflicts lower income and minority populations. When over one quarter to one-third of the voting public becomes obese, they will be able to demand treatment, displacing the needs of other groups seeking federal and state assistance.

The Surgeon General's report estimated the costs of obesity to be $117 billion a year in 2001 and asserted that half of these costs are associated with treating the comorbidities of obesity.[1] Of these, the largest proportion of costs is associated with the treatment of diabetes.[21] The growing prevalence of both obesity and diabetes in children and teens, as well as younger adults, suggests that these costs will continue to grow rapidly and will make an ever-larger contribution to total health care costs nationally. Sturm reported that obesity outranks both smoking and drinking in its deleterious effects on health and health costs,[22] but public health policy and medical insurance policies have yet to react to these facts. A study in a large health maintenance organization (HMO) also documents significantly higher costs for physician visits, hospital visits, and medications for its morbidly obese members versus the normal weight members enrolled in the HMO's Northern California Region.[23]

One compelling reason to treat obesity is that we know very little about how to prevent it. The only way to decrease the increasing expenses associated with treating a population that is becoming increasingly obese is to decrease

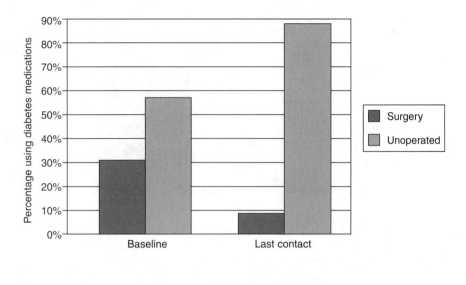

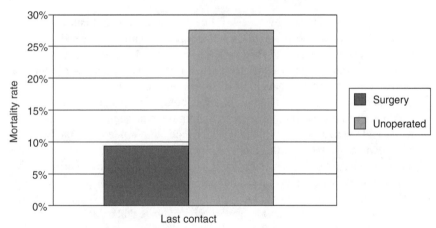

FIGURE 1–2   Morbidly obese, diabetic patients treated by gastric bypass show a significant decrease in their use of medications to treat their diabetes and a significant decrease in mortality over a 5-year followup period when compared to similar patients without surgical therapy. Note that the mortality reported here includes perioperative mortality and more years of followup in the surgically treated patients, yet it is dramatically lower in the surgery group. (Adapted from MacDonald et al.[19])

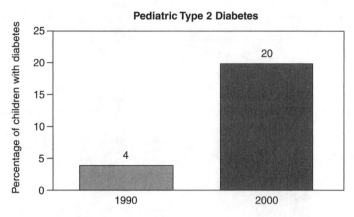

FIGURE 1–3   Prevalence of type 2 diabetes in the pediatric population is rising while the prevalence of type 1 diabetes is proportionally decreasing. (Adapted from American Diabetes Association.[8])

the prevalence of obesity by successful medical and surgical treatment of this disease. States have proposed to the CDC various community-based interventions to prevent obesity, and funding specifically for these programs or related purposes is being made available to states. It is unfortunate that the funding for the National Health and Nutrition Examination Survey (NHANES) is inadequate to provide state by state baseline data both prior to and after these interventions so that we might have clearer and more consistent insight into what works and what does not. What may undermine our confidence in the data that will become available in the future is uneven data collection and evaluation methodology. Also, the primary focus of many of these interventions is on physical activity and not on the moderation of food intake or portion control. The reluctance to focus on portion control is regrettable because treatment studies in both adults[24–29] and children[30,31] clearly indicate that a dual focus on both caloric restriction and exercise will be necessary. It is also naïve not to fund public interventions that warn the public on the dangers of large portion intake, especially because many fast food advertisements try to entice customers by specifically promising them larger portions.

Dr. Marion Nestle's book, *Food Politics,*[32] identifies numerous ways in which food marketers target children and adults to influence their food choices and eating behavior. Her description of the strategies used inside elementary and secondary schools is particularly chilling. One business, Channel One, contracts to provide televisions and computers to schools by requiring that school children view 2 minutes of commercial messages each school day with food industry advertising making up a significant proportion of the advertisers (Ref. 32, p. 189). The business model of Channel One apparently relies heavily on the sales of this advertising time to food companies and other advertisers, so in effect, taxpayers are providing their children as marketing targets so that Channel One's profit goals are met. There is evidence that children trust the advertisers and believe those companies have their interests in mind (Ref. 32, p. 190).

The roots of this problem have to do with the way our nation's schools are funded. School district budgets have not kept pace with the high costs of educational materials. Also, most administrators have very limited budgets at their disposal for the development of their educational curriculum and related materials. There is also widespread acceptance of advertising in schools, both overt and covert. School administrators, teachers, and parents may not be aware of the extent to which they are mortgaging the health and well being of school children when they allow commercial interests to shape their children's food choices within schools. On the other hand, however, data unequivocally demonstrating the deleterious effects of these marketing strategies on the health of children are lacking. The growing prevalence of obesity and type 2 diabetes among children and teens (see Figures 1–1 and 1–3) is considered to be indirect but inconclusive proof.

In some school districts, fast food companies have taken over school food service operations. These developments are not seen as injurious to the health of students by most school administrators but are viewed as a mechanism for the schools to raise money. Many schools welcome the elimination of a school food service operation that is costly and inconvenient for schools to run. Asking a fast food company to take over the school food service operation eliminates the burden of providing meals that children like and will actually eat. Nutritional considerations are the least of school administrators' concerns as they are pressured to focus on basic skills to help students pass national quality standard testing. The idea that nutrition, physical activity, and weight management can and should integrate classroom teachings with school cafeteria offerings and the physical education program, and should coordinate with health messages delivered throughout the school, has not caught hold. Yet children and teens are interested in nutrition and exercise—or at least dieting, weight management, and sports performance. These subject areas offer rich opportunities to strengthen skills and build knowledge in both science and mathematics.

Vending machines provide easy access to both candy and soda for children to consume throughout the school day. According to one report, as of 2000, soda companies established highly lucrative "pouring contracts" with at least 200 school districts in 33 states (Ref. 29, p. 204). Pouring contracts are exclusive contractual arrangements between school districts and soda companies that generate significant revenues—large amounts of discretionary dollars—for cash-strapped schools. The word "discretionary" is key, in that school administrators have few discretionary dollars at their disposal, therefore they highly prize the funds made available through these pouring contracts. The contracts vary considerably from one school district to another in size and contractual details. An essential element of a pouring contract is a commitment on the part of the school district to sell only one brand of soda in all school vending machines and to display only that brand's logo on vending machines and perhaps elsewhere (e.g., the soda company's logo may appear on the scoreboard in the gym, on the school's athletic field scoreboards, playing field, or on student T-shirts). Most contracts call for an upfront lump sum payment to the school district followed by additional annual payments made by the soda distributorship to the school system for the duration of the contract. It is not unusual for pouring contracts to provide additional cash bonuses of increasing size if soda sales reach certain target volumes; in short, the school budget benefits from selling more soda to children.

Between 1985 and 1997, milk sales to school districts declined by nearly 30% and soda sales increased by a staggering 1100% (Ref. 30, pp. 198–199). The sodas consumed by school children are regular sugar sodas, providing approximately 10 teaspoons of sugar or 150 calories per 12-ounce can—in addition to caffeine. In some locations, the 12-ounce can, once considered standard in vending machines, is being replaced by the larger 20-ounce soda size that delivers 250 calories per serving and even more caffeine. Fast food restaurants and vendors in movie theaters, zoos, and amusement parks offer sodas as large as 64 ounces, which deliver as much as 800 calories, depending on how much ice is in the cup. This number of calories can represent half or more of the total daily calories required by a young teenage girl or boy who spends most of his or her leisure time sitting in front of a television, video game, or computer instead of engaged in physical activity. The same is true for adults who consume these beverages. It is worth remembering that calories from soda deliver only calories and offer nothing else of nutritional value.

Although it is certainly unnecessary and undesirable to do so, with careful planning it is possible to include one 12-ounce can of soda in the daily diet of an active child or adult without compromising nutritional status. Yet, it is increasingly questionable whether our nation's children and adults are sufficiently active. There are also data suggesting that most children, and even most adults, are consuming more than one 12-ounce can of soda each day. Few children walk to school and many adults do not consider it safe to walk anywhere in their communities. Most schools have reduced or eliminated what used to be daily physical activity programs. Several studies associate nutrient-poor soda consumption with childhood obesity. Obesity is a consequence, however, of varying combinations of insufficient energy expenditure and excessive caloric intake in children, just as it is in adults. More such studies are needed to determine why prevalence rates for obesity and diabetes are rising so quickly in children and adolescents and to determine how best to reverse these trends.

PREVENTION AND TREATMENT OF OBESITY

Complicating strategies to treat and prevent childhood obesity is the question of whether or not the problem can be solved without addressing the obesity of their parents, which is fast becoming ubiquitous. Overweight and obesity among adults of childbearing age is rapidly increasing. The prevention of obesity in children may ultimately depend on the behavior of their parents and caregivers who are their role models. It may also depend on the cultivation of improved parenting skills in high-risk populations, since parental neglect has been found to be a strong predictor of obesity.[35] The long-term studies of successful treatment of pediatric obesity have engaged the child's entire family—especially the parents or caregivers—in the treatment process.[33,34] In some of the most important studies to date, only children whose parents were willing and engaged participants in the treatment process were accepted to those studies. This may well have contributed to the promising results that have persisted over the long term.[33,34] Indeed, several studies point to the unique role of parents in fostering positive eating and exercise behaviors of their children.[37–39] Such studies point to the critical positive influence of parental behavior. In other words, it is highly likely that parents must effectively model the very behaviors they hope their children will adopt.[37] An even more striking corollary finding in these studies is that admonishing children to behave in a way that parents do not themselves behave has a negative impact on the behavior of the children. Several other studies examined this dissonance between parental behavior and parental preaching and how it impacts the behavior of children.[38,39] The implication of these findings is that prevention of obesity in children may well be linked to treatment in adults, where "treatment" is broadly defined to mean teaching parents to adopt and consistently display healthful personal eating and exercise habits. One provocative study of the treatment of childhood obesity produced better results when the parents of overweight children were targeted rather than targeting the children directly.[36]

Prevention and treatment of obesity among children is made more difficult by a high prevalence of major depression among overweight teens. An analysis conducted by Shape Up America! of NHANES III data in teens between the ages of 15 and 19 years showed a strikingly high proportion of teens in the 95th gender- and age-specific BMI percentile and above who met the clinical diagnostic criteria (American Psychological Association's *Diagnostic and Statistical Manual of Mental Disorders,* 4th ed. [DSM-IV] criteria) for major depression. Among the heaviest children, 20% of boys and 30% of girls, as compared to 0% and 6% of the thinnest boys and girls, respectively, met diagnostic criteria for major depression (Figure 1–4).

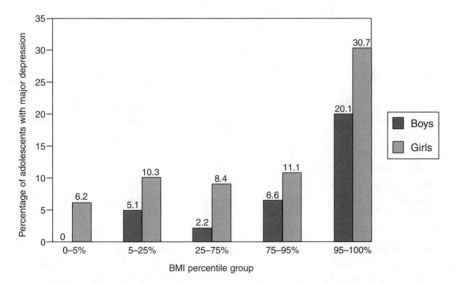

FIGURE 1–4   Shape Up America! analysis of NHANES III data concerning the prevalence of major depression in adolescents between the ages of 15 and 19 years when divided by BMI percentile.

Focus group research by Shape Up America! has revealed that health care providers who serve the obese pediatric population in the Washington, DC, metropolitan area perceive a strong connection between depression and obesity in teens.[40] Depression is linked to physical inactivity, inappropriate use of food and other behaviors that encourage and promote obesity. It may contribute to the persistence of obesity into adulthood observed among the majority of teenagers whose BMI falls at the 95th percentile or above.[12]

ROLE OF THE CLINICIAN

There is evidence that physicians do not intervene with their overweight and obese patients. Reviews of multiple medical specialty groups demonstrated that most subspecialty physicians are not sure how to assess and treat obesity.[41] This lack of preparation of medical professionals for dealing with the most prevalent nutritional problem in America is a reflection of the fact that a formal course in nutrition or equivalent nutrition education remains absent from the curriculum of the large majority of the nation's medical schools despite sporadic efforts since the 1950s[42–44] to remedy this problem. The medical school curriculum is in part shaped by the questions on national exams. Thus a greater emphasis on nutrition and obesity in the exams needs to be promoted as part of the solution to this problem. Another contributing factor is the dearth of properly trained clinical nutrition faculty who can organize and champion the inclusion of a formal course in nutrition.

Despite the failure of physicians to intervene, there is also encouraging evidence that when they do intervene, physicians can have a positive impact on the behaviors of their patients. In one study[44] the self-reported attempts of patients to improve their eating and exercise behaviors increased by 50% when encouraged by their physician to make those lifestyle changes.

BARRIERS TO TREATMENT

As the science demonstrating the effectiveness of weight reduction in the prevention and management of diabetes and other comorbidities of obesity continues to strengthen, more attention can be directed to the question of the cost of treatment and the likely benefits that can be achieved outside of the clinical research center where these important studies were conducted. There is a serious institutional impediment to collecting the necessary outcomes and cost data, and that is the refusal of insurance companies to reimburse for the costs associated with the diagnosis and treatment of obesity. Although a diagnostic code for obesity does exist the criteria for its use are scientifically out of date, and insurance companies usually refuse to cover costs associated with the obesity diagnostic code.[46] Documentation of the true costs of treating obesity becomes impossible as physicians seek alternative codes for the comorbidities of obesity for which they can be reimbursed. Martin et al. have published a detailed analysis of this problem.[47]

It is regrettable that the US Surgeon General and other public health leaders have failed to decry this unjust denial of coverage to the obese and morbidly obese populations. It must be addressed if we are to remove this formidable barrier to the collection of valid obesity treatment costs and outcomes data in response to the demand for suitable cost benefit analyses. Leadership on this issue is sorely needed, but may have to await awareness that the escalating health care costs are heavily driven by the growing epidemic of diabetes which, in turn, is being driven by the obesity epidemic.

The NIH and the CDC have slowly begun to assume leadership roles. Zhang and his colleagues from the Division of Diabetes Translation of the CDC recently published a review of the cost-effectiveness of interventions for reducing body weight 4%, documenting that both medical and surgical treatment of the obese and the morbidly obese are some of the most cost-effective treatments that have been analyzed under the US Public Health Department criteria.[48] The NIH also has reviewed published data and produced guidelines for the treatment of obesity.[9] Additionally, the NIH dedicated more than $80 million for a 5-year period starting in 2000 to determine if the medical–behavioral treatment of obesity in people with diabetes would reduce the known mortality and morbidity of this disease. In 2003, NIH is scheduled to choose four to six Obesity Surgery Research Centers in an attempt to develop multicenter studies that will help determine the most appropriate treatment protocols for applying obesity surgery to the obese population and how to improve the procedures that are used. Establishing the scientific basis of how surgical treatments work should also help the development of more precise medical treatments. The CDC also continues to follow the incidence of diseases and consequences in the US population. These studies have steadily identified obesity as the major public health problem the US faces in this new millennium.[3,4,50] For the first time in 2003, the CDC reported the odds ratio of adults with a BMI > 40 kg/m^2 (the definition of morbid obesity) having diabetes,[7,36] hypertension,[6,37] asthma,[4,39] and fair or poor health[4,19] as compared to adults with normal weights,[50] furthering the argument that the morbidly obese need to be offered bariatric surgery to reduce the expense of these diseases and their associated mortality.

SUMMARY

The key reason for treating overweight and obesity is that the prevalence of obesity is growing in all age groups. This means that not only is it impacting parents, it is also afflicting their children and teens. Obesity is driving the tremendous growth in prevalence of type 2 diabetes, which, in turn, is a primary driver of escalating health care costs. In adults, the striking success of the Diabetes Prevention Program[16] shows that weight loss combined with lifestyle change that includes increases in physical activity can be accomplished and is central to diabetes prevention in high risk overweight individuals. For morbidly obese individuals, bariatric surgery decreases the early mortality associated with the development of diabetes.

We know less about obesity prevention than we do about obesity treatment, but the prevention of obesity in children will most likely require the planning, cooperation, and role modeling of their parents. This is because parental eating and exercise behaviors exert a profound influence on the eating and exercise behavior of their children. The treatment of adult obesity in which comprehensive lifestyle change is accomplished becomes a cornerstone of prevention once it is appreciated that children need positive parental role models who themselves demonstrate, as well as nurture, a healthy lifestyle in their children. The vast majority of US parents are themselves overweight, obese, or morbidly obese. This is now a fact of American life that is impacting the lifestyle, weight, and health of children.

We will continue to hear demands to account for the costs and properly evaluate the benefits of treating obesity, but we will be unable to respond to those demands until health care professionals are able to consistently use appropriate obesity diagnostic and treatment codes. Evaluating the true costs and benefits of treating obesity requires that physicians and other allied health care professionals can openly diagnose and treat obesity, and be compensated appropriately for their time. Currently, insurance coverage infrequently covers the cost of obesity treatment. Leadership and political will is needed to remove the barriers to insurance coverage. Morbidly obese patients are frequently denied coverage for bariatric surgery even though this procedure consistently produces dramatic and enduring weight loss. For the patient with uncomplicated obesity, insurance coverage is unlikely until one or more of the obesity comorbidities such as hypertension or diabetes develops. With respect to the treatment of obesity, we delude ourselves that the failure to cover the cost of treatment is someone else's problem. As more and more obese patients fall ill, miss work, lose wages, require treatment, and die prematurely, obesity is the central public health problem of the 21st century. Until we know how to prevent it, treating obesity is our only choice.

REFERENCES

1. US Department of Health and Human Services, Public Health Service, Office of the Surgeon General. The Surgeon General's call to action to prevent and decrease overweight and obesity 2001. Available at: http://www.surgeongeneral.gov/library. Accessed July 1, 2003.
2. Shape Up America! and American Obesity Association. *Guidance for Treatment of Adult Obesity.* Washington, DC: Shape Up America!, 1998–2001.
3. Flegal KM, Carroll MD, Ogden CL, Johnson CL. Prevalence and trends in obesity among US adults, 1999–2000. *JAMA* 2002;288:1723–1727.
4. Ogden CL, Flegal KM, Carroll MD, Johnson CL. Prevalence and trends in overweight among US children and adolescents, 1999–2000. *JAMA* 2002;288:1728–1732.
5. Shape Up America! Press Release dated December 6, 1994. Dr. C. Everett Koop launches a new "crusade" to combat obesity in America. Available at: http://www.shapeup.org/dated/120694.htm. Accessed July 1, 2003.
6. McGinnis JM, Foege WH. Actual causes of death in the United States. *JAMA* 1993;270(18):2207–2212.
7. Allison DB, Fontaine KR, Manson JE, Stevens J, Van Itallie TB. Annual deaths attributable to obesity in the United States. *JAMA* 1999;282(16):1530–1538.

8. American Diabetes Association: Type 2 diabetes in children and adolescents. *Diabetes Care* 2000;23(3):381–398.

9. NIH Conference. Gastrointestinal surgery for severe obesity. Consensus Development Conference Panel. *Ann Intern Med* 1991;115:956–961.

10. World Health Organization. Obesity: preventing and managing the global epidemic. Geneva: WHO, 1998.

11. Strauss RS, Pollack HA. Epidemic increase in childhood overweight, 1986–1998 *JAMA*, 2001; 286:2845–2848.

12. Whitaker RC, Wright JA, Pepe MS, Seidel KD, Dietz WH. Predicting obesity in young adulthood from childhood and parental obesity. *N Engl J Med* 1997;337(13):869–873.

13. Dietz WH. Health consequences of obesity in youth: childhood predictors of adult disease. *Pediatrics* 1998;101(Suppl):518–525.

14. Sinha R, Fisch G, Teague B, et al. Prevalence of impaired glucose tolerance among children and adolescents with marked obesity. *N Engl J Med* 2002;346:802–810.

15. Centers for Disease Control and Prevention. Diabetes: disabling, deadly, and on the rise 2002. Available at: http://www.cdc.gov/diabetes/pubs/glance.htm. Accessed July 1, 2003.

16. Diabetes Prevention Program Research Group. Reduction in the incidence of type 2 diabetes with lifestyle intervention or metformin. *N Engl J Med* 2002;346:393–403.

17. Sjostrom LV. Morbidity of severely obese subjects. *Am J Clin Nutr* 1992;55:508S–515S.

18. Pories W, Swanson MS, MacDonald KG, et al. Who would have thought it? An operation proves to be the most effective therapy for adult-onset diabetes mellitus. *Ann Surg.* 1995;222(3):339–352.

19. MacDonald KG Jr, Long SD, Swanson MS, et al. The gastric bypass operation reduces the progression and mortality of non-insulin-dependent diabetes mellitus. *J Gastrointest Surg* 1997;1:213–220.

20. Freedman DS, Khan LK, Serdula MK, Galuska DA, Dietz WH. Trends and correlates of class 3 obesity in the United States from 1990 through 2000. *JAMA* 2002;288:1758–1761.

21. Wolf AM, Colditz GA. Current estimates of the economic cost of obesity in the United States. *Obes Res* 1998;6(2):97–106.

22. Sturm R. The effects of obesity, smoking, and drinking on medical problems and costs. *Health Aff (Millwood)* 2002;21:245–253.

23. Quesenberry CP, Caan B, Jacobson A. Obesity, health services use, and health care costs among members of a health maintenance organization. *Arch Intern Med* 1998;158(5):466–472.

24. Blair SN. Evidence for success of exercise in weight loss and control. *Ann Intern Med* 1993;119:702–706.

25. Wing RR. Behavioral treatment of severe obesity. *Am J Clin Nutr* 1992;55:545S–551S.

26. Perri MG, Sears SF, Clark JE. Strategies for improving maintenance of weight loss. Toward a continuous care model of obesity management. *Diabetes Care* 1993;16:200–209.

27. Pavlou KN, Krey S, Steffee WP. Exercise as an adjunct to weight loss and maintenance in moderately obese subjects. *Am J Clin Nutr* 1989;49:1115–1123.

28. Pavlou KN, Whatley JE, Jannace PW, et al. Physical activity as a supplement to a weight-loss dietary regimen. *Am J Clin Nutr* 1989;49:1110–1114.

29. Dyer RG. Traditional treatment of obesity: Does it work? *Baillieres Clin Endocrinol Metab* 1994;8:661–685.

30. Epstein LH. Exercise in the treatment of childhood obesity. *Int J Obes Relat Metab Disord* 1995;19(Suppl 4):S117–S121.

31. Epstein LH, Coleman KJ, Myers MD. Exercise in treating obesity in children and adolescents. *Med Sci Sports Exerc* 1996;28(4):428–435.

32. Nestle M. Food Politics: *How the Food Industry Influences Nutrition and Health*. Berkeley and Los Angeles, CA: University of California Press, 2002.

33. Epstein LH, Valoski A, Wing RR, McCurley J. Ten-year outcomes of behavioral family-based treatment for childhood obesity. *Health Psychol* 1994;13(5):373–383.

34. Epstein LH, Valoski A, Wing RR, McCurley J. Ten-year follow-up of behavioral, family-based treatment for obese children. *JAMA* 1990;264(19):2519–2523.

35. Lissau I, Sorensen TI. Parental neglect during childhood and increased risk of obesity in young adulthood. *Lancet* 1994;343:324–327.

36. Golan M, Weizman A, Apter A, Fainaru M. Parents as the exclusive agents of change in the treatment of childhood obesity. *Am J Clin Nutr* 1998;67(6):1130–1135.

37. Fisher JO, Mitchell DC, Smickiklas-Wright H, Birch LL. Parental influences on young girls' fruit and vegetable, micronutrient, and fat intakes. *J Am Diet Assoc* 2002;102(1):58–64.

38. Birch LL, Davison KK. Family environmental factors influencing the developing behavioral controls of food intake and childhood overweight. *Pediatr Clin North Am* 2001;48(4):893–907.

39. Fisher JO, Birch LL. Eating in the absence of hunger and overweight in girls from 5 to 7 years of age. *Am J Clin Nutr* 2002;76(1):226–231.

40. Diabesity focus group data collected by Shape Up America! in January 2001 and reported at March 2001 Conference on Diabesity in America. Conference proceedings available at http://www.shapeup.org. Accessed July 1, 2003.

41. Kristeller JL, Hoerr RA. Physician attitudes toward managing obesity: Differences among six specialty groups. *Prev Med* 1997;26:542–549.

42. Intersociety Professional Nutrition Education Consortium. Bringing physician nutrition specialists into the mainstream: rationale for the Intersociety Professional Nutrition Education consortium. *Am J Clin Nutr* 1998;68:894–898.

43. Heimburger DC, Stallings VA, Routzahn R. Survey of physician clinical nutrition training programs. *Am J Clin Nutr* 1998;68:1174–1179.

44. Heimburger DC, Intersociety Professional Nutrition Education Consortium. Physician nutrition specialist track: If we build it, they will come? *Am J Clin Nutr* 2000;71:1048–1053.

45. US Department of Health and Human Services. Physician advice and individual behaviors about cardiovascular risk reduction. *MMWR Morb Mortal Wkly Report* 1999;48(4):74–77.

46. Martin, LF, White S, Lindstrom W Jr. Cost-benefit analysis for the treatment of severe obesity. *World J Surg* 1998;22:1008–1017.

47. Martin LF, Robinson A, Moore BJ. The socioeconomic issues affecting the treatment of obesity in the new millennium. *Pharmacoeconomics* 2000;18:335–353.

48. Zhang P, Wang G, Narayan KMV. Cost-effectiveness of interventions for reducing body weight. In: Medeiros-Neto G, Halpern A, Bouchard C, eds. *Progress in Obesity Research 9*. Eastleigh, UK: John Libbey & Co. Ltd., 2003:579–584.

49. Gold MR, Siegel JE Russell LB, Weinstein MC, eds: Cost-Effectiveness in Health and Medicine. New York, Oxford University Press, 1996.

50. Mokdad AH, Ford ES, Bowman BA, et al. Prevalence of obesity, diabetes, and obesity-related health risk factors, 2001. *JAMA* 2003;289:76–79.

THE EVOLUTION OF SURGERY FOR MORBID OBESITY

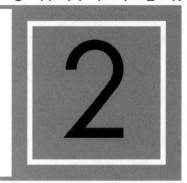

LOUIS F. MARTIN

After World War II, food rationing ended, able-bodied men returned to plant and harvest the crops of our farmlands, and diversion of manufacturing and raw materials for the war effort was no longer necessary. Therefore, in the late 1940s and early 1950s there suddenly was a significant increase in food production. Food was available to the public at the lowest prices in a decade. Advances in mechanization and military tested processes were made available to improve commercial canning, freezing, and storing, and transporting food to all regions of the United States. This marked the beginning of a period in American history where, for the first time, food was plentiful, and for nearly everyone, affordable. Poor nutritional intake became nonexistent except for the poorest class of citizens in isolated areas like Appalachia or the inner-city ghettos.

Related to these improvements in the availability and the cost of common food items, for the first time, in the early 1950s, American and some European physicians regularly began seeing hugely obese people, often with medical problems directly related to their massive obesity. University medical centers (in the midwest especially) were being referred patients who weighed more than 400, and sometimes more than 500, pounds. These individuals had developed Pickwickian syndrome (obesity–hypoventilation syndrome), severe venous stasis of the lower extremities with recurrent bouts of cellulitis, heart failure, deep venous thrombosis, pulmonary emboli, diabetes, hypertension, and degenerative arthritis in all their weight-bearing joints. Many of these patients had surgical problems due, at least in part, to their obesity, such as gallstones (formed during periods of weight loss from dieting or semistarvation followed by large gains in weight at harvest season when cheap food became available again); inguinal, umbilical, and incisional hernias; and obesity-related malignancies such as ovarian, breast, prostate, and colon cancer. Operating room tables and instruments, x-ray tables, hospital beds, and most standard hospital items, such as wheel chairs, stretchers, and chairs in waiting areas, were not sturdy or large enough to accommodate these people. Surgeons in the 1950s recognized that these massively obese people were untreatable unless an effective treatment for their obesity could be created and began designing surgical procedures for these patients to specifically help them lose weight.

Experience soon demonstrated that these morbidly obese individuals (a term developed for this disease by Dr. J. Payne to help insurance companies understand why surgical treatment was necessary because so many had premature deaths before they reached an age of 40 to 50 years) were refractory to diet and available drug therapy, leading to the evolution of surgical management. The initial operations to treat obesity evolved from the years of clinical experience general surgeons had accumulated treating patients with iatrogenically induced "short-gut" syndrome, a condition seen after extirpation of substantial segments of the small intestine as a consequence of acute thrombosis of the arterial or venous systems leading to necrosis. Almost all patients who had significant sections of their small intestine removed lost weight because the total area of the absorptive surface area of the small intestine was decreased causing "malabsorption" and "maldigestion." Because different sections of the small bowel preferentially absorb certain vitamins, minerals, bile salts, fats, and other substances, when these specific segments are lost, then certain disease states, such as iron-deficiency anemia, calcium-oxalate kidney stones, cholesterol gallstones, and vitamin K deficiency, are more likely to develop. When the length of the intestine was removed to treat a section where ischemia and/or necrosis had developed, the patient usually had postoperative diarrhea and could develop low protein, vitamin, and mineral levels, if there was insufficient surface area left to absorb the digested food elements. Often this insufficiency was overcome by the remaining bowel increasing its absorptive surface by increasing the height and number of individual villi (the absorbing fingers of the bowels' inner surface). During the time of this transition, however, massively obese patients could sustain themselves much better than similar aged patients of normal weight because obese individuals have the reserve caloric stores in their extra fat mass and their increased muscle mass, which developed to move their extra weight around their environment (see Chapter 3 to learn more about how the body responds to semistarvation and differences identified in this response between morbidly obese and normal weight individuals). Even after the transition occurs, the shortened length of the bowel left after major resections usually means that a portion of any average-size meal will not be absorbed, so the patient will have some diarrhea after each meal. This produces a negative social circumstance where the individual has to have a bathroom available soon after a meal ends. This also limits most patients who have major bowel resections from overeating if they want to have a job and a social life.

Several surgeons in different university medical centers, made the intellectual leap from considering the short-gut syndrome as a major liability for everyone who experienced it, to the point where they considered creating the short-gut syndrome to treat the massively obese patients admitted to their hospitals with otherwise untreatable problems. It took approximately 15 years to have this concept—where the surgeon would deliberately create malabsorption or maldigestion by an operation—evolve before it became acceptable to a group of surgeons outside the initial group of innovators. Less than 10 years after the concept of creating a short-gut syndrome to treat morbid obesity became acceptable, a large number of patients had already received this type of operation and it became obvious that the severity of complications that could develop after the procedure eliminated this "first-generation" operation from clinical practice. This type of cycle continues to repeat itself with the introduction of each new phase of bariatric surgery although the control mechanisms and the length of the cycles suggest we are learning as we progress.

As experience with the short-gut syndrome accumulated after World War II, several different surgeons in the 1950s, in different countries and without knowledge of each other, began designing operations to treat massive obesity and its associated medical problems. Typically, a few patients were treated in each hospital with the support of their medical and surgical colleagues. The medical community then waited to judge the success of these initial experiments. This was in an era before Institutional Review Boards (IRBs) existed. IRBs were created, in the 1970s, to oversee and monitor experimental treatments to help protect the rights of the patients who volunteered to participate in these treatments. The federal government has developed an extensive set of guidelines through the National Institutes of Health (NIH) to ensure that patients are informed of the risks, known or unknown, associated with clinical trials that the patients are being asked to accept. Although, in hindsight, some would judge these attempts at developing a surgical solution for morbid obesity crude by today's standards, it was an entirely different era with different standards, and these surgeons were the first group of physicians trying to help a group of people that still suffers from exceptional discrimination by the general public, the media, many aspects of our health care system, and the federal government.

Dr. Richard L. Varco, a surgeon at the University of Minnesota, probably performed the first jejunoileal bypass in 1953, to produce malabsorption in a massively obese patient to induce weight loss (Figure 2–1).[1,2] This procedure consisted of an end-to-end jejunoileostomy with the distal end of the bypassed small bowel separately anastomosed to the cecum to drain it. At about the same time, Dr. Victor Henriksson of Gothenburg, Sweden, probably performed a similar type small-bowel malabsorptive operation, but he resected the small bowel that was excluded from the digestive pathway. Henriksson's operation eliminated the "safety net" of reversibility if complications developed.[1] Neither surgeon published the details or the outcome of their patients.

Some of the first experimental work on the role of different sections of the gastrointestinal (GI) tract on the absorption of nutrients, vitamins, and minerals was performed to help determine which sections of the small bowel were least important for digestion of essential nutrients and, therefore, could be "bypassed" to create a shortened, intestinal, digestive pathway with minimal side effects. Much of this information, which helped surgeons decide how the bowel could be altered to produce weight loss with the fewest consequences from malabsorption and maldigestion, originated at the University of Minnesota. In 1954, Kremen et al.[3] published a research article comparing the effects of bypassing various portions of the small intestine. In this paper, they also reported

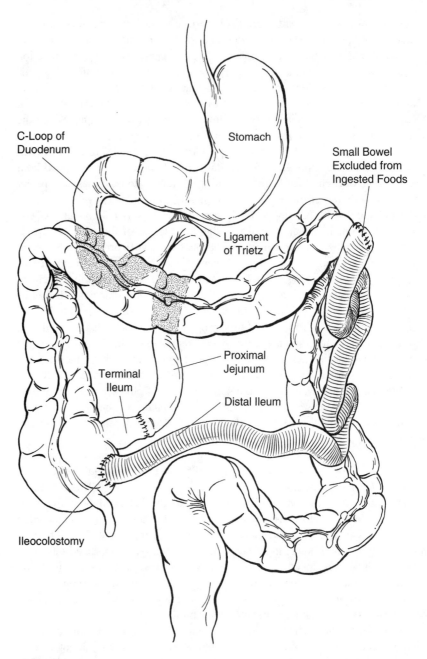

FIGURE 2–1   The first malabsorption procedure preformed by Dr. Richard Varco in 1953 at the University of Minnesota to treat morbid obesity.

the results of a patient upon whom they had performed an end-to-end je-junoileal bypass to treat obesity, similar to what Varco had done. Their paper was the first publication of bariatric surgery in the medical literature. These US surgeons envisioned that this procedure would be reversed when the patient reached ideal body weight, limiting the potential for complications.

Several surgeons, including Payne and DeWind,[4,5] Sherman and collegues,[6] and Lewis et al.,[7,8] performed variations of small-bowel bypasses on a series of 10 to 100 patients in the late 1950s through the 1960s. The history of this evolution of the small-bowel bypass is described extensively in several review articles[9,10] and book chapters.[1,2] The essential lessons learned during this period were that the proximal 35 to 50 cm (11.8 to 19.7 inches) of jejunum can accomplish nutrient absorption in the vast majority of people and in virtually all obese people; preserving the last 5 to 10 cm (2 to 3.9 inches) of ileum, especially maintaining the ileocecal value, substantially decreases complications and inconveniences associated with electrolyte imbalances, diarrhea, and the development of gallstones and nephrolithiasis; and when the bypassed segment of the small bowel is left with a closed proximal stump, bacterial overgrowth can occur in this bypassed segment. If the bypassed segment is brought out to the skin as an ostomy, where it can be flushed with nutrients or connected to the biliary system where bacteriostatic fluids and pancreatic enzymes are continuously flushed down the limb, then bacterial overgrowth can be prevented. Initially, however, surgeons worried more about nutrient reflux into the bypassed segment decreasing the weight loss associated with the procedure. Only later as complications accumulated in the large number of patients who underwent small-bowel bypasses in the late 1960s and early 1970s, was it speculated that the bacteria that washed back into the bypassed small bowel might be absorbed into the mesenteric venous circulation and produce inflammation in the liver and other problems.

Payne and DeWind[5] are credited with originating the most popular form of the small-bowel bypass, the "14 + 4" jejunoileal bypass that was the "standard" operation for the 15 to 20 years that this form of malabsorptive procedure was routinely performed (Figure 2–2). They divided the jejunum 35 cm (14 inches) past the ligament of Treitz and connected the proximal jejunum in an end-to-side manner 10 cm (4 inches) from the ileocecal, leaving the 300 to 500 cm (118.1 to 196.9 inches) of distal jejunum and proximal ileum bypassed. This procedure produced significant weight loss in the vast majority of people it was performed on. It was relatively easy to perform, even in the most morbidly obese (superobese) patients, because the technical procedures were performed on the readily accessible midgut. Diarrhea was the primary negative consequence of this procedure. A bowel movement usually occurred within 30 minutes of food ingestion.

It was the reflux of bacteria into the bypassed small bowel that ultimately led to the abandonment of all of these first-generation malabsorption procedures. The wall of the bypassed, nonfunctioning small bowel became atrophic, probably allowing for bacterial translocation through the bowel wall into the portal venous system causing stimulation of the Kupffer cells in the liver and the celiac lymphatics. Subsequent cytokine stimulation or other mechanisms, such as gut alcohol production and absorption, led to acute hepatic failure, at times, and death ensued in approximately 5% of patients in the first postoperative year. Other symptoms suggesting an autoimmune mechanism caused by cytokine stimulation included arthralgias, fevers, cutaneous eruptions and progressive hepatic injury and fibrosis. Possibly 50% of patients who had these early variations of jejunoileal bypass developed cirrhosis within 25 years of

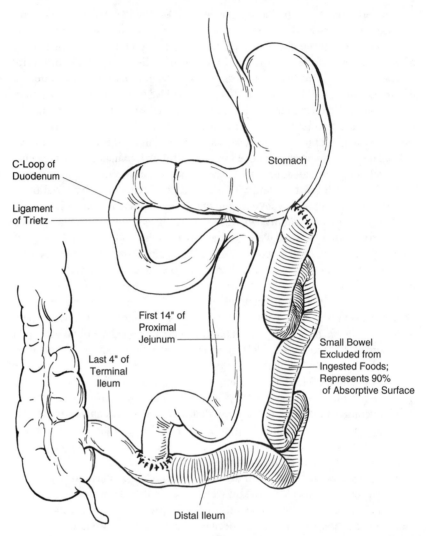

FIGURE 2–2   The "14 + 4" jejunoileal bypass created by Payne and DeWind in the mid-1960s.

the procedure. Thus, what appeared to be a very effective weight loss operation had to be abandoned 30 years after it was initially described due to an unacceptable rate of complications that were identified by the persistence of the bariatric surgeons who followed their patients over the course of the patients lives, as opposed to the usual 30 to 90 days postoperatively that insurance companies allow surgeons to follow patients before they begin refusing to reimburse the surgeon for their medical care.

Although these very thoughtful and innovative surgeons, and others like them, began responding empathetically to the problems with which these massively obese patients were presenting by trying to design operations that would be effective in helping people lose weight, this field of bariatric medicine (the treatment of the obese) remains a problematic area. This is primarily the result of long-term patient followup to document both the consequences and the long-term weight-loss results of operations that alter the gastrointestinal tract to help people lose weight.

The history of the rise in popularity of the small-bowel bypass as a surgical treatment of obesity and then its discrediting once the total list of the consequences of the procedure became known, over a 20-year period, illustrates why the federal government and the medical insurance industry need to assume greater responsibility for the collection of long-term data after surgical procedures. This is especially important now that mechanisms for obtaining the cost-effectiveness of various treatments have been established by the US Public Health Service.[11] The collection of this type of data enables comparisons of medical versus surgical treatments for a specific disease, as well as of the results of the treatments and their effects on changes in patients' quality of life over time. Then, as a society, we can decide whether it is more cost-effective to treat a morbidly obese person at age 30 years with a bariatric procedure or to withhold this type of treatment and pay for the consequences of the complications of the comorbid problems associated with morbid obesity, which might include a heart attack, a stroke, knee or hip joint replacement, early disability retirement from work because of osteoarthritis of the back, or a combination of these problems. It is illogical and unethical to refuse to pay for surgical treatment of morbid obesity, which is one of the most cost-effective treatments when evaluated by formal cost-effectiveness analyses as outlined by the US Public Health Service.[12]

As reports of the complications of the jejunoileal bypass accumulated in the 1970s, other bariatric operations, such as the gastric bypass and the various forms of gastroplasties, began to take center stage as safer, although technically more challenging, procedures.[10] Despite the problems that developed with the small-bowel bypasses, the concept of developing an effective malabsorption operation was never totally abandoned. The creative energy for this concept, however, left the United States as a consequence of our medical malpractice laws.[13] Even under the guidance of IRBs, developing procedures are not immune to malpractice risks. Our legal system also acts more like a sledgehammer than a surgical blade. Once a certain type of procedure is associated with complications, all similar procedures can be condemned in court.

An Italian surgeon, Dr. Nicola Scopinaro, developed the first popular "second-generation" malabsorptive procedure known as a "biliopancreatic bypass."[14] His group has studied its outcomes and the physiological consequences of this procedure since the mid-1970s. His important innovation was to start the malabsorptive limb in the proximal duodenum so that the limb was continually flushed with bacteriostatic bile and pancreatic juices to limit stasis and the accumulation of colonic flora in toxic amounts. This limb was labeled the "biliopancreatic" limb, and the small bowel segment that carried food to where the two limbs joined was labeled the "enteric" limb. The segment after the two limbs was connected was labeled the "common channel" (Figure 2–3). The length of the common channel is important because nutrient digestion and absorption essentially occur only in this segment after the biliary and pancreatic juices mix with ingested food. Through trial and error, significant modifications of the procedure have occurred so that it now includes a partial horizontal gastrectomy to both limit food intake modestly and separate the two limbs by closing the duodenal stump. Also, a 200-cm (78.7-inch)–long Roux-en-Y gastrojejunostomy is created by dividing the ileum 250 cm (98.4 inches) from the ileocecal valve and then reanastomosing the long proximal biliopancreatic limb of duodenum, jejunum, and proximal ileum to the last 50 cm (19.6 inches) of terminal ileum in an end-to-side manner to create a short 50-cm (19.6-inch)–long common channel.

The group has used this approach to surgically treat more than 2500 patients and has followed them for more than 20 years. During the followup period, no patient has developed the hepatic failure, arthralgias, nephrolithiasis, cutaneous eruptions, or impaired mentation that was seen with the first-

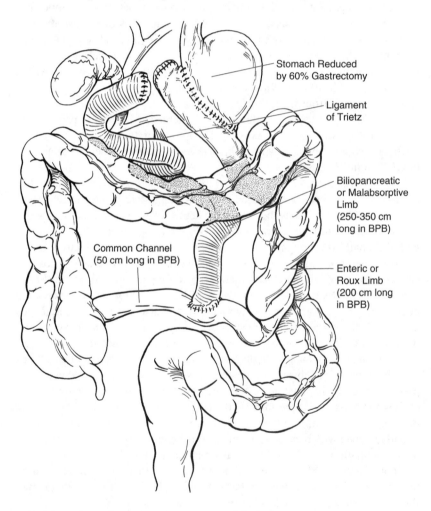

FIGURE 2–3 The biliopancreatic bypass (BPB) developed by Dr. Nicola Scopinaro in Genoa, Italy, in the 1970s.

generation of malabsorptive procedures.[15] The biliopancreatic bypass still causes diarrhea, flatulence, and stomal ulcers in the enteric, Roux limb. Some patients cannot tolerate the procedure because it produces anemia, bone demineralization, and protein malabsorption, and because it requires an unusual level of compliance with oral supplementation of doses of minerals (especially iron and calcium), vitamins (especially vitamins D and B_{12}), and protein at levels greater than recommended by the FDA.

Another second-generation malabsorption procedure evolved in Quebec under the direction of Dr. Picard Marceau and his colleagues at Lavall University, the biliopancreatic diversion with duodenal switch.[16] They decided to preserve the pylorus of the stomach and keep the first portion of the duodenum in the enteric limb of the procedure by dividing the duodenum just proximal to where the common bile duct passes posterior to it at the junction of the first and second portions of the duodenum (Figure 2–4). They also decreased the size of the stomach by more than 60% by removing the greater curvature of the fundus, corpus, and antrum as a sleeve gastrectomy, which allowed for vitamin B_{12} absorption because food still comes in contact with intrinsic factor made in the stomach. This type of gastrectomy also decreases the incidence of the "dumping" phenomenon because the pylorus is still present to hold gastric contents until the right osmotic concentration is produced for absorption without the irritation of hyperosmotic fluids being released into the ileum. It also eliminates stomal ulcers in the small bowel because the acid produced by the stomach exits into the first portion of the duodenum, which produces bicarbonate to neutralize it before it enters the jejunum or ileum, which are not designed to accept an acid load. They used a longer length for their common channel (100 cm [39.4 inches]) to help increase protein absorption.

In Chapter 12, Dr. Marceau relates his experiences with more than 500 patients treated in the last 10 to 15 years. Patients who choose these types of procedures must be intelligent enough to monitor their protein intake, keeping it greater than 65 to 80 g/d, and to supplement their diet with vitamins, minerals, and antidiarrheal agents. Many surgeons in the United States still resist considering using the biliopancreatic bypass as a primary operation because of negative lay press and legal responses to malabsorptive procedures that bypass the majority of the small bowel. Some surgeons, however, have enthusiastically used these procedures. These include the Hess brothers in Ohio,[17] and more recently, Dr. Michael Garriger in New York City,[18] who has completed a series of these procedures laparoscopically with his associates at the Mount Sinai Hospital.

Another use for malabsorptive type procedures was designed by Dr. Henry Buchwald at the University of Minnesota.[19] In a 5-year prospective study supported by the NIH, he demonstrated that if the terminal ileum (the portion of the small bowel where most lipids are absorbed) was bypassed, patients with genetic hyperlipidemia would have serum lipid levels return to normal values. His team was also the first to show that the thickness of atherosclerotic plaques seen on coronary artery angiograms would actually be reduced in size, decreasing the percentage of blockage in the arteries by keeping lipid levels normalized in these patients.[20] Therefore, coronary artery disease is reversible with

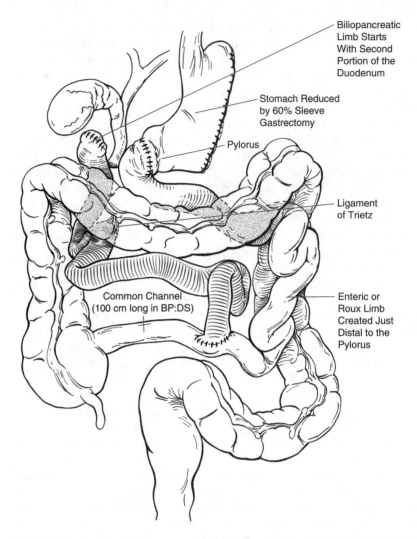

Biliopancreatic
Limb Starts
With Second
Portion of the
Duodenum

Stomach Reduced
by 60% Sleeve
Gastrectomy

Pylorus

Ligament
of Trietz

Common Channel
(100 cm long in BP:DS)

Enteric or
Roux Limb
Created Just
Distal to the
Pylorus

FIGURE 2–4   The biliopancreatic diversion with duodenal switch (BP:DS) developed by Dr. Picard Marceau at Lavall University.

the right treatment to eliminate elevated lipid levels. This procedure, the ileal bypass, which diverts foods from the final 150-cm (59.1-inch) segment of the ileum before the ileocecal valve by dividing the ileum at this point and then anastomosing the enteric limb of the bowel directly into the colon in an end-to-side manner that does not usually result in significant weight loss (Figure 2–5). It also has very few associated complications, probably because the segment of bowel that is bypassed is relatively short. The indications for this operation have become much more limited with the development of the lipid-lowering drugs (the statins) in the last decade, although it is still used if someone is allergic to these medications or has developed recurrent pancreatitis from hyperlipidemia not controlled by the statins.

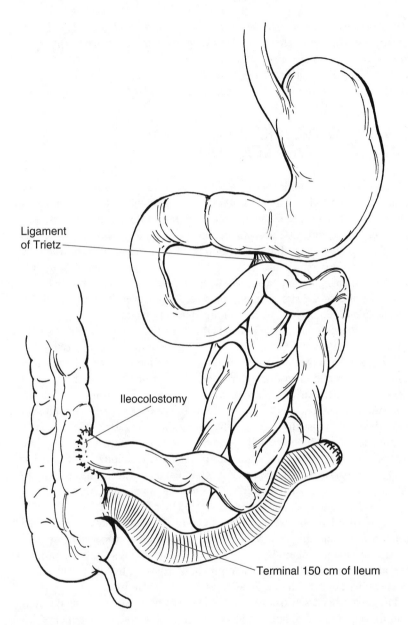

Ligament of Trietz

Ileocolostomy

Terminal 150 cm of Ileum

FIGURE 2–5   The ileal bypass developed by Dr. Henry Buchwald to treat familial hyperlipidemia.

When Dr. Buchwald has a morbidly obese patient who also has high lipid levels, he usually combines the ileal bypass with a vertical banded gastroplasty (described in the "Restrictive Procedures" section of this chapter and in Chapter 10), which is a pure restrictive bariatric procedure (personal communication, June 2002). He worries that an ileal bypass combined with a gastric bypass might lead to unacceptable nutritional deficiencies. No randomized control trial

(RCT) has been conducted that confirms or denies his theory. He has heard from other surgeons that they have successfully combined the ileal bypass with a gastric bypass. These isolated reports do not have the necessary followup to guarantee the safety of this approach or to define how bariatric procedures should be combined with medical and/or surgical treatment of familial hyperlipidemia.

COMBINED RESTRICTIVE–MALABSORPTIVE PROCEDURES

While numerous surgical groups were trying to perfect a "malabsorptive" operation to treat morbid obesity in the 1960s, the complications these operations produced stimulated other surgeons to try entirely different approaches. The first procedure to gain wide acceptance other than small-bowel bypasses was a procedure created by Dr. Edward Mason at the University of Iowa, which he labeled a "gastric bypass," and first described it in 1966 (Figure 2–6).[21] This procedure primarily caused patients to decrease their initial food intake by restricting the size of the stomach and the size of the outlet from the restricted gastric segment, rather than by causing malabsorption and diarrhea.

The small proximal gastric pouch is then attached to the jejunum, usually 20 to 150 cm (7.9 to 59.1 inches) from the ligament of Treitz, bypassing the distal stomach, all of the duodenum, and a portion of the jejunum from the flow of nutrients. This eliminates the pylorus from its role in regulating the osmotic content of the gastric effluent, which can lead to dumping. When the pylorus is removed or bypassed, a hyperosmotic meal is transported to the small bowel without the dilution usually produced by the addition of gastric juices such as hydrochloric acid. When the small bowel is exposed to irritating hyperosmotic solutions, such as maple syrup, a complex physiologic reaction is produced that usually includes sweating, tachycardia, abdominal pain with cramps leading to diarrhea, general malaise, and a variety of other less-common symptoms, such as arrhythmias, headache, and other neurologic symptoms.

The gastric bypass also produces vitamin B_{12} deficiency because food does not pass the antrum to allow attachment of intrinsic factor (that is secreted in the antrum) to the vitamin B_{12} contained in various foods so that vitamin B_{12} can be absorbed. Iron deficiency is common after gastric bypass because iron is most readily absorbed in the duodenum, which is also bypassed.

The gastric bypass also closes off the majority of the stomach and the duodenum from traditional diagnostic tests such as endoscopic inspection and radiologic examinations with barium meals. This concerns many physicians because of the frequency of complaints of midepigastric pain in the population in general. There is the potential problem of a patient developing a gastric malignancy or ulcer disease that would escape early detection. Because the gastric bypass has been used as a bariatric treatment for more than 35 years without the development of either of these phenomena occurring more often in postoperative patients than in the general population, these concerns seem less important. Peptic ulcer disease is probably less common after gastric bypass because within 3 months of the procedure, the mass of acid-secreting cells in

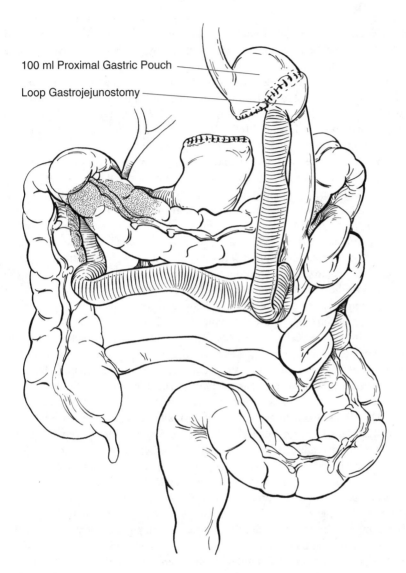

100 ml Proximal Gastric Pouch

Loop Gastrojejunostomy

FIGURE 2–6   The initial gastric bypass developed by Dr. Edward Mason in 1966.

the corpus of the stomach has significantly decreased as a consequence of diminished stimulation from direct contact with food and no antral distention.

Within 10 years of its introduction, the gastric bypass became the dominant bariatric procedure performed by American bariatric surgeons, who, until the late 1990s, performed the majority of the bariatric operations in the
world. This evolution occurred because the patients who were treated with gastric bypass had far fewer postoperative complications than did patients with
small-bowel bypass, making it far easier to take care of them postoperatively.
Also, the primary features of the procedure, the restricted size of the proximal

stomach, a small anastomosis (10 to 14 mm [0.4 to 0.6 inches] wide) between the new pouch and the small intestine, and the short section of bypassed small bowel, did not appear to have to be precisely defined to achieve reliable weight loss of approximately 45.4 kg (100 lb) in the first postoperative year. Although the gastric pouch was initially described as being as big as 100 to 150 mL in volume, it was easiest to divide the stomach above the connection of the short gastric vessels to the spleen to decrease the risk of injuring the spleen. When this is done, the pouch is usually less than 50 mL and can be made as small as 10 to 15 mL without increasing the complication rates. In fact, the smaller pouch size improves weight loss and typically eliminates acid secretion cells from the upper pouch (because those cells are all located more distally). The incidence of ulcer developing in the attached small bowel (poststomal ulcer), which is not usually exposed to acid, decreases. Additionally, in the early 1970s, surgical stapling devices became available on the commercial market making it much easier to perform the gastric division and leading to the generic term of "gastric stapling" procedures that would incorporate both the gastric bypass and "gastroplasty" procedures that used these new devices, which were invented in the Soviet Union. Alden[22] introduced the stapler as a method of separating the two gastric pouches and suggested that when the staplers were used, the stomach did not have to be completely divided into two separate structures, as initially described by Mason.[21] It was also assumed that the leak rate for the gastrojejunostomy might be lower if the stomach was not divided (this assumption was never directly tested in an RCT and is now generally believed not to be true because the leak rate for divided versus nondivided gastric pouches for gastric bypass is similar in all modern series).

The 1970s also witnessed the first use of an RCT to compare two bariatric procedures. Dr. Ward Griffen (when he was chairman at the University of Kentucky) performed an RCT comparing jejunoileal bypass to gastric bypass.[23] He also altered Dr. Mason's initial concept by converting the loop gastrojejunostomy to a Roux-en-Y gastrojejunostomy (Figure 2–7). This eliminated bile-induced gastritis in the proximal pouch and esophagitis, along with the esophageal and gastric dysphagia that can result from long-term bile exposure. The complication rate was significantly lower after gastric bypass versus jejunoileal bypass in this RCT, yet the weight loss outcomes were similar. Buckwalter[24] soon after reported similar results from a nonrandomized comparison of the two procedures. Thus, both patient groups—those who accepted a randomized surgical protocol and those who demanded to choose which procedure was performed on them—had similar results with the gastric bypass, demonstrating equal weight loss outcomes with significantly lower complication rates.

Numerous additional modifications to the gastric bypass were proposed in the 1980s and early 1990s without any specific feature achieving widespread popular acceptance among bariatric surgeons because the basic features of the operation produced such consistent results that more specific modifications of technique could not be shown to produce significantly improved outcomes. The only RCT to specifically test different design modifications of a standard gastric bypass that appears to improve results in a select subpopulation of morbidly obese patients was completed by Dr. Robert Brolin and colleagues at the

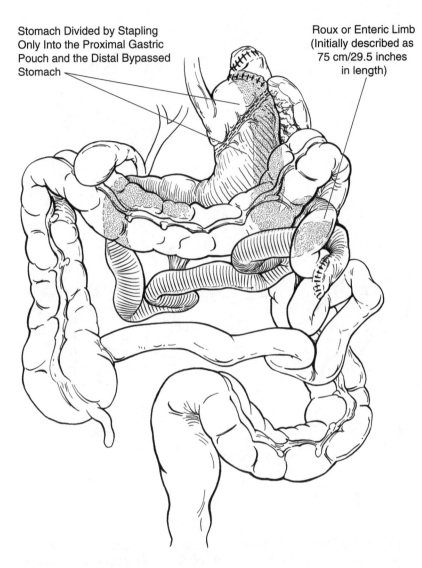

Stomach Divided by Stapling
Only Into the Proximal Gastric
Pouch and the Distal Bypassed
Stomach

Roux or Enteric Limb
(Initially described as
75 cm/29.5 inches
in length)

FIGURE 2–7   The Roux-en-Y gastric bypass suggested by Dr. Ward Griffen uses a stomach stapler to segment the stomach without separating it into two divided segments and brings the Roux limb retrocolic and retrogastric.

state medical school in New Brunswick, NJ.[25] In "superobese patients" (defined as greater than or equal to 90.7 kg [200 lb] overweight for this comparison), his grouped tested whether a Roux limb length of 150 cm (59.1 inches) would produce better weight loss than a more standard Roux limb length of 75 cm (29.5 inches). In a small group of patients, Brolin demonstrated a difference in weight loss that was significant but still less than 10% of the initial weight of the patients (7%) at 2 years postoperation using a "long-limb" gastric bypass (Figure 2–8).

Although surgeons in the 1980s and early 1990s tried various Roux limb

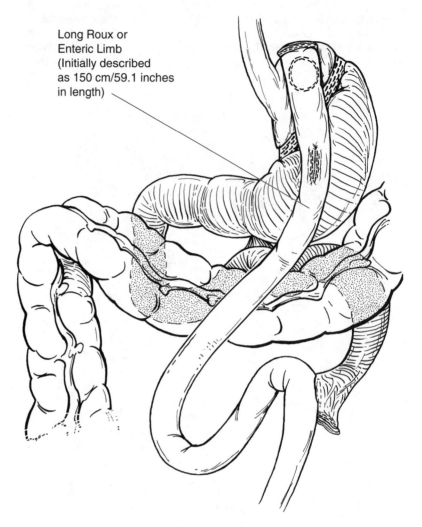

Long Roux or
Enteric Limb
(Initially described
as 150 cm/59.1 inches
in length)

FIGURE 2–8   The long limb gastric procedure demonstrating the use of the various "stapled" anastomosis and the Roux limb brought up antecolic and antegastric.

lengths, the literature on biliopancreatic bypass has convinced most bariatric surgeons that malabsorption is controlled more by how short the "common channel" is, rather than the length of the "enteric" or "biliopancreatic" limbs (see Figure 2–3). Surgeons who worry that superobese patients need a more drastic operation initially often recommend the use of a "distal" gastric bypass (Figure 2–9) where the connection between the enteric and biliopancreatic limbs are placed more distally; typically at 150 cm (59.1 inches) from the ileocecal valve. This increases the incidence of protein and vitamin malabsorption, especially in noncompliant patients who will not maintain a high-protein diet supplemented by extra vitamins, calcium, and iron, and who require more intensive postoperative monitoring. Because there has been no large-series RCT comparing whether a distal gastric bypass for the superobese routinely produces better weight loss without increasing the complication rate, most bariatric surgeons choose to use less-drastic initial operations and then revise unsuccessful patients to more drastic procedures until more information is available (see Chapter 16).

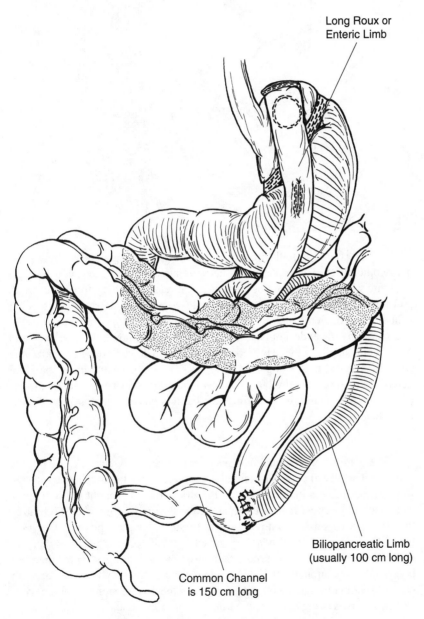

Long Roux or
Enteric Limb

Biliopancreatic Limb
(usually 100 cm long)

Common Channel
is 150 cm long

FIGURE 2–9   A distal gastric bypass with a 150-cm (59.1-inch)–long common channel. The Roux limb here is retrocolic and antegastric.

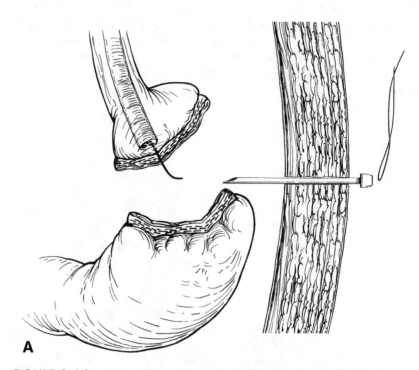

A

FIGURE 2–10   The pull-through method of performing a gastric bypass laparoscopically. **A.** The endoscope is inserted into the blind gastric pouch where the snare will be pushed out of the pouch and released by electrocautery. **B.** A pull-through wire from a percutaneous endoscopic gastrostomy (PEG) tube kit is inserted through the abdominal wall by using a 16-gauge catheter or needle, and snared by the endoscopist to be pulled out of the mouth. **C.** The anvil end of a circular stapling device is prepared to be pulled down into the gastric pouch from the surgical field using the pull-wire. The larynx usually has to be lifted anteriorly to allow the anvil to slide down the esophagus behind it and the endotracheal tube within it (sometimes the balloon has to be deflated on the endotracheal tube).

There are other technical features of creating a Roux-en-Y gastric bypass that do not appear to make substantial differences to the long-term outcome results. These features include whether the Roux limb is brought up to the gastric pouch in a retrocolic versus an antecolic position, or whether the limb is then brought up further in a retrogastric versus antegastric position (see Figures 2–7, 2–8, and 2–9). When the stomach is totally divided into two separate parts, the Roux limb can be brought up retrocolic and retrogastric but then can be available for an anterior, side-to-side gastrojejunostomy because the limb can be brought through the opening created by the divided stomach. Even without the stomach being divided, the limb can often be brought anterior through the bare area over the caudate lobe of the liver. These features allow the sur-

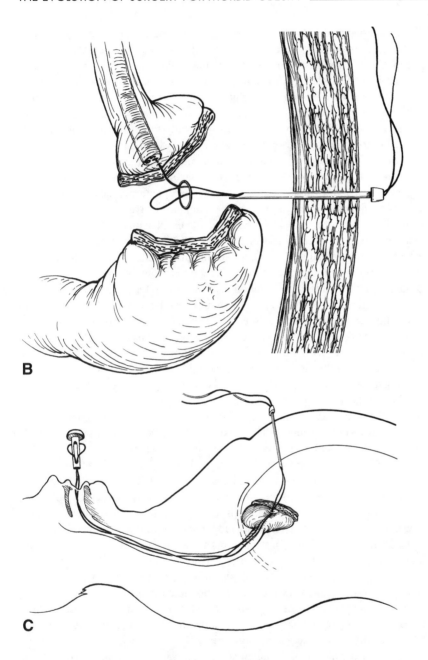

B

C

geon multiple choices based on the length of the mesentery and any adhesions that may be present from prior events.

The innovation that has generated the most interest in bariatric surgery to surgeons since the introduction of stapling devices is the ability to complete bariatric procedures laparoscopically. Several groups in America and Sweden attempted to use laparoscopic techniques to perform gastric bypasses in the 1990s.

The first group to develop a practice largely devoted to performing gastric bypasses laparoscopically were Drs. Allan Wittgrove and G. Wes Clark in San Diego, CA.[26,27] The gastric bypass is technically difficult to perform, especially on morbidly obese patients in whom standard-length stapling devices can be too short to reach the deep intraabdominal spaces of the morbidly obese patients. Wittgrove and Clark managed to use the first-generation of stapling instruments specifically developed to be used laparoscopically to develop a technique that worked in the vast majority of patients they attempted it on. They used an innovative transoral passage of the anvil of a circular stapler endoscopically to create their gastrojejunostomy (Figure 2–10). They used a "pull-wire" initially designed to place gastrostomy tubes, using endoscopic techniques to help create the gastrojejunostomy. In the pull-wire technique for gastrostomy tube placement, the gastrostomy tube is pulled down the esophagus into the stomach and then out through the abdominal wall after the pull-wire is passed transcutaneously through the abdominal wall through a needle placed into the stomach by an assistant working with the endoscopist. The wire is snared in the stomach by the endoscopist, then pulled out the mouth and attached to the gastrostomy tube, and then pulled down as described above to bring the tube into position from the inside to the outside. For a laparoscopic gastric bypass, the anvil of the circular stapler is pulled down the esophagus after the edoscopist uses the pull wire to encircle the anvil by passing the wire up the shaft of the anvil then out the side of the shaft and over the mushroom cap of the anvil. (Figure 10 shows the anvil being pulled into the gastric pouch, ready to complete the gastrojejunostomy.) Once the shaft of the anvil is pulled out of the gastric pouch (while the mushroom top stays in the pouch), the circular stapler is passed through the abdominal wall into the Roux limb of the jejunum. The spike end of the stapler is pushed out of the limb and into the shaft of the anvil to complete the gastrojejunostomy.

Once Wittgrove and Clark demonstrated that laparoscopic techniques did not increase the complication rate (Chapter 9 discusses how laparoscopic techniques decrease certain postoperative complications) and produced weight loss similar to gastric bypass by laparotomy, other surgical groups demonstrated that modifications of their laparoscopic technique produced equally good results. Torre and Scott[28] demonstrated that the anvil can be placed transabdominally without the aid of the endoscopy. Hiaga and colleagues[29] showed that the gastrojejunostomy and jejunojejunostomy can be handsewn within the same 90-minute framework that others complete this procedure laparoscopically using staplers. Schauer's group showed that a linear stapler followed by hand sewing the openings produced results similar to that of Wittgrove and Clark's technique for the gastrojejunostomy.[30]

Significantly, most of the laparoscopic innovations in technique have been pioneered by surgeons in private practice rather than surgeons in university settings. Most of the innovations for transforming the gastric bypass and biliopancreatic bypass to laparoscopic techniques have occurred in the United States in spite of problems with malpractice laws, while many other advances in laparoscopic techniques for other common abdominal surgical procedures have been made in Europe. The Europeans' (excluding Scopinaro) lack of enthusiasm for using any type of malabsorption procedure was largely responsible for this difference in the recent evolution of the surgical technique as it relates to the gastric bypass and biliopancreatic bypass.

RESTRICTIVE PROCEDURES

Even as Mason and his colleagues at the University of Iowa introduced gastric bypass as a bariatric treatment in the late 1960s, they worried that the procedure produced significant physiologic changes in the gastrointestinal tract. Mason was concerned that the full significance of these changes would not be known for 30 years. Almost 40 years later, gastric bypass has become the dominant bariatric procedure in the United States, as it has consistently produced good weight loss outcomes without the disastrous complications produced by the jejunoileal bypass. Mason and others, however, struggled in the early 1970s to create even safer, more physiologic bariatric procedures. Along with Dr. Kenneth Printen, Dr. Mason developed the concept of a purely restrictive operation, limiting food intake by decreasing the size of the gastric pouch above a restricted gastric outlet, rather than creating malabsorption or diverting the flow of nutrients into nonphysiologic routes.[31]

They published their initial results over a 2-year period, using a gastroplasty in 1973, where they divided the stomach horizontally leaving a narrow gastrogastrostomy opening (10 to 12 mm [3.9 to 4.7 inches]) on the greater curvature of the stomach (Figure 2–11).[31] This procedure was unable to consistently induce or maintain weight loss because of the upper pouch enlarging and becoming more muscular as it modified to adjust to the restriction, and/or because of the stoma enlarging so that food passed without restriction into the lower portion of the stomach. All throughout the 1970s, variations on this theme were attempted without success.[10] This extensive experimentation, with some patients receiving multiple revisions, was another major factor in turning the medical insurance industry against bariatric surgery, in addition to the complications they were having to pay for as a result of jejunoileal bypass surgery. The 1970s ended the era where surgeons dictated what procedures they performed and ended their ability to price new procedures at levels they suggested. Insurance companies demanded the right to preapprove elective surgical procedures and severely restricted the number of policies that qualified for bariatric surgery as part of their evolution into the "managed care" era that still dominates the insurance field.[32]

The medical profession, especially surgeons, lost a major chance to manage its own destiny when it accepted the largess of the government paying for procedures in the new Medicaid and Medicare programs without initiating an evaluation program to credential or certify which procedures, especially new procedures, were effective. The Medicaid and Medicare programs initiated in the late 1960s were initially treated by physicians with suspicion. By the 1970s, however, they were being used as a source of unregulated expansion, especially in university medical centers where human experimentation took off in several areas.[33] Bariatric surgeons, along with cardiac surgeons, ophthalmol-

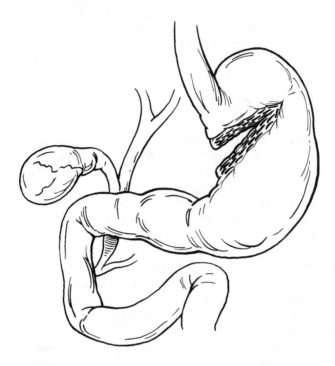

FIGURE 2–11   The original Mason gastroplasty.

ogists, orthopedists, and urologists, created many new effective operations, but also generated enormous expenses. Creativity without adequate measures to separate and regulate effective and ineffective procedures led to commercial insurance programs trying to eliminate their participation in any trials involving new surgical procedures. Only recently has the government tried to reestablish mechanisms for surgical experimentation to occur outside the walls of government institutions such as the NIH, or outside of the approval process of FDA trials, where the company completing the trial usually pays for all surgical costs. Some new medical implant devices have been approved after a trial where the patients themselves had to pay the costs of their surgical procedure.[34] Medicare patients can now use their insurance benefits to become participants in many FDA trials. It is hoped that other insurance companies will also follow this policy.

This decade of experimentation did result in the development of two different groups developing gastroplasties that produced stable, long-term weight loss results by the mid-1980s. Dr. Henry Laws demonstrated that a silastic ring wrapped around the outside of the stomal outlet of a vertically, rather than a horizontally, placed staple line gastroplasty could serve as a permanent restrictive devise to create a small proximal gastric pouch with a stable, small gastric outlet (Figure 2–12).[35] Dr. Mason also created a similar type vertically stapled gastroplasty that was made technically easier by using a circular stapler to create a circular hole through the stomach at a predetermined point near the lesser curvature defined by using a bougie (Figure 2–13A)[36] and by measuring the distance from the esophagogastric junction. An angled stapling instrument could then be passed through the hole along the bougie toward the esophagogastric junction to create a standard-sized pouch, which was restricted by sewing a strip of 1.5-cm (0.6-inch)–wide polypropylene mesh through the gastric window and the lesser curvature mesentery to itself to create a permanent ring 12 mm (0.5 inches) in diameter (Figure 2–13) as the restricted neostoma at the end of the vertical tube created by the stapler. Alternatively, a linear stapling device that has the capacity to place four to six rows of staples and then cut parallel in the middle of the rows can be used to divide the vertical pouch from the rest of the fundus (Figure 2–13B). This approach creates a more permanent scar than placing staples without cutting the pouch off from the rest of the stomach.

Eckhout and Willbanks[37] worked with the Autosuture Stapling Company to create a notched stapler to modify Laws' procedure so as to make it easier to perform, with more consistent results using the silastic ring. Some surgeons found that the polypropylene mesh used by Mason caused excessive granulation tissue and obstruction, with the liver attaching itself to the mesh and flattening the outlet.

Several surgeons have been able to perform vertical-banded gastroplasties laparoscopically. The easiest way is probably that described by Champion in which a wedge of fundus is removed to create the vertical gastric tube before placing a band or ring around the distal outlet (Figure 2–14).[38] With advances in instrument design, even easier techniques may become available. Over the last 20 years, it has become obvious that this technique works because a lesser curvature tube of stomach has the best muscular support and stays functionally stable. Although the permanent band or ring also keeps the neostoma from enlarging, adhesions, especially to polypropylene mesh, can lead to

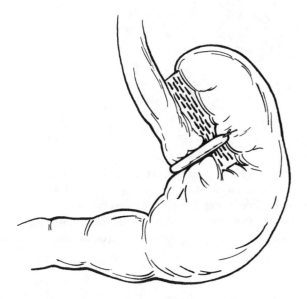

FIGURE 2–12   The silastic ring gastroplasty.

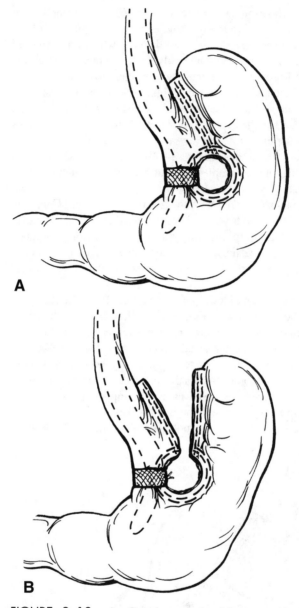

FIGURE 2–13   **A.** Creation of the Mason vertical-banded gastroplasty (VBG) with bougie in the esophagus and stomach to help calibrate the width of the pouch by dispensing the line of staples tightly against the tube. **B.** VBG modified by dividing the pouch from the rest of the stomach to eliminate the possibility of a late staple rupture leading to failure of the procedure.

stomal obstruction and in some instances, to erosion of the medical device (material) into the stomach lumen.

GASTRIC BANDING

In the mid-1970s, Angelchik began using a band wrapped around the distal esophagus to treat gastroesophageal reflux disease.[39] His band was a composite of several materials glued together that was sewed to itself and left just above the esophagogastric junction without imbricating tissue around it to keep it in place. His band frequently moved up on the esophagus toward the chest or came apart, relocating in numerous intraabdominal positions, causing complications. The failure of the initial model to stay together led to its removal from the market until a better design was created in the late 1990s.

This idea was transferred to bariatric surgery where several different surgical groups began experimenting with band placement in the late 1970s and early 1980s to duplicate the success of restrictive gastroplasties without having to cut or staple the stomach. Dr. Molina described this approach where he used a permanent gastric band made of polypropylene mesh to wrap around the upper stomach (Figure 2–15).[40] This produces a permanent, nonadjustable gastric band sewn to itself, creating a small proximal gastric pouch just below the esophagogastric junction. Molina's approach is associated with a low initial complication rate because it is a clean procedure with no intestinal perforations and can be done quickly through a small 8- to 10-cm (3.1- to 3.9-inch) upper midline incision in the abdomen. His technique has not been adapted for use in many other centers because there are almost no published long-term data and because it is completed as an outpatient procedure with very little preoperative patient preparation or followup. Fewer than 3 days are spent to complete the whole program except for telephone followup. This is against the standards set and maintained by most other bariatric surgeons (see Chapter 6). Many other bariatric surgeons have converted one or more of the patients initially treated by Molina and his colleagues to more accepted bariatric procedures.

Kuzmak[41] and Hellers[42] developed a solution to the largest problem encountered with vertical-banded gastroplasties or nonadjustable gastric bands almost simultaneously. They connected a band with a balloon lining 330 degrees of its inside arc to tubing that could be connected to an access port reservoir similar to those used for parenteral infusion therapy, which could be left subcutaneously placed on the muscle wall. This access port lays below the subcutaneous fat on the rectus muscle but can be accessed by a needle and syringe to infuse saline under fluoroscopic guidance. The band designed by Kuzmak was modified to use a buckling device to close and lock itself, while the Heller band had tabs to sew together to fix it. Both bands were then imbricated in a tube of stomach sewn over the band to prevent its movement (Figure 2–16).

This was initially an expensive curiosity, but with the explosion of laparoscopic surgery that occurred in the early 1990s, these bands were ideally designed for laparoscopic placement. The technical features to determine the best anatomic approach and method of securing the band in a position where

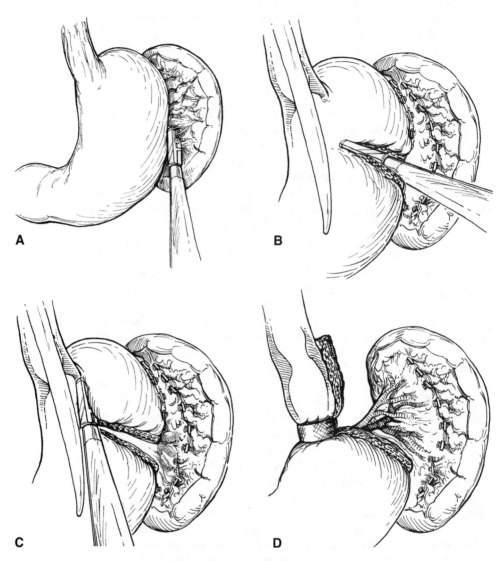

FIGURE 2–14 Laparoscopic vertical-banded gastroplasty as initially described by Dr. Ken Champion by (**A**) removing the short, gastric vessels connecting the greater curvature of the stomach to the spleen; (**B**) beginning to wedge out the upper-left corner of the fundus and corpus to create the vertical tube of the gastroplasty; and (**C**) completing the vertical part of the excision with the bougie in place to define the width of the tunnel. **D.** The completed procedure with the band wrapped around the outlet of the vertical gastroplasty. Omentum can be sewn over the band and outlet to decrease adhesions to the liver.

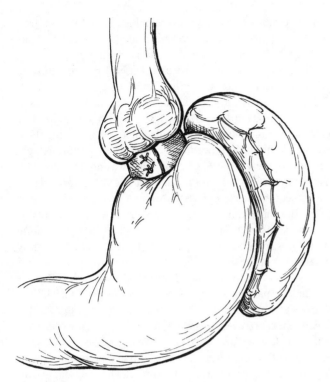

FIGURE 2–15   The Molina nonadjustable gastric band made out of polypropylene mesh.

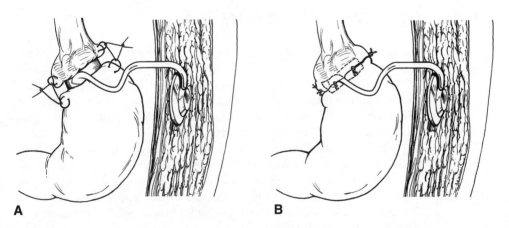

FIGURE 2–16   Adjustable gastric band. **A.** Band wrapped around stomach and connected to subcutaneously placed reservoir so that the inner balloon can be adjusted. **B.** Stomach sewn over the band to imbricate it in place in its own tunnel.

the size and shape of the proximal gastric pouch remained constant took most of the 1990s to solve. Kuzmak entered a relationship with the BioEnterics Corporation, a division of INAMED Corporation (Santa Barbara, CA). His band completed several FDA-monitored trials and was released for general use in June 2001.[34] Heller's band has been produced by Obtech, Inc. of Switzerland, and is mainly available in Western Europe. Obtech was purchased by Johnson & Johnson (New Brunswick, NJ) in June 2002. More than 100,000 adjustable bands have been placed laparoscopically worldwide since 1993, making it the most common laparoscopic bariatric procedure now routinely performed, except in the United States. In the United States, the band was not available until June 2001, so that open gastric bypass is the most commonly performed procedure, although laparoscopic gastric bypass is running a close second now. The popularity of the adjustable band stems, in part, from its reversibility. It can be removed and the stomach resumes its original shape and size within days. It is also initially less invasive and is associated with a lower mortality rate, probably only 10% that of the other bariatric procedures that open the GI tract. However, the band has had to be revised, replaced by a more effective operation, or has not helped patients using it lose at least 10% of their initial body weight in 10 to 40% of patients who have used it, especially in the US trials that used relatively inexperienced laparoscopic surgeons.[34] As experience with how to place the band, when and how to adjust it, and how to train its users to work effectively with it improves, the overall outcome results should improve, approaching those reported by surgical teams who have used it in over 500 patients with excellent results.[43]

EXPERIMENTAL APPROACHES

The percentage of morbidly obese patients who have accepted a bariatric surgical therapy for treatment of their obesity and its comorbid medical problems is still less than 10% of those eligible for treatment. This is because surgical therapies hurt and cause at least significant short-term disabilities, and because all the therapies described so far in this chapter alter the function of the gastrointestinal tract, either causing diarrhea, or pain, or both, if one overeats.

All the major pharmaceutical companies are trying to develop medications that will decrease nutrient absorption, decrease appetite, or increase metabolic rate. At some point, all of us can imagine that our genes will be tested for defects and that remedies will be available to correct most of the alterations that cause specific diseases, including obesity. In the meantime, numerous new surgical avenues are being pursued.

Scientists have postulated for years that the brain rather than the stomach should be the source of the restriction to eating. Only one surgical attempt has been made in humans. This approach was based on scientific observations in animals that appetite can be stimulated and occasionally suppressed by creating lesions in the lateral hypothalamus of the brain. Similar lesions in humans after strokes or tumor formation suggest similar results are possible. In 1974, Quaade reported that electrocoagulation of sites in the lateral hypothalamus using stereotaxic stimulation produced small but significant transient reduction in caloric intake and body weight in 3 of 5 treated patients.[44]

Several investigators have tried electrical stimulation of the neural or muscular complexes in the stomach to create gastric paresis or vagally induced satiety (Figure 2–17); this is discussed in Chapter 13. The long history of the successful use of pacemakers for cardiac problems without discernible side effects has given the pacemaker companies latitude to try their technology on a number of other medical problems, including stimulation of the diaphragm to improve respiratory function in quadriplegia, control of seizures, pain control, and gastric stimulation of paresis secondary to diabetic neuropathy. Attempts to use electrical stimulation of the stomach to decrease weight evolved from the experience of pacing the stomach in diabetics. In diabetics who have lost intrinsic pacemaker function in the stomach, externally derived pacing can improve appetite at low levels but can cause nausea at higher levels. Other innovations will be tested because the number of people desiring relatively safe, noninvasive therapies is in the millions and very few therapies have worked.

FURTHER EVOLUTION OF BARIATRIC SURGICAL PROCEDURES

The evolution of laparoscopic techniques to bariatric surgery has created a new wave of enthusiasm for bariatric surgery in general. Attention is now focused

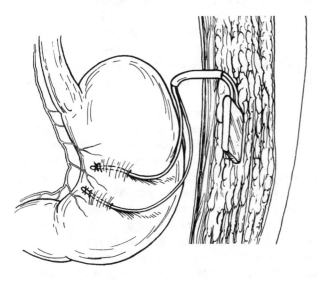

FIGURE 2–17   Implantable Gastric Stimulator (IGS) with two bipolar implantable leads above and below the pes anserinus connected to a battery stimulator placed in the subcutaneous fat. In an FDA-monitored trial, Transneuronix Inc. (Fort Lee, NJ) created various methods of retrograde gastric electrical stimulation (pacing) to determine whether tachygastria is an effective treatment for the morbidly obese. The settings for when and how the battery fires to create the stimulation via the pacing wires can be changed by a computer program using radio frequency signaling.

on the newer, less invasive procedures, as well as on how the medical profession and the medical insurance industry treat morbidly obese individuals. Open surgical procedures to the abdomen usually keep patients out of work from 3 to 10 weeks and require up to 4 to 6 months for a complete return to all preoperative social and work functions. This limits these types of procedures to people who have the social and economic support to be able to take this time off.

Prior to the introduction of laparoscopic bariatric techniques, fewer than 1% of the people who were eligible to have a bariatric procedure to treat their morbid obesity and its comorbid medical problems completed a preoperative evaluation and proceeded with operative therapy in a given calendar year in the United States. The introduction of laparoscopic surgical techniques allows a portion of the population to return to work within 1 week of surgery and allows the vast majority of patients to return to full activities in under 3 months. This has greatly increased the demands for this type of surgery (probably 4- to 10-fold).

The demand currently outstrips the capacity of surgeons trained to perform these difficult laparoscopic procedures in morbidly obese patients. Increased demand by morbidly obese patients for laparoscopic procedures has stimulated more general surgeons to enter the field of bariatric surgery, especially younger surgeons who are learning these techniques as a routine part of their training. Older bariatric surgeons, who trained before laparoscopic techniques were developed in the late 1980s and 1990s, are left to try to service the population of patients who are not candidates for laparoscopic surgery (i.e., those with prior upper abdominal operations with adhesions or the superobese, where instruments are still too short to reach), to learn these new techniques at their own expense (time away from their practice, expensive course work including hands-on training, and the frustration facing the senior surgeons placed back in a dependent, learning role), or to recruit newly trained surgeons to their practices.

These older surgeons have publicly worried that the newer surgeons are too "technique" oriented. Fewer than half of the university teaching programs in general surgery had multidisciplinary teams practicing bariatric surgery in the late 1990s and the nature of the teaching programs allow the resident trainees little participation in this type of activity. Tension exists between newly trained surgeons who want to practice laparoscopic bariatric surgery part time as one component of a laparoscopic practice and these older surgeons who feel that this type of practice demands a full-time commitment with a dedicated support structure in a specialized office environment (see Chapter 6).

The medical insurance industry has felt the pressure from morbidly obese patients demanding access to surgical treatments. When fewer patients were interested, it was easier to deny access to surgical treatment because it rarely became an issue in contracting with companies. The issue never came up or was often brushed aside as too expensive or experimental to include in a contract. The "patient rights" movement and media attention makes these arguments look politically incorrect and unethical, particularly in light of the other procedures they pay for that are the result of morbid obesity causing comorbid disease, such as joint replacement, back surgery, tracheostomy for sleep apnea, peritoneal shunts for pseudotumor cerebri, and skin grafts for venous stasis ulcers. The recent publication of *Guidelines for Obesity Treatments* by the NIH[45] and the World Health Organization (WHO),[46] who both endorse bariatric surgery for morbidly obese patients, has further increased the pressure to include the therapies in medical insurance contracts. Businesses are at risk for discrimination, class action, or wrongful death suits if they ignore these recommendations.

Increased patient demand has also stimulated the medical manufacturing market. Large companies that make surgical stapling devices, such as Johnson & Johnson and Tyco, and many other smaller companies, see this market expanding exponentially over the next several years. Once these companies make a decision to enter this type of market, they increase the pressure on the medical insurance industry to change benefits by bringing more political and advertising pressure. They also bring their expertise to training more surgeons to perform these difficult tasks and to designing instruments that will be easier to use.

The number of people that will have laparoscopic bariatric surgery will obviously increase. The challenge to the medical profession, the insurance industry, and their regulations will be to see that this can be done safely. Various surgical associations have already created guidelines to help hospitals and their credentialing boards identify what components are necessary to create a safe bariatric surgical program. The American Society for Bariatric Surgery (ASBS) and the Society of American Gastrointestinal Endoscopic Surgeons (SAGES) jointly cooperated to release guidelines to help hospitals credential bariatric surgeons in 2001.[47] This is an instance where an organization that represents the established bariatric surgeons cooperated with an organization that represents the leading edge of laparoscopic surgeons to establish safeguards for patients and the medical profession to allow this field to evolve. The oldest, centralized surgical organization, the American College of Surgeons, also published its own guidelines for this type of practice in 2001.[48]

Mortality for bariatric operations is usually 1% or less unless the surgeon is operating mostly on patients who are superobese (usually those 200% above ideal body weight or who have a body mass index >60 kg/m^2) or those who are on Medicaid or indigent, in whom higher levels of mortality and morbidity are expected.[49] The increased mortality associated with lower socioeconomic status is assumed to be caused by the greater level of disease burden, both medical and psychiatric, that these individuals must display before they qualify for surgical treatment in our society. Similar to many other difficult operations, surgeons and hospitals that are performing bariatric procedures (high-volume centers) frequently have fewer complications and deaths because treatment of these high-risk patients is more routine.[50] The difficulty of most bariatric operations causes the initial learning curve to be steep, with more complications occurring in the surgeon's first 100 cases than in the subsequent group of 100 cases. Fewer morbidly obese people will die or have serious complications if bariatric operations are restricted to high-volume centers that could be labeled "Centers of Excellence" similar to organ transplantation centers. To date, however, neither the insurance industry nor the state or federal government have been willing to establish criteria for Bariatric Centers of Excellence based on outcome criteria modeled after the credentialing of trauma centers and transplant centers. It is not clear how bariatric treatments will evolve in this new century, but the field can expect to be discredited again if the mortality rate or the morbidity rates for procedures witnesses a sharp rise because too many inexperienced surgeons attempt to perform bariatric procedures infrequently.

REFERENCES

1. Buchwald H, Rucker RD. The rise and fall of jejunoileal bypass. In: Nelson RL, Nyhus LM, eds. *Surgery of the Small Intestine*. Norwalk, CT: Appleton Century Crofts, 1987:529–541.
2. Deitel M. Jejunocolic and jejunoileal bypass: a historical perspective. In: Deitel M, ed. *Surgery for the Morbidly Obese Patient*. Philadelphia: Lea & Febiger, 1988:81–89.
3. Kremen AJ, Linner LH, Nelson CH. An experimental evaluation of the nutritional importance of proximal and distal small intestine. *Ann Surg* 1954;140:439–444.
4. Payne JH, DeWind LT, Commons RR. Metabolic observations in patients with jejunocolic shunts. *Am J Surg* 1963;106:272–289.
5. Payne JH, DeWind LT. Surgical treatment of obesity. *Am J Surg* 1969;118:141–147.
6. Sherman CD, May AG, Nye W. Clinical and metabolic studies following bowel bypassing for obesity. *Ann N Y Acad Sci* 1965;131:614–622.
7. Lewis LA, Turnbull RB, Page LH. "Short-circuiting" of the small intestine. *JAMA* 1962;182:77–79.
8. Lewis LA, Turnbull RB, Page LH. Effects of jejunocolic shunt on obesity; serum lipoproteins, lipids, and electrolytes. *Arch Intern Med* 1966;117:4–16.
9. O'Leary JP. Gastrointestinal malabsorptive procedures. *Am J Clin Nutr* 1992;5S:567S–570S.
10. Buchwald H. Evolution of operative procedures for the management of morbid obesity. *Obes Surg* 2002;12:705–717.
11. Martin, LF, White S, Lindstrom W Jr. Cost-benefit analysis for the treatment of severe obesity. *World J Surg* 1998;22:1008–1017.
12. Zhang P, Wang G, Narayan KMV. Cost-effectiveness of interventions for reducing body weight. In: Medeiros-Neto G, Halpern A, Bouchard C, eds. *Progress in Obesity Research 9*. Eastleigh, UK: John Libbey & Co. Ltd., 2003:579–584.
13. Casey BE, Civello KC, Martin LF, O'Leary JP. Medical malpractice risk associated with bariatric surgery. *Obes Surg* 1998;8:158–159.
14. Scopinaro N, Gianetta E, Civalleri D. Biliopancreatic bypass for obesity: I. Initial experiences in man. *Br J Surg* 1979;66:618–620.
15. Scopinaro N, Adami GF, Marinari GM, et al. Biliopancreatic diversion: two decades of experience. In: Deital M, Cowan SM Jr, eds. *Update: Surgery for the Morbidly Obese Patient*. Toronto, Canada: FD-Communications, 2000:227–228.
16. Marceau P, Biron S, Bourque R-A, et al. Biliopancreatic diversion with a new type of gastrectomy. *Obes Surg* 1993;3:29–35.
17. Hess DW, Hess DS. Biliopancreatic diversion with a duodenal switch. *Obes Surg* 1998;8:267–282.
18. Ren CJ, Patterson E, Gagner M. Early results of laparoscopic biliopancreatic diversion with duodenal switch: a case series of 40 consecutive patients. *Obes Surg* 2000;10:514–523.
19. Buchwald H, Varco RL. A bypass operation for obese hyperlipidemia patients. *Surgery* 1971;70:62–70.

20. Buchwald H, Varco RL, Matts JP, et al. Effect of partial ileal bypass surgery on mortality and morbidity from coronary artery disease in patients with hypercholesterolemia. Report of the Program on the Surgical Control of the Hyperlipidemias (POSCH). *N Engl J Med* 1990;323:946–955.

21. Mason EE, Ito C. Gastric bypass in obesity. *Surg Clin North Am* 1967;47:1845–1852.

22. Alden JF. Gastric and jejunoileal bypass: A comparison in the treatment of morbid obesity. *Arch Surg* 1977;112:799–806.

23. Griffen WO, Young VL, Stevenson CC. A prospective comparison of gastric and jejunoileal bypass procedures for morbid obesity. *Ann Surg* 1977;186:500–507.

24. Buckwalter JA. Clinical trial of jejunoileal and gastric bypass for the treatment of obesity: four-year progress report. *Am Surg* 1980;46:377–381.

25. Brolin RE, Kenler HA, Gorman JH, Cody RP. Long-limb gastric bypass in the superobese. A prospective randomized study. *Ann Surg* 1992;21:387–395.

26. Wittgrove AC, Clark GW, Tremblay LJ. Laparoscopic gastric bypass, Roux-en-Y: Preliminary report of five cases. *Obes Surg* 1994;4:435–437.

27. Wittgrove AC, Clark GW. Laparoscopic gastric bypass, Roux-en-Y 500 patients: technique and results, with 3–60 month follow-up. *Obes Surg* 2000;10:233–239.

28. de la Torre RA, Scott JS. Laparoscopic Roux-en-Y gastric bypass: A totally intra-abdominal approach—technique and preliminary report. *Obes Surg* 1999;9:492–497.

29. Higa KD, Boone KB, Ho T. Laparoscopic Roux-en-Y gastric bypass for morbid obesity in 850 patients: Technique and follow-up. *Arch Surg* 2000;135:1029.

30. Schauer PR, Ikramuddin S, Gourash W, et al. Outcomes after laparoscopic Roux-en-Y gastric bypass for morbid obesity. *Ann Surg* 2000;232:515–529.

31. Printen KJ, Mason EE. Gastric surgery for relief of morbid obesity. *Arch Surg* 1973;106:428–431.

32. Lauve RM, Martin LF. What surgeons need to know to help patients receive quality medical care in managed care settings. *Am J Surg* 1997;174:452–458.

33. Martin LF, O'Leary JP. The surgeon's role in improving medical care in the managed care era. *Am J Surg* 1997;174:294–296.

34. Martin LF, Smits GJ, Greenstein RJ. Laparoscopic adjustable gastric banding to treat morbid obesity: 3-year efficacy and 5-year safety data from the US multicenter trials. (*submitted*)

35. Laws HL, Piatadosi S. Superior gastric reduction procedure for morbid obesity. A prospective, randomized trial. *Am J Surg* 1981;193:334–336.

36. Mason EE. Vertical banded gastroplasty. *Arch Surg* 1982;117:701–706.

37. Eckhout GV, Willbanks OL, Moore JT. Vertical ring gastroplasty for obesity: five-year experience with 1463 patients. *Am J Surg* 1986;152:413–416.

38. Champion JK. Laparoscopic vertical banded gastroplasty. In: Cohen RV, Libanori H, Schiavon A, Schauer P, eds. *Videolaparoscopic Approach to Morbid Obesity.* Via Letera Medical Publishers (*in press*).

39. Angelchik JP, Cohen R. A new surgical procedure for the treatment of gastroesophageal reflux and hiatal hernia. *Surg Gynecol Obstet* 1979;148:246–249.

40. Oria HE. Gastric banding for morbid obesity. *Eur J Gastroenterol Hepatol* 1999;11:105–114.

41. Kuzmak LI. Silicone gastric banding: A simple and effective operation for morbid obesity. *Contemp Surg* 1986;28:13–18.

42. Forsell P, Hallberg D, Hellers G. Gastric banding for morbid obesity: Initial experience with a new adjustable band. *Obes Surg* 1993;3:369–374.

43. O'Brien PE, Brown WA, Smith A, McMurrick PJ, Stephens M. Prospective study

of laparoscopically placed, adjustable band in the treatment of morbid obesity. *Br J Surg* 1999;86:113–118.

44. Quaade F, Vaernet K, Larsson S. Stereotaxic stimulation and electrocoagulation of the lateral hypothalamus in obese humans. *Acta Neurochir (Wien)* 1974;30:1111–1117.

45. North American Association for the Study of Obesity (NAASO) and the National Heart, Lung, and Blood Institute (NHLBI). *Clinical Guidelines on the Identification, Evaluation, and Treatment of Overweight and Obesity in Adults. The Evidence Report.* NIH Publ #98–4083. Rockville, MD: US Government Printing Office, 1998.

46. World Health Organization. Obesity: Preventing and managing the global epidemic. Geneva: WHO, 1998.

47. SAGES. *Guidelines for Laparoscopic and Conventional Surgical Treatment of Morbid Obesity.* Society of American Gastrointestinal Endoscopic Surgeons (SAGES), Los Angeles, CA, 2002.

48. Committee on Emerging Surgical Technology and Innovation. ACS recommendations for facilities performing bariatric surgery. *Bull Am Coll Surg* 2000;85:20–23.

49. Martin LF, Tan T-L, Holmes PA, Becker DA, Horn J, Bixler EO. Preoperative insurance status influences postoperative complication rates for gastric bypass. *Am J Surg* 1991;161:625–634.

50. Luft HS, Bunker JP, Enthoren AC. Should operations be regionalized? The empirical relationship between surgical volume and mortality. *N Engl J Med* 1979;301:1364–1369.

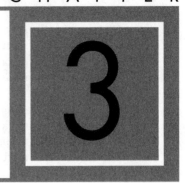

THE PHYSIOLOGY OF THE BRAIN, THE GUT, AND THE FAT CELLS IN THE MORBIDLY OBESE

FRANK L. GREENWAY / SCOTT E. GREENWAY / WILLIAM J. RAUM

The surgical treatment of obesity originated from observations made on nutrient absorption in patients who lost segments of their small bowel from disease and from animal experiments designed to define which segments (determining minimal lengths) of the small bowel were required to maintain homeostasis of body protein, vitamin, and mineral stores. Over the last 30 years, the evolution of bariatric surgery has focused more on improvements in technique and instrumentation than on advances related to the physiologic functions of the central nervous system, the gastrointestinal tract, and the host of hormones, proteins, neuropeptides, and other substances that have been identified that influence appetite, satiety, energy expenditure, and the regulation of the subcutaneous and visceral fat stores. Basic scientists and the government agencies that support the majority of their research have also underused the unique model that surgical treatment of morbid obesity provided during the last 20 years, where important research has identified numerous new substances and genes that affect the above physiologic functions. The National Institutes of Health is making an effort to improve the scientific understanding of how bariatric operations work by specifically funding four to six bariatric research centers over the next 5 years and having these centers collect tissue and blood, which will be made available to other centers with grants to pursue relevant research hypotheses. Because obesity appears posed to become the number one public health problem in the United States, and eventually the world, focusing attention on the factors that determine why certain bariatric procedures are successful not only helps to improve the outcomes of surgical treatment, but helps us understand the physiology of obesity. This should lead us to a more focused attempt to develop medications that will duplicate the success of these surgical procedures and eliminate the need for such invasive treatment.

Because the literature on the physiology of the brain, gut, and fat cells spans volumes, this chapter focuses on the aspects that impact body weight regulation in the morbidly obese and, in particular, those aspects related to efforts to surgically treat the disease by altering these interactions. The treatment of morbid obesity has included hypothalamic surgery, regional fat removal and surgical interventions on the intestinal tract. This chapter approaches the problem from these vantage points. This chapter is not intended to be an exhaustive review of the literature.

THE BRAIN

Integration and Hypothalamic Obesity

The laws of thermodynamics tell us that obesity, a state of excess stored energy, results from an excess in energy intake relative to energy expenditure. That is, more food or calories are consumed than are burned. The brain is the integrator of signals controlling energy intake and energy expenditure. More specifically, a section of the brain, the hypothalamus, with the rest of the autonomic nervous system is an important element in control of energy balance. A balance between two components of this system, the parasympathetic and sympathetic provide an unconscious control of many systems including the cardiovascular, respiratory, digestive, and other body systems. Destruction or chemical inhibition of one component tends to lead to increased activity of the other. In fact, it has been stated that all types of obesity known result in abnormally low sympathetic activity.[1]

The relationship of the autonomic nervous system to the control of body weight can be seen in rodent experiments with surgically induced hypothalamic lesions or in humans with hypothalamic injury from trauma or brain infarcts.[2] Destruction of one area of the hypothalamus (medial) increases parasympathetic activity and vagal nerve firing while, at the same time, decreasing the firing of sympathetic nerves. Increased vagal activity, characteristic of ventromedial hypothalamic injury, triggers pancreatic islet insulin release, causing increased food intake and eventually leads to obesity. In rodent experiments where vagal stimulation of the pancreatic islet cells was blocked, hypothalamic injury did not cause obesity.[3] The importance of the role played by hyperinsulinemia in the etiology of hypothalamic obesity has also been demonstrated through the successful treatment of hypothalamic obesity in humans with somatostatin, a hormone that inhibits insulin secretion. Lustig et al. demonstrated that children with hypothalamic obesity are sensitive to insulin and that decreasing the early phase of insulin secretion with somatostatin causes weight loss.[4]

Not only does ventromedial hypothalamic injury increase parasympathetic activity, but it also decreases the firing rate (activity) of sympathetic nerves. Just as increased parasympathetic activity increases food intake, decreased sympathetic activity decreases energy expenditure. This dual effect of the autonomic nervous system to increase food intake while decreasing energy expenditure gives the autonomic nervous system a prominent place in the control of body weight. These observations in hypothalamic obesity give clues to the properties of an effective treatment strategy. One could postulate that effective obesity treatments should alter the autonomic nervous system in an opposite direction to that seen with hypothalamic obesity.

In fact, injury to the ventrolateral hypothalamus in animals has been accompanied by weight loss caused by a reduction in food intake and an increase in energy expenditure, the opposite of lesions in the ventromedial hypothalamus.[5] This is also true in humans.[6] These observations led to an attempt to treat morbid obesity in a human with a lesion in the ventromedial hypothalamus.[7] This attempt was only temporarily successful, but was done unilaterally. The irreversible nature of bilateral hypothalamic lesioning in humans discouraged an attempt of this more radical approach.

Hypothalamic injury is a convenient obesity model to study and, through its use, much has been learned about the physiology of weight regulation. It is a rare cause of obesity, however. A review of the medical literature in 1975 revealed less than 100 reported cases.[8] One could legitimately ask if the changes taking place in hypothalamic injury have any relationship to the more common variety of obesity. Peterson et al. performed careful tests of autonomic nervous system function in 56 healthy men with varying percentages of overweight. They found that there was a depression in the sympathetic nervous system activity associated with obesity, but, unlike hypothalamic obesity, there was a depression of parasympathetic activity as well.[9] Most obesity is caused by several factors of variable influence on overall energy balance. Experimentally induced obesity can aid in isolating those factors and the conditions that influence their expression.

Vagus Nerve and the Parasympathetic System

Moving down from the hypothlamus, parasympathetic activity conducted through the vagus has been studied by severing the vagal nerve (truncal vagotomy). Kral and Gortz reported a series of 21 morbidly obese subjects who underwent a bilateral truncal vagotomy. The average weight loss was 20 kg (44.1 lb), although the range of weight loss varied from 0 to 50 kg (0 to 110.2 lb).[10] Those who lost weight had a decrease in food and liquid intake.[11] The bariatric procedure, vertical-banded gastroplasty (VBG), with and without truncal vagotomy, was compared in 69 patients. At 5 years of followup, 34 subjects with vertical-banded gastroplasty lost significantly less weight (21 kg [46.3 lb]) than did the 25 subjects with the addition of truncal vagotomy (33 kg [72.8 lb]).[12] These studies suggest that the vagal nerve seems to be playing a role in the physiology of morbid obesity.

The Sympathetic System

The documented increase of sympathetic activity in the obese has been further explored by testing the system with overfeeding and underfeeding. Underfeeding by 10% reduces energy expenditure by 6 to 8 kcal/kg of fat-free mass per day. Overfeeding increases energy expenditure to the same degree. Whether obese or of normal body weight, the human body defends its usual weight.[13] Therefore, reducing calorie intake decreases calories burned and prevents weight loss, while increasing intake increases calories burned and prevents weight gain. This study, suggesting that usual weight is defended, has been used to explain why the maintenance of medically induced weight loss has been so poor.[14] Because energy expenditure is primarily affected by the sympathetic nervous system, these observations indicate that dysregulation of the sympathetic nervous system is a key, if not essential, step in the development of morbid obesity.

The primary transmitters of information within the sympathetic nervous system are the catecholamines epinephrine, norepinephrine, and dopamine. These neurotransmitters can be stimulated or inhibited and measured. Drugs with similar activity can be given to mimic effects of the sympathetic nervous system. More dramatic weight loss can be accomplished through fasting or very-low-calorie dieting and their effect on the sympathetic nervous system noted. Total and modified fasting is commonly associated with postural hypotension, a symptom mediated by decreased activity of the sympathetic nervous system.[15] During a 400 kcal/d diet, the postural blood pressure drop was associated with a statistically significant decrease in norepinephrine, further implicating decreased sympathetic nervous system activity.[16] Bray presented evidence of a reciprocal relationship between food intake and sympathetic nervous system activity.[17] This may explain the robust effect of caffeine and ephedrine which caused a 17.5% weight loss over 6 months of which 75% was attributed to a decrease in food intake while 25% was attributable to an increase in energy expenditure.[18,19]

Neuropeptides

Although the autonomic nervous system is a major participant in the mechanisms controlling body weight at the level of the brain, other brain systems are also involved. Three examples are neuropeptide Y, orexins, and the melanocortin-4 receptors.

Neuropeptide Y (NPY) stimulates appetite and inhibits thermogenesis, the heat generated by burning calories. Injection of NPY into the paraventricular nucleus of the rat hypothalamus causes the most potent central appetite stimulation known. NPY levels increase during starvation to counter this loss of calories by stimulating appetite and decreasing calories lost through the generation of heat. Leptin and insulin secretion, to be discussed more below, fall during starvation and may help to stimulate the rise in NPY.

Orexins are found in the lateral hypothalamus and increase food intake in response to fasting or hypoglycemia, while α-melanocyte–stimulating hormone,

TABLE 3–1. PEPTIDES AFFECTING FOOD INTAKE CENTRALLY	
INCREASE FOOD INTAKE	DECREASE FOOD INTAKE
Beta-endorphin	Alpha-melancocyte–stimulating hormone
Dynorphin	Apolipoprotein A-IV
Galanin	Calcitonin
Ghrelin	Cocaine amphetamine-regulated transcript
Growth hormone-releasing hormone	Corticotrophin-releasing hormone
Melanin-concentrating hormone	Cyclo-Histadine-proline
Neuropeptide Y	Glucagon-like peptide-1
Orexin	Insulin
	Neurotensin
	Urocortin

acting on the melanocortin-4 receptor, inhibits food intake and results in weight loss.[20] The melanocortin-4 receptor has special relevance to morbid obesity by being the most common single gene defect cause of the disease in humans.[21]

Glucocorticoids also play an important role in obesity and although they are not neuropeptides, their secretion is controlled by the peptides corticotrophin-releasing hormone and adrenocorticotropic hormone (ACTH). Glucocorticoids, usually referred to (inaccurately) as just "steroids," are secreted from the adrenal glands. There are many pharmacologic agents available that mimic the effects of the steroids secreted by the adrenal glands, including hydrocortisone, prednisone, and dexamethasone. Increased levels of glucocorticoids (from the adrenals or given as drugs) result in Cushings syndrome and the development of central obesity. Adrenalectomy, when performed in rodents, removes the major source of glucocorticoid secretion and increases sympathetic activity that reverses or prevents the progression of obesity.[22] The autonomic nervous system, related neuropeptides and glucocorticoids are primary participants in the central nervous system control of body weight. All compounds that increase sympathetic tone reduce food intake, thus linking the autonomic nervous system to these compounds[17] (Table 3–1).

THE GUT

The gut is presumed to play an important role in morbid obesity, because all of the successful treatments for morbid obesity are surgical interventions on the gastrointestinal tract.[23] There are many gastrointestinal hormones known to impact feeding. All, with the exception of ghrelin, decrease food intake (Table 3–2). Although more gut hormones impacting food intake are continually being discovered, the most interesting gastrointestinal hormones from the standpoint of this discussion are those that change or have the potential to change with the gastrointestinal surgeries used to treat morbid obesity. The hormones derived from the bypassed upper intestinal tract, in general, decrease, while those derived from the distal gastrointestinal tract increase.[23]

INCREASE FOOD INTAKE	DECREASE FOOD INTAKE
Ghrelin	Amylin
	Apolipoprotein A-IV
	Bombesin
	Cholecystokinin
	Cyclo-histadine-proline
	Enterostatin
	Gastric inhibitory polypeptide
	Gastrin-releasing peptide
	Glucagon
	Glucagon-like peptide-1
	Insulin
	Motilin
	Neuromedin
	Neurotensin
	Pancreatic polypeptide
	Peptide YY
	Somatomedin

TABLE 3–2. GASTROINTESTINAL HORMONE AFFECTING FEEDING

Hormones Decreased by Obesity Bypass Operations

MOTILIN

Motilin, a hormone from the upper gastrointestinal tract, is decreased in obese individuals compared to lean.[24] Being an upper gastrointestinal hormone, it is decreased in the postoperative period after gastric or intestinal bypass surgery.[25] Twenty years following intestinal bypass surgery, motilin levels were elevated as compared to nonoperated controls.[26] Because motilin levels do not correlate with weight loss, motilin appears to be playing a minor role in the success of gastrointestinal bypass surgery.

PANCREATIC POLYPEPTIDE

Pancreatic polypeptide has a similar pattern to motilin. It is depressed in obese subjects.[27] After bypass surgery, it is further reduced. Twenty years after intestinal bypass, however, it is at levels above those in nonoperated obese controls. Thus, pancreatic polypeptide would also appear to play a minor role in the success of gastrointestinal bypass surgery for obesity.

GASTRIC INHIBITORY POLYPEPTIDE

Gastric inhibitory polypeptide (GIP), another upper gastrointestinal hormone, may have a more substantial role to play in the mechanism of weight loss after gastrointestinal bypass surgery. Obesity is associated with elevated GIP levels that do not decrease with food restriction or medical weight loss,[28] but do fall after bypass surgery.[25] Inhibition of GIP secretion in rodents prevents obesity.[29] However, elevated levels are seen 20 years after intestinal bypass[25] and successful maintenance of a lower body weight, confounding the long-term role of gastric inhibitory polypeptide in the mechanism of bypass-induced weight loss.

GHRELIN

Ghrelin is a recently discovered circulating gastrointestinal peptide hormone, and the only one demonstrated to increase food intake in humans. It is produced by the stomach, stimulates growth hormone secretion, and causes hyperphagia in rats that results in obesity.[30,31] In humans, ghrelin levels increase prior to meals, and ghrelin administration stimulates food intake.[32] These actions suggest that ghrelin may be the signal for meal initiation. Although ghrelin levels are lower in the obese subjects, they do not decrease normally after a meal as they do in lean subjects.[32] A dietary-induced 17% reduction of body weight increases 24-hour plasma ghrelin by 24%. This elevation of ghrelin has been postulated to induce weight regain. However, a 36% weight loss following gastric bypass operations for obesity decreased 24-hour plasma ghrelin by 77% as compared to normal weight controls, and by 72% as compared to obese controls.[33] Thus, ghrelin levels increased after nonsurgical weight loss, but decreased following surgically induced weight loss. These observations support the concept that ghrelin plays an important role in the weight loss produced by obesity bypass operations.

Hormones Increased by Obesity Bypass Operations

Because gastrointestinal hormones generally inhibit food intake, those that increase after obesity bypass operations are more likely to be involved in the mechanism of weight loss. Enteroglucagon, cholecystokinin, and neurotensin increase after gastric bypass surgery. Enteroglucagon is a prime candidate to explain the dramatic therapeutic effect that the bypass operations have upon diabetes. Neurotensin has been postulated to participate with vasoactive intestinal peptide in the dumping syndrome (diarrhea, flushing, tachycardia) that may occur with the ingestion of sugar or fat after gastric bypass. This noxious response to foods with high sugar or fat content tends to reduce intake and aids in overall caloric reduction.

ENTEROGLUCAGON-GLP-1 AND DIABETES

Gastric bypass corrects elevated fasting plasma glucose, insulin, and glycosylated hemoglobin, and normalizes the intravenous glucose tolerance test. In the longest-term studies (14 years) normal blood sugars were maintained in 91% of the patients.[34,35] In fact, 121 (82.9%) of 146 patients with diabetes and 150 (99%) of 152 patients with asymptomatic diabetes (impaired glucose tolerance) undergoing the gastric bypass developed normal blood sugars with complete normalization of their glucose metabolism.[34,36] When morbidly obese patients undergoing gastric bypass were compared with morbidly obese controls, the gastric bypass gave a 30-fold decrease in the risk of developing diabetes.[37] Gastric bypass also decreased the need for medication to treat diabetes from 31% to 8.6% of 154 patients, as compared to 78 morbidly obese unoperated controls whose medication requirement for diabetes increased from 56.4% to 87.5%.[38]

Resolution of diabetes is also observed following the biliopancreatic diversion (BPD) procedure. After a minimum 1-year followup of 1773 patients undergoing BPD, 248 (14%) with preoperative, mild, untreated hyperglycemia, 108 (6.1%) with diabetes treated with oral hypoglycemic agents, and 32 (1.8%) with diabetes requiring insulin, experienced normalization of glucose, insulin levels, and insulin sensitivity, and were free of the need for diabetic medications.[39] By using the duodenal switch, a variation of the BPD, 69 of 72 diabetic patients attained normal blood sugars and eliminated the need for diabetic medications.[40]

The gastric bypass also prevents subsequent development of diabetes.[34,41] Of 61 morbidly obese patients without diabetes, 50 underwent a gastric bypass and 11 acted as unoperated controls. After 8 years, 6 (55%) of the 11 controls developed diabetes but after 10.2 years, none of the patients having the gastric bypass developed diabetes.[41] The gastric bypass also reduced diabetes-related mortality from 28% in the control group to 9% in the surgically treated group. For every year of followup, the chance of dying was 4.5% for the control group versus 1% in the gastric bypass group.[36,38]

Although the mechanism of the dramatic effect conferred by bypass procedures for obesity on diabetes is not known, hypotheses include weight reduction, decreased caloric intake, and increased delivery of undigested chyme to the distal small intestine. Weight loss cannot be the whole explanation because euglycemia can be attained within 10 days postoperatively after the gastric bypass, well before any significant weight loss occurs.[34,36,38] Serum glucose normalized in patients with diabetes 1 month after the BPD when they still had more than 80% of their excess weight. Even after significant weight loss, these patients are still obese.[42] Leptin, insulin, glucose, and insulin resistance were reduced in six gastric bypass patients at a stable weight, as compared to six unoperated controls matched for weight, body fat, and lean body mass. Therefore, it would appear that the effect of gastric bypass on diabetes is a result of a decreased caloric intake or increased delivery of undigested chyme to the distal small intestine.[36]

Pories et al. described a patient who had a stomach full of food when the abdomen was opened in the operating room to perform a gastric bypass. The stomach was closed and operation canceled. This subject received the same postoperative diet as subjects undergoing the gastric bypass. The drop in glucose and insulin was identical to postoperative patients following the gastric bypass. This study paradigm is similar to pair-feeding experiments in animals and suggests that calorie restriction is sufficient to explain the improvement in diabetes during the early postoperative period of active weight loss.[34]

In similar studies, we measured insulin, leptin, glucagon, glucose, and cortisol levels in subjects matched with similar fat loss who were treated with a low-calorie liquid diet, gastric bypass, and BPD.[43] Insulin and leptin levels fell rapidly in all three groups, and correlated best with decrease in fat mass, and were not significantly different from one another.

In general, bypass operations reduce fat mass and the levels of glucose and insulin more than restrictive procedures such as vertical-banded gastroplasty or adjustable silicone banding. The greater reduction in weight and subsequent improvement in diabetes may be a result of changes in gut hormones that do not occur in purely restrictive procedure or nonsurgical weight loss. It has been reported that gastric bypass changes gut hormone profiles to a greater degree than restrictive obesity operations.[44] Enteroglucagon, a hormone secreted by the distal small intestine, is increased after bypass surgery.[25] Enteroglucagon and glucagon-like peptide 1 (GLP-1) are the same compound and are formed in the small bowel. In mammals, there is one gene responsible for the production of the 160-amino acid peptide proglucagon, which contains both glucagon and GLP-1. Glucagon (amino acids 33 to 61) is secreted by the pancreas and enteroglucagon–GLP-1 (amino acids 78 to 107) is secreted by the terminal ileum in response to a mixed meal.[44] Enteroglucagon–GLP-1 decreases the rate of glucose production by the liver and increases insulin production.[25] Twenty years after intestinal bypass surgery, glucose and insulin responses were like that of lean controls, but were accompanied by large increases of GLP-1 and gastric inhibitory polypeptide.[46]

Higher enteroglucagon-GLP-1 levels occur after bypass procedures for obesity than in those that are only restrictive in nature. The reason for the higher enteroglucagon-GLP-1 levels with bypass surgery may be explained by the more rapid presentation of the meal to the distal ileum where enteroglucagon-GLP-1 is secreted.[45] Enteroglucagon–GLP-1 inhibits pancreatic glucagon secretion, a hormone that raises the blood glucose level, and stimulates insulin secretion, a hormone that lowers the blood glucose level. Enteroglucagon increases insulin sensitivity, prolongs gastric emptying and decreases intestinal motility.[46]

Glucose disposal is increased after intestinal bypass. Oral and intravenous glucose tolerance is normalized.[48] Enteroglucagon–GLP-1 is the most potent of the incretins, gut peptides that stimulate insulin release.[49] The overproduction of glucose in type II diabetes contributes to insulin resistance through hyperglucagonemia.[50] Enteroglucagon–GLP-1 infusions in patients with poorly controlled diabetes stimulate insulin secretion, decrease blood glucagon levels, and slow gastric emptying.[51] Because the bypass procedures for obesity increase enteroglucagon–GLP-1 and because enteroglucagon–GLP-1 improves diabetes, enteroglucagon–GLP-1 is likely to be responsible for the improvement of diabetes with bypass obesity surgery as compared to purely restrictive obesity surgical procedures.

CHOLECYSTOKININ

Cholecystokinin (CCK) was recognized to decrease food intake in the early 1970s.[52] Rats lacking the CCK-A receptor are obese, but the same is not true for mice. There are two CCK receptor types, and the A receptor is thought to mediate the effect on food intake. Only recently was it learned that A receptors are not present in the human pancreas, as they are in rodents. This knowledge has enabled the development of CCK-A agonists for safe use in humans. These agonists will help in defining the role that increased CCK after bypass operations might have. Studies in humans show that CCK regulates meal size, but whether this is a short-term effect that dissipates with time is not yet known.[53]

NEUROTENSIN

Neurotensin is elevated in patients following bypass surgery and increases further with the symptoms of the dumping syndrome.[54,55] Somatostatin and pectin, when given as a treatment, improve the symptoms of dumping syndrome and decrease levels of neurotensin.[55,56]

APOLIPOPROTEIN A-IV AND PEPTIDE YY

Apolipoprotein (apo) A-IV is synthesized in the small intestine, is stimulated by chylomicron (fat from a meal) formation, and inhibits food intake centrally. Infusion of the small intestine with lipid (chylomicrons) stimulates apo A-IV in the entire small intestine to a greater degree than infusion into the proximal gut. The decrease in food intake associated with the delivery of lipid to the distal small bowel is termed the ileal brake and is thought to be mediated by peptide YY (PYY). PYY is synthesized in the ileum and colon by endocrine cells and is released by certain lipids like long-chain fatty acids. PYY stimulates apo A-IV synthesis and secretion. Intestinal lymph collected during active lipid absorption and injected in other animals suppresses their food intake, an effect thought to be caused by apo A-IV.[58] PYY is elevated after obesity bypass surgery, and serum from rats after obesity bypass surgery inhibits food intake. Therefore, it is likely that PYY and apo A-IV play an active role in the mechanism of obesity bypass related weight loss.[26,59]

ENTEROSTATIN

Obesity bypass surgery decreases the preference for fat.[60] Enterostatin is the 5-amino acid activation peptide cleaved from the pancreatic peptide procolipase during fat digestion, and decreases food intake and body weight by decreasing fat ingestion.[61] Enterostatin has been difficult to measure and the effect of obesity bypass surgery on enterostatin blood levels is not known. Nevertheless, enterostatin is a likely candidate to be involved in the mechanisms related to food preference after obesity bypass surgery.

FAT CELLS

The fat cell is being increasingly appreciated as an endocrine organ and not just a passive reservoir for storing calories. This appreciation was stimulated by the discovery of leptin, a cytokine (class of peptide) made by the fat cell

TABLE 3–3. PRODUCTS FROM FAT CELLS AFFECTING ENERGY BALANCE	
DECREASE FOOD INTAKE	ASSOCIATED WITH INSULIN RESISTANCE
Adiponectin	Acetylation stimulating protein
Ciliary neurotrophic factor	Interleukin-6
Leptin	Plasminogen activator inhibitor-1
Oleoylestrone	Resistin
	Tumor necrosis factor-α

with actions in the central nervous system. Other cytokines, proteins and fats are secreted by fat cells and have effects on energy balance (Table 3–3).

Proteins from Fat Cells

LEPTIN

Mice and humans lacking leptin become massively obese, and replacement of leptin reverses this obesity.[62,63] Rodents lacking the receptor for leptin in the brain also become massively obese.[64] Based upon these observations, leptin gave promise of being an effective obesity treatment. Although this promise has not been realized, leptin legitimized obesity as a physiologic problem worthy of study, rather than as a condition caused only by sloth and gluttony. Leptin is now felt to signal the sufficiency of food intake, with low levels stimulating intake, while high levels do very little.[65]

ACETYLATION-STIMULATING PROTEIN

Acetylation-stimulating protein (ASP) is produced by fat cells through the interaction of complement factor C3, factor B, and adipsin. Mice lacking adipsin have lower body fat and increased insulin sensitivity despite a higher food intake. To prevent the accumulation of fat, energy expenditure must increase to balance the higher food intake.[66] Therefore, ASP and adipsin may inhibit energy expenditure. Rodents that undergo obesity bypass surgery have a greater energy expenditure per unit of lean body mass and have greater insulin sensitivity than do weight-matched controls,[36,66] but adipsin and ASP were not measured in these studies. Whether there is any relationship between acetylation stimulating protein and obesity bypass operations is unknown.

ADIPONECTIN

Adiponectin is another fat cell protein that is derived by cleavage from complement-related protein 30. Adiponectin is associated with insulin sensitivity and is decreased in obesity.[67] Adiponectin administration increases fatty acid oxidation in muscle and causes weight loss in mice consuming a high fat and high sucrose diet without changing food intake.[68] Thus, adiponectin would have the opposite effect of ASP on energy expenditure.

RESISTIN

Resistin is a newly discovered fat cell factor that is downregulated by peroxisome proliferator-activator receptor (PPAR)-γ and elevated in obesity and insulin resistance.[69] Because resistin is decreased in rodent obesity models and increased by insulin sensitizing drugs (opposing effects), the role of resistin in the obesity and insulin resistance has been questioned.[70]

OTHER FAT CELL PROTEINS

Tumor necrosis factor-α is also a fat-cell product that is associated with insulin resistance through the serine phosphorylation of insulin receptor substrate (IRS)-1.[71] Plasminogen activator inhibitor-1 is produced particularly by omental fat cells and may be responsible for the elevated levels associated with insulin resistance and the tendency toward atherothrombosis.[72] Interleukin-6 is also a product of fat cells and is postulated, as a proinflammatory cytokine, to be involved in the link between obesity and atherosclerosis.[73]

Lipids from Fat Cells

OLEOYL-ESTRONE

Oleoyl-estrone is a fatty acid, oleic acid with the estrogen estrone linked through an ester bond at the 3 position of the estrone molecule. The compound is produced by fat cells, secreted into the bloodstream, and carried on high-density lipoprotein particles.[74] Daily oral, gavage administration of oleoyl-estrone to Wistar rats induces fat loss with preservation of lean tissue. This weight loss was partially the result of a reduction in food intake and partly the result of maintained energy expenditure. Thus, oleoyl-estrone depletes fat reserves without lowering energy expenditure.[75] Oleoyl-estrone has been postulated to be the feedback signal from fat tissue to the brain informing the body of the amount of fat present. There is a close relationship of body fat mass with circulating oleoyl-estrone in humans. Obese women have abnormally low oleoyl-estrone levels consistent with deficient oleoyl-estrone signaling the presence of adequate fat stores.[76] A spermine-coupled cholesterol metabolite from the dogfish shark is a powerful appetite suppressant that at a sufficient dose can cause rats to starve themselves to death with food available in the cage. This compound has a structural similarity to oleoyl-estrone, and like oleoyl-estrone, acts centrally, suggesting that similar receptors may be involved.[77]

CONCLUSIONS

The brain, gut, and fat cells are all involved in the physiology of morbid obesity. Most of what we know of this physiology is a result of observations made in animals and humans after obesity bypass operations. Unlike the purely restrictive obesity operation, obesity bypass surgery appears to alter physiology so that a 30 to 40% loss of initial body weight is maintained for more than a decade. Although ghrelin appears to be important in the weight loss associated with gastric bypass, and enteroglucagon–GLP-1 appears to be important in the dramatic improvement of diabetes seen with obesity bypass surgery, there may be many other mechanisms that have yet to be elucidated. Although there is evidence from animals that bypass surgery increases energy expenditure per unit of lean body mass, the role the sympathetic nervous system may play in the physiology of the weight loss in humans having obesity bypass procedures has yet to be explored. Even though more is known about the gut and its influence on obesity bypass surgery, the role that apo A-IV may have on food intake or that enterostatin may have on macronutrient selection has yet to be explored. The relationship between the fat cell and the physiology of morbid obesity is suggested by lower levels of oleoylestrone in obese women, but the influence of obesity bypass surgery on oleoylestrone levels has yet to be studied.

Morbid obesity is an increasing public health problem in the United States. Obesity bypass surgery is an effective treatment that alters physiology. Therefore, obesity bypass surgery offers an excellent model for determining the physiologic mechanisms underpinning morbid obesity. There is much to be learned, but discovering the mechanisms may allow better treatments. The role of obesity surgery in the treatment of obesity and its comorbid conditions, which is now so important, may be eliminated if the physiologic mechanisms which contribute to its long term success are understood and can be manipulated medically. We have seen the surgical treatment of peptic ulcer disease be essentially replaced by the antibiotic treatment of *Helicobacter pylori*. Defining the physiology of morbid obesity through understanding the mechanisms behind the success of obesity bypass surgery holds promise of developing a medical treatment for the disease that may make these operations unnecessary.

REFERENCES

1. Bray GA. Obesity, a disorder of nutrient partitioning: the MONA LISA hypothesis. *J Nutr* 1991;121:1146–1162.
2. Bray GA. Autonomic and endocrine factors in the regulation of food intake. *Brain Res Bull* 1985;14:505–510.
3. Inoue S, Bray GA, Mullen YS. Transplantation of pancreatic beta-cells prevents development of hypothalamic obesity in rats. *Am J Physiol* 1978;235:E266–E271.
4. Lustig RH, Rose SR, Burghen GA, et al. Hypothalamic obesity caused by cranial insult in children: altered glucose and insulin dynamics and reversal by a somatostatin agonist. *J Pediatr* 1999;135:162–168.
5. Keesey RE, Corbett SW, Hirvonen MD, Kaufman LN. Heat production and body weight changes following lateral hypothalamic lesions. *Physiol Behav* 1984;32:309–317.
6. Kamalian N, Keesey RE, ZuRhein GM. Lateral hypothalamic demyelination and cachexia in a case of "malignant" multiple sclerosis. *Neurology* 1975;25:25–30.
7. Quaade F, Vaernet K, Larsson S. Stereotaxic stimulation and electrocoagulation of the lateral hypothalamus in obese humans. *Acta Neurochir (Wien)* 1974;30:111–117.
8. Bray GA, Gallagher TF Jr. Manifestations of hypothalamic obesity in man: a com-

prehensive investigation of eight patients and a review of the literature. *Medicine (Baltimore)* 1975;54:301–330.

9. Peterson HR, Rothschild M, Weinberg CR, Fell RD, McLeish KR, Pfeifer MA. Body fat and the activity of the autonomic nervous system. *N Engl J Med* 1988;318:1077–1083.

10. Kral JG, Gortz L. Truncal vagotomy in morbid obesity. *Int J Obes* 1981;5:431–435.

11. Gortz L, Bjorkman AC, Andersson H, Kral JG. Truncal vagotomy reduces food and liquid intake in man. *Physiol Behav* 1990;48:779–781.

12. Kral JG, Gortz L, Hermansson G, Wallin GS. Gastroplasty for obesity: long-term weight loss improved by vagotomy. *World J Surg* 1993;17:75–78; discussion 79.

13. Leibel RL, Rosenbaum M, Hirsch J. Changes in energy expenditure resulting from altered body weight. *N Engl J Med* 1995;332:621–628.

14. Jeffery RW, Drewnowski A, Epstein LH, et al. Long-term maintenance of weight loss: current status. *Health Psychol* 2000;19:5–16.

15. Johnson D, Drenick EJ. Therapeutic fasting in morbid obesity. *Arch Intern Med* 1977;137:1381–1382.

16. DeHaven J, Sherwin R, Hendler R, Felig P. Nitrogen and sodium balance and sympathetic nervous system activity in obese subjects treated with a low-calorie protein or mixed diet. *N Engl J Med* 1980;302:477–482.

17. Bray GA. Reciprocal relation of food intake and sympathetic activity: experimental observations and clinical implications. *Int J Obes Relat Metab Disord* 2000;24(Suppl 2):S8–S17.

18. Astrup A, Breum L, Toubro S, Hein P, Quaade F. The effect and safety of an ephedrine/caffeine compound compared to ephedrine, caffeine and placebo in obese subjects on an energy restricted diet. A double-blind trial. *Int J Obes Relat Metab Disord* 1992;16:269–277.

19. Astrup A, Toubro S, Christensen NJ, Quaade F. Pharmacology of thermogenic drugs. *Am J Clin Nutr* 1992;55:246S–248S.

20. Williams G, Harrold JA, Cutler DJ. The hypothalamus and the regulation of energy homeostasis: lifting the lid on a black box. *Proc Nutr Soc* 2000;59:385–396.

21. Mergen M, Mergen H, Ozata M, Oner R, Oner C. A novel melanocortin 4 receptor (MC4R) gene mutation associated with morbid obesity. *J Clin Endocrinol Metab* 2001;86:3448.

22. Bray GA. Food intake, sympathetic activity, and adrenal steroids. *Brain Res Bull* 1993;32:537–541.

23. Greenway FL. Surgery for obesity. *Endocrinol Metab Clin North Am* 1996;25:1005–1027.

24. Pieramico O, Malfertheiner P, Nelson DK, Glasbrenner B, Ditschuneit H. Interdigestive gastroduodenal motility and cycling of putative regulatory hormones in severe obesity. *Scand J Gastroenterol* 1992;27:538–544.

25. Sarson DL, Scopinaro N, Bloom SR. Gut hormone changes after jejunoileal (JIB) or biliopancreatic (BPB) bypass surgery for morbid obesity. *Int J Obes* 1981;5:471–480.

26. Naslund E, Gryback P, Hellstrom PM, et al. Gastrointestinal hormones and gastric emptying 20 years after jejunoileal bypass for massive obesity. *Int J Obes Relat Metab Disord* 1997;21:387–392.

27. Lieverse RJ, Masclee AA, Jansen JB, Lamers CB. Plasma cholecystokinin and pancreatic polypeptide secretion in response to bombesin, meal ingestion and modified sham feeding in lean and obese persons. *Int J Obes Relat Metab Disord* 1994;18:123–127.

28. Jones IR, Owens DR, Luzio SD, Hayes TM. Obesity is associated with increased

post-prandial GIP levels which are not reduced by dietary restriction and weight loss. *Diabete Metab* 1989;15:11–22.

29. Miyawaki K, Yamada Y, Ban N, et al. Inhibition of gastric inhibitory polypeptide signaling prevents obesity. *Nat Med* 2002;8:738–742.

30. Kojima M, Hosoda H, Date Y, Nakazato M, Matsuo H, Kangawa K. Ghrelin is a growth-hormone-releasing acylated peptide from stomach. *Nature* 1999;402:656–660.

31. Wren AM, Small CJ, Abbott CR, et al. Ghrelin causes hyperphagia and obesity in rats. *Diabetes* 2001;50:2540–2547.

32. English PJ, Ghatei MA, Malik IA, Bloom SR, Wilding JP. Food fails to suppress ghrelin levels in obese humans. *J Clin Endocrinol Metab* 2002;87:2984.

33. Cummings DE, Weigle DS, Frayo RS, et al. Plasma ghrelin levels after diet-induced weight loss or gastric bypass surgery. *N Engl J Med* 2002;346:1623–1630.

34. Pories WJ, Swanson MS, MacDonald KG, et al. Who would have thought it? An operation proves to be the most effective therapy for adult-onset diabetes mellitus. *Ann Surg* 1995;222:339–350; discussion 350–352.

35. Pories WJ, MacDonald KG Jr, Flickinger EG, et al. Is type II diabetes mellitus (NIDDM) a surgical disease? *Ann Surg* 1992;215:633–642; discussion 643.

36. Hickey MS, Pories WJ, MacDonald KG Jr, et al. A new paradigm for type 2 diabetes mellitus: could it be a disease of the foregut? *Ann Surg* 1998;227:637–643; discussion 643–644.

37. Saad MF, Knowler WC, Pettitt DJ, Nelson RG, Mott DM, Bennett PH. Sequential changes in serum insulin concentration during development of non-insulin-dependent diabetes. *Lancet* 1989;1:1356–1359.

38. MacDonald KG Jr, Long SD, Swanson MS, et al. The gastric bypass operation reduces the progression and mortality of non-insulin-dependent diabetes mellitus. *J Gastrointest Surg* 1997;1:213–220.

39. Scopinaro N, Adami GF, Marinari GM, et al. Biliopancreatic diversion. *World J Surg* 1998;22:936–946.

40. Marceau P, Hould FS, Simard S, et al. Biliopancreatic diversion with duodenal switch. *World J Surg* 1998;22:947–954.

41. Long SD, O'Brien K, MacDonald KG Jr, et al. Weight loss in severely obese subjects prevents the progression of impaired glucose tolerance to type II diabetes. A longitudinal interventional study. *Diabetes Care* 1994;17:372–375.

42. Scopinaro N, Gianetta E, Adami GF, et al. Biliopancreatic diversion for obesity at eighteen years. *Surgery* 1996;119:261–268.

43. Wall DB, Raum WJ, Klein Sr. Medical or surgical treatment of morbid obesity: effect on fat loss, leptin, insulin, and other hormone levels. *Endocrinology* 2000;2060:499. (Abstract)

44. Sugerman HJ, Starkey JV, Birkenhauer R. A randomized prospective trial of gastric bypass versus vertical banded gastroplasty for morbid obesity and their effects on sweets versus non-sweets eaters. *Ann Surg* 1987;205:613–624.

45. Orskov C. Glucagon-like peptide-1, a new hormone of the entero-insular axis. *Diabetologia* 1992;35:701–711.

46. Naslund E, Backman L, Holst JJ, Theodorsson E, Hellstrom PM. Importance of small bowel peptides for the improved glucose metabolism 20 years after jejunoileal bypass for obesity. *Obes Surg* 1998;8:253–260.

47. Mason EE. Ileal [correction of ilial] transposition and enteroglucagon/GLP-1 in obesity (and diabetic?) surgery. *Obes Surg* 1999;9:223–228.

48. Rehfeld JF, Lauritsen KB, Holst JJ. Increased glucose disposal after jejunoileostomy. *Diabetologia* 1979;16:31–34.

49. Kreymann B, Williams G, Ghatei MA, Bloom SR. Glucagon-like peptide-1 7–36: a physiological incretin in man. *Lancet* 1987;2:1300–1304.

50. Baron AD, Schaeffer L, Shragg P, Kolterman OG. Role of hyperglucagonemia in maintenance of increased rates of hepatic glucose output in type II diabetics. *Diabetes* 1987;36:274–283.

51. Willms B, Werner J, Holst JJ, Orskov C, Creutzfeldt W, Nauck MA. Gastric emptying, glucose responses, and insulin secretion after a liquid test meal: effects of exogenous glucagon-like peptide-1 (GLP-1)-(7–36) amide in type 2 (noninsulin-dependent) diabetic patients. *J Clin Endocrinol Metab* 1996;81:327–332.

52. Gibbs J, Young RC, Smith GP. Cholecystokinin elicits satiety in rats with open gastric fistulas. *Nature* 1973;245:323–325.

53. Moran TH. Cholecystokinin and satiety: current perspectives. *Nutrition* 2000;16:858–865.

54. Lawaetz O, Blackburn AM, Bloom SR, Aritas Y, Ralphs DN. Gut hormone profile and gastric emptying in the dumping syndrome. A hypothesis concerning the pathogenesis. *Scand J Gastroenterol* 1983;18:73–80.

55. Yamashita Y, Toge T, Adrian TE. Gastrointestinal hormone in dumping syndrome and reflux esophagitis after gastric surgery. *J Smooth Muscle Res* 1997;33:37–48.

56. Richards WO, Geer R, O'Dorisio TM, et al. Octreotide acetate induces fasting small bowel motility in patients with dumping syndrome. *J Surg Res* 1990;49:483–487.

57. Lawaetz O, Blackburn AM, Bloom SR, Aritas Y, Ralphs DN. Effect of pectin on gastric emptying and gut hormone release in the dumping syndrome. *Scand J Gastroenterol* 1983;18:327–336.

58. Tso P, Liu M, Kalogeris TJ, Thomson AB. The role of apolipoprotein A-IV in the regulation of food intake. *Annu Rev Nutr* 2001;21:231–254.

59. Atkinson RL, Brent EL. Appetite suppressant activity in plasma of rats after intestinal bypass surgery. *Am J Physiol* 1982;243:R60–R64.

60. Atkinson RL, Brent EL, Whipple JH. Altered dietary preference for fat and sucrose after intestinal bypass surgery in rats. *Int J Obes* 1982;6:499–506.

61. Erlanson-Albertsson C, York D. Enterostatin—a peptide regulating fat intake. *Obes Res* 1997;5:360–372.

62. Zhang Y, Proenca R, Maffei M, Barone M, Leopold L, Friedman JM. Positional cloning of the mouse obese gene and its human homologue. *Nature* 1994;372:425–432.

63. Farooqi IS, Jebb SA, Langmack G, et al. Effects of recombinant leptin therapy in a child with congenital leptin deficiency. *N Engl J Med* 1999;341:879–884.

64. Maffei M, Fei H, Lee GH, et al. Increased expression in adipocytes of ob RNA in mice with lesions of the hypothalamus and with mutations at the db locus. *Proc Natl Acad Sci USA* 1995;92:6957–6960.

65. Rosenbaum M, Leibel RL. The role of leptin in human physiology. *N Engl J Med* 1999;341:913–915.

66. Havel PJ. Peripheral signals conveying metabolic information to the brain: short-term and long-term regulation of food intake and energy homeostasis. *Exp Biol Med (Maywood)* 2001;226:963–977.

67. Weyer C, Funahashi T, Tanaka S, et al. Hypoadiponectinemia in obesity and type 2 diabetes: close association with insulin resistance and hyperinsulinemia. *J Clin Endocrinol Metab* 2001;86:1930–1935.

68. Fruebis J, Tsao TS, Javorschi S, et al. Proteolytic cleavage product of 30-kDa adipocyte complement-related protein increases fatty acid oxidation in muscle and causes weight loss in mice. *Proc Natl Acad Sci USA* 2001;98:2005–2010.

69. Steppan CM, Bailey ST, Bhat S, et al. The hormone resistin links obesity to diabetes. *Nature* 2001;409:307–312.

70. Way JM, Gorgun CZ, Tong Q, et al. Adipose tissue resistin expression is severely suppressed in obesity and stimulated by peroxisome proliferator-activated receptor gamma agonists. *J Biol Chem* 2001;276:25651–25653.

71. Sykiotis GP, Papavassiliou AG. Serine phosphorylation of insulin receptor substrate-1: a novel target for the reversal of insulin resistance. *Mol Endocrinol* 2001;15:1864–1869.

72. Juhan-Vague I, Alessi MC, Morange PE. Hypofibrinolysis and increased PAI-1 are linked to atherothrombosis via insulin resistance and obesity. *Ann Med* 2000;32(Suppl 1):78–84.

73. Yudkin JS, Kumari M, Humphries SE, Mohamed-Ali V. Inflammation, obesity, stress and coronary heart disease: is interleukin-6 the link? *Atherosclerosis* 2000;148:209–214.

74. Fernandez-Real JM, Sanchis D, Ricart W, et al. Plasma oestrone-fatty acid ester levels are correlated with body fat mass in humans. *Clin Endocrinol (Oxf)* 1999;50:253–260.

75. del Mar Grasa M, Cabot C, Esteve M, et al. Daily oral oleoyl-estrone gavage induces a dose-dependent loss of fat in Wistar rats. *Obes Res* 2001;9:202–209.

76. Cabot C, Masanes R, Bullo M, et al. Plasma acyl-estrone levels are altered in obese women. *Endocr Res* 2000;26:465–476.

77. Zasloff M, Williams JI, Chen Q, et al. A spermine-coupled cholesterol metabolite from the shark with potent appetite suppressant and antidiabetic properties. *Int J Obes Relat Metab Disord* 2001;25:689–697.

PSYCHOLOGICAL FACTORS CONTRIBUTING TO THE DEVELOPMENT OF OBESITY AND THE CONDITIONS THAT MUST BE TREATED PREOPERATIVELY

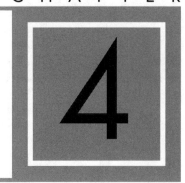

F. MERRITT AYAD

William James argued that in some ways, a given human being is like all other human beings, like some other people in certain respects, and like no other person in some ways. This axiom certainly applies to obese humans. They are like all other obese people in that they have too much body fat, and they need food, water, sleep, relationships, exercise, and meaning in their lives. They are like some other obese people in that they are of a certain gender, race, culture, socioeconomic status, activity level, comorbid disease group(s), and general health level. And they are like no other person in terms of their unique blend of genes, life experiences, habits, and chance. Predicting bariatric surgery outcomes is not simple, and it is far from precise. Human beings are too complex and variable for us to presage treatment results with certainty. We can speak of risk factors for poor outcomes, or enabling factors for good ones, but we have all been fooled by our own predictions. Patients with poor prognoses have surprised us with their unexpected successes, just as people with good prognoses have stunned us with their failures.

In the morbidly obese population there is a great deal of overlap between somatic and psychological disorders. In some cases we treat one clinical domain, when another is the real culprit. For example, a patient with undiagnosed sleep apnea may present with symptoms of irritability, fatigue, concentration problems, and loss of interest in previously enjoyed activities. A mental health professional may give that patient a diagnosis of depression. Later, the patient has a sleep study and is diagnosed with sleep apnea, and is then treated with a continuous positive-air-pressure device. Miraculously, the patient's attitude improves, the patient's energy level increases, and the patient begins to perform many activities that the patient had been avoiding. Other patients have both sleep apnea and clinical depression, and must be treated for both.

Sometimes patients show different sides of themselves to different clinicians. A patient may tell one interviewer that they do not eat in response to emotions, but then endorse questionnaire items which acknowledge the association between dysphoric states of mind and an increase in their consumption of certain foods. When a patient has orthopedic problems with chronic pain, sleep problems, mood problems, and significant recent losses, it requires the collaborative effort of several clinicians in order to prioritize and integrate interventions. The need for a multidisciplinary team cannot be overemphasized. There is no place for turf wars when treating morbidly obese patients who have pathology in many clinical domains, and who are requesting an invasive therapeutic option that will acutely destabilize some of these domains in return for significant improvements over a longer duration of time (as long as an adverse event does not lead to an untimely death or major complication). Often someone from one discipline obtains vital information that will help a clinician in another specialty to clarify their diagnostic thinking. A comprehensive bariatric medicine clinic would ideally have at least one of each of the following: a surgeon; an internal medicine physician or endocrinologist; a psychiatrist and/or a psychologist; a social worker; a nurse; and an exercise physiologist. Having a pain specialist as a consultant is also a great asset.

This chapter first addresses the interaction of biological, psychological, and social variables in morbid obesity. Next, the dynamics of families, individuals, and couples commonly associated with obesity are described. Finally, the common psychiatric conditions that are best treated presurgically are discussed.

BIOLOGICAL, PSYCHOLOGICAL AND SOCIAL VARIABLES

It should be said from the outset that the effort to distinguish the psychological from biological and social is in and of itself artificial. We have come a long way since Descartes separated the mind and the body in his 17th century writings. We now have no doubt that learning is processed at the neurochemical level throughout the life span, and that during certain critical periods of development, our brain structures are myelinated, shaped, and changed by experiences. If, for example, a mother misinterprets cues from her infant, and repeatedly feeds the child when the child is not hungry, there are biological, psychological, and social sequelae of this interaction. The developing child may go on to eat when the child is not hungry, may engage in maladaptive battles for control with others throughout life, or may have difficulty in regulating emotions. The year 2000 Surgeon General's report by Dr. David Satcher was entitled the "Decade of Behavior." Dr. Satcher expressed his view that Americans need to work together for the next 10 years to increase awareness of the millions of untreated Americans who have behavioral disorders. His research found that smoking, alcohol abuse, obesity, unprotected sex, drug abuse, suicide, violence, and mental illness were taking a huge toll on the American people. Dr. Satcher stated that, "Mind and body are inseparable. . . . [E]veryday language tends to encourage the misperception that mental health or mental illness is unrelated to physical health and physical illness. In fact, the two are inseparable." Mental disorders are reflected in physical changes in the brain. The report views mental health/mental illness as well as somatic health/somatic disease as points on continua, just as many researchers view stress as ranging from exciting challenges, to everyday hassles, to disease-producing phenomena.

Eating

The consumption of food involves biological, psychological, and social processes. We must ingest calories to fuel the machine of life. We must find the right combination of macronutrients (e.g., proteins, carbohydrates, fats, and fiber) and micronutrients (e.g., vitamins, minerals) for our age, activity level, and medical status. Some theories of human development purport that an infant first gets to know and love the mother's breast and its milk, and only later realizes that there is a person who has many functions, needs, desires, and behaviors other than feeding him or her. Nevertheless, feeding remains associated with love, affection, and nurturing for most of us. Food is one of the most powerful reinforcers, as well as one of the most sought after pleasures on the planet. We have all heard a wonderful dish described as being "better than sex!" When people travel, celebrate, socialize, or romance, they want fabulous food. It is no wonder that many obese patients often resent the admonitions to refrain from the pleasures they see others enjoying.

Kesten has described the important links between culture, spirituality, and food.[1] Culture creates strong emotional ties to food. Mexican, Italian, Thai, French, Chinese, Greek, Lebanese, Creole, and all the other cultural foods one can think of have long histories and traditions that unite people. In most countries, food is a vital aspect of social interchange. Spiritual belief plays a significant role in many eating traditions. For example, Jews have Kosher dietary laws, Catholics renew their faith with bread and wine symbolizing the blood and flesh of Christ, Muslims honor food for its divine essence, and Japanese have tea rituals that renew the spirit. Most religions and cultural traditions encourage cooking with love, and many implicitly or explicitly allude to the healing aspects of nourishment. Hippocrates once said, "let food be your medicine and medicine be your food," clearly endorsing the importance of a healthy and balanced diet. What may be "healthy" for a given individual may be detrimental to the health of someone else. There are hundreds of "healthy diets" on the market. The average consumer does not know how to sift the informational wheat from the chaff. Diets that lead to short-term weight loss may not be sufficiently balanced for long-term health maintenance. Some of our patients hear "deprivation" when the word "diet" is uttered and are doomed to rebel against any plan that leaves them feeling deprived. Some do better with concepts such as "healthful eating" or "balanced eating plan." While the notion of making our eating behavior one of several "healthy lifestyle choices" may sound easy, it surely is not.

In a fascinating article, Kesten speaks of the "enlightened diet."[1] Her thesis is that the American quest for the "best diet" is misguided. She suggests that "integrated nutrition" is what all humans need. She addresses four domains of nutrition: *biological nutrition,* which prevents or reverses physical ailments; *psychological nutrition,* which deals with the powerful associations and meanings linked to eating, and with how emotions affect food choices and vice versa; *spiritual nutrition,* which allows us to reunite with the spiritual meaning of food (i.e., mindfulness, appreciation, gratitude, and love); and *social nutrition,* which deals with the benefits that come from eating in a socially supportive environment, and the sense of continuity that comes from connections between our heritage and food. Most diets neglect one or more of these domains, and in so doing create the need to deviate from them. Kesten points out *Webster's* definition of enlightened, which is "freed from ignorance and misinformation" and argues that the effort to understand the multidimensional healing powers of food is fundamental to achieving the health and balance which comes from integrated and enlightened eating.[1]

Stress

How individuals cope with stress is related to the development of both obesity and psychological disorders. We live in very stressful times. Between 1984 and 1998 there were 29,000 research articles published on stress and coping.[2] Swindle et al. found that the number of Americans who reported feeling on the verge of a "nervous breakdown" increased from 18.9% in 1957 to 26.4% in 1996, with the largest increase being since 1976.[3] In recent years, Americans have struggled with the AIDS epidemic; ubiquitous crime; death and disability related to illicit drugs; floods; fires; the Columbine incident and others like it; the tragedy surrounding the terrorist attacks of September 11, 2001; the stock market crash, which has decimated the life savings of millions of Americans; priests who sexually abused a horrifyingly large number of children; and greed and corruption at some of the highest levels of business (e.g., Enron, World-Com). Scientists have identified ecological problems such as global warming, ozone depletion, acid rain, and deforestation, which will significantly reduce the quality of life for untold numbers of earth's inhabitants in the future. Human overpopulation and overconsumption created and maintains these problems. The American dream of life, liberty, and the pursuit of happiness has evolved into the American myth that one can "have it all," and that anyone can be "number one!" Consumers expect more and more, but want to do less and less to obtain it. They do not want to be responsible for any bad outcome associated with their purchases. It is no longer "buyer beware." We want someone else to blame for our poor choices. Also, the axiomatic belief that "you get what you pay for," has been replaced by our tendency to believe we can obtain higher quality at bargain basement prices because we know how to "shop." The tension that grows between consumers' unrealistic expectations and economic reality creates a great deal of instability in our country, as well as the gulf that separates the "haves" from the "have nots." Our culture of entitlement leads too many people to focus on short-term gratifications to the detriment of long-term planning for the individual, the family, the country, and the planet.

Currently, we are witnessing increases in health care technology that promise high-priced treatments for both rare and common diseases while more than 44 million Americans have no health insurance and cannot afford adequate health care. While most families require multiple wage earners, the divorce rate remains at 50%. Stress is a very important biological-psychological-social variable to assess when working with the morbidly obese. Hans Selye's pioneering work has remained essential to our understanding of stress.[4] He found that mild, brief, and controllable degrees of stress ("eustress") could be perceived as pleasant or exciting and could lead to growth and development. It was, however, the more severe, protracted or uncontrollable states of stress ("distress") that led to disease states. He went on to say that extended distress could lead to anxiety, hypervigilance, ulcers, immunosuppression, and melancholic depression. Hypersecretion of cortisol is associated with some of these disorders. Since Selye's original work, other medical conditions, such as stroke, heart disease, cancer, lower respiratory diseases, rheumatoid arthritis, and asthma, have been found to be caused or exacerbated by stress. More recent research on the neuroendocrine aspects of stress has found that excessive release of corticotropin-releasing hormone may be implicated in the development of panic attacks,[5,6] obsessive compulsive disorder,[7] and alcohol abuse.[8] Disease causes stress, and stress causes disease. Chronic stress can be embedded in lifestyle choices such as career (e.g., workaholics, middle managers, emergency work of various types, child protection workers, and dangerous professions such as police work). All people experience injury, illness, loss, suffering, and death during the course of life. How we perceive events activates the hypothalamic–pituitary–adrenal (HPA) axis differently, and each person has coping behaviors related to activation of this neuroendocrine stress-response system. The central nervous system mediates arousal, vigilance, and mobilization during an emergency. In some individuals, the HPA axis fails to readjust after exposure to a traumatic stressor or chronic stress (i.e., neuroendocrine dysregulation). Failure to readjust may result in immune dysfunction, hypertension, ulcer, or neurobehavioral problems. To deal with a stressful event, most of us have eaten too much and/or made a poor food choice at one time or another. A subgroup of morbidly obese patients uses food to deal with stress habitually and excessively. While the ingestion of mood altering foods brings temporary relief from stress, excessive reliance on these foods usually weakens the body over time as a consequence of the development of obesity, adult onset diabetes, and atherosclerosis, which then makes the individual even more vulnerable to stress in the future.

Tennen et al. summarized studies dealing with stress, alcohol consumption, and coping.[9] There are three general categories of coping: "problem-focused coping," where the person does something to try to change the situation; "emotion-focused coping," where the person deals with the emotional reaction to the stressor; and "avoidant-coping," where the person turns his or her attention away from the stressful situation. Emotion-focused and avoidant-coping approaches best predicted alcohol consumption levels and alcohol-related problems. It would useful to apply this model to morbidly obese patients, using food instead of alcohol as the dependent variable.

Contemporary research of the psychological processes used in coping and adaptation is about to make a quantum leap. In the past, there was insufficient communication between researchers and clinicians. Many studies were flawed by response biases, inaccurate recall by subjects, and the general limitations associated with cross-sectional experimental designs. There were many problems with having patients complete lengthy surveys retrospectively. Following the microanalytic process-oriented research design outlined by Lazarus,[10] Tennen and colleagues[9] developed a "daily process approach" to coping research. They proposed study designs using personal digital assistant (PDA) technology, which prompts subjects for specific entries of responses at fixed times in the day, and allows them to enter data whenever they engage in maladaptive coping behavior (e.g., drinking alcohol or eating five doughnuts). This enables researchers to prospectively track the rapidly fluctuating processes, such as mood and coping, much closer to their real-time occurrences. This approach is idiographic in that it studies the unfolding relations among variables within an individual, and nomothetic in that it will then look for the sturdy relationships among variables across individuals or subgroups of subjects.

Sleep

Sleep function is strongly tied to stress, somatic illness, and psychiatric disorders. Sleep disorders contribute to fatigue, which decreases energy expenditure and often leads to weight gain. Chronic insomnia affects up to 40% of adults in a given year, and 10% of adults complain of moderate to severe sleep problems.[11] There are more than 80 recognized conditions that can affect sleep and waking behavior.[12] Obstructive sleep apnea usually prompts an obese patient's referral to a sleep disorders center. Sleep disturbance is correlated with fatigue-related accidents, decreased productivity, increased absenteeism, poorer health, reduced quality of life, and somatic and psychiatric disorders. Obesity, hypertension, and the male gender are the three characteristics most commonly associated with sleep apnea.

Like stress and depression, insomnia can be a cause or a result of a medical disorder. Epidemiological studies indicate that one-third to one-half of people with chronic insomnia suffer from mood or anxiety disorders. Depressed patients frequently report early morning awakening with an inability to return to sleep. Soldatos found that depressed patients are two to three times as likely to suffer from insomnia as non-depressed people.[13] Ford and Kamerow reported that subjects with insomnia had a greatly increased risk of redeveloping a new episode of major depression one year later.[14] Barnes et al. studied a geriatric population over a 2-year period and found that sleep disturbance was the best predictor for development of depression.[15] Roth emphasized that depression can cause insomnia or insomnia can cause depression.[16]

Manic patients report decreased need for sleep, and insomnia often precedes a manic episode. Anxious patients report that ruminations and dysphoric thoughts interfere with sleep or preclude restful sleep. Panic disorder patients report nocturnal panic attacks. Posttraumatic stress disorder patients may have sleep disrupted by flashbacks, intrusive recollections of the traumatic event, or recurrent dreams of the trauma. Hypersomnia is more common in seasonal affective disorder patients, or bipolar depressed phase patients.[17] Patients with eating disorders, usually with a prior history of sleep walking,[18] are more likely to experience a phenomenon called "sleep eating." The sleep eater typically gets up after sleep onset and eats large amounts of high-calorie foods. The percentage of morbidly obese who sleep eat ranges from 9 to 27%.[19] Recent research has discovered that morning phototherapy suppresses nocturnal sleep eating.[20]

The National Center on Sleep Disorders reports that as many as 18 million Americans (4% of middle-aged males, and 2% of middle-aged females) have a disorder called sleep apnea. This condition contributes to the development of hypertension, heart attack, and stroke, and is listed as a major comorbid condition associated with obesity. Apnea is a Greek word meaning "want of breath" or "without breath." There are three types of sleep apnea: obstructive, central, and mixed. The most common one is obstructive sleep apnea. Risk factors for the development of obstructive sleep apnea are being male, overweight, having hypertension, and older than age 40 years. Some obese people have an excess amount of tissue in the throat that narrows the airway and causes heavy snoring, periods of not breathing (i.e., apneic events), and frequent arousals. Use of alcohol increases the frequency and duration of breathing pauses. Sleep apnea is also associated with the development of the following conditions: depression; sexual dysfunction; and learning and memory difficulties. Morbidly obese patients, especially men and superobese women, need to be questioned about their sleep habits; many are treated for sleep apnea and depression concurrently.

Exercise

The lack of regular exercise is an important biological-psychological-social variable in the development and maintenance of obesity. Any sound weight-loss program must include an exercise component tailored to the strengths and limitations of each patient. Taylor et al. conducted an extensive review of the literature on the benefits of exercise.[21] They found that regular exercise increases academic performance; assertiveness; confidence; emotional stability; independence; intellectual functioning; internal locus of control; memory; mood; perception; positive body image; self-control; sexual satisfaction; work efficiency; and well-being. They also found that exercise decreases absenteeism from work; alcohol abuse; anger; anxiety; confusion; depression; dysmenorrhea; headaches; hostility; phobias; stress response; tension; and work errors. Willis and Campbell stated that, ". . . an exercise program that capitalizes on positive emotions, such as fun, joy, self-satisfaction, confidence, pride, enthusiasm, and excitement, has a decided advantage over one that focuses solely on health benefits or physiological outcomes."[22] They go on to attribute the high dropout rates associated with traditional fitness programs to a lack of attention to the factors that contribute to a positive emotional response in a given individual's prescription for exercise.

Additionally, our clinic has found that it is important for obese patients to have more than one form of exercise to choose from. Having a repertoire of exercises to choose from reduces boredom and eventual discontinuance. Also, if an exercise is contingent on good weather or an available partner, then the absence of either will limit exercise. Because of childhood teasing or failure experiences in sports or physical education at school, a subgroup of our obese patients have become averse to any type of exercise. With these patients, we suggest that they pair an exercise with something else they enjoy doing regularly. For example, if a patient loves to watch a particular television program or read certain types of literature, we suggest that they pair a tolerable exercise (e.g., stationary bike or treadmill) with watching the program or reading. For patients who love to shop, we suggest that they take a brisk walk in an air conditioned shopping mall, and then reward themselves by browsing in a store that caught their interest. Some of our patients with chronic pain have been surprised by their ability to perform water aerobics and feel better. Patients with severe orthopedic conditions, however, may benefit most from consultation with a physical or occupational therapist who prescribes exercises which allow them to safely work around their deficits. Some of these patients report that the coaching aspect of the therapy motivates them to do more for themselves, just as some of our healthier obese patients talk about the benefits of a personal trainer.

Pain

Another important biological-psychological-social variable that occurs in the majority of morbidly obese people and that must be placed on a continuum and studied is pain. Increased breast size in women and waist size in men are often associated with the development of back pain. Many obese patients experience physical pain related to injuries, previous surgery, joint degeneration, and/or neuromuscular problems. Sometimes the injury and pain precede the development of obesity, and sometimes the orthopedic condition and concomitant pain are a result of obesity. There is also a subgroup of patients who have pain conditions attributable to both pre- and postobesity factors. In all these cases, the mobility problems related to pain usually exacerbate the obesity due to decreased energy expenditure. Pain perception comes from multiple areas of the brain working in concert.[23] Memory plays an important role in all pain experience. Short-term memory is based on a biochemical–electrical impulse system, whereas long-term memory is created through protein synthesis. Affective response to pain is related to both desire and expectation. When a sense of loss is related to the pain in terms of health status, independence, quality of life, self-worth, or bonds with others, then the affective component is exponentially increased. Thus, the meanings the person ascribes to the pain, including the person's values, cultural beliefs about pain, and previous experiences with it combine to form the person's unique pain experience.

Pain can lead to depression. Depression is known to worsen the experience of pain. Some physicians trivialize the pain that morbidly obese people experience by telling them that the only way to treat their pain is for them to lose weight while not providing their patients with a reliable way to lose weight. The message the patient receives is that the physician will not treat their pain because they are fat and unworthy of treatment.

Binge Eating

Currently, obesity is classified as a disorder in physical medicine, but not in psychiatry. Obesity is classified as a general medical condition in the International Classification of Diseases (ICD-10). In the *Diagnostic and Statistical Manual of Mental Disorders–Fourth Edition Text Revision* (DSM-IV-TR),[24] the eating disorders that are formally classified are anorexia nervosa, bulimia nervosa, and eating disorders not otherwise specified. Binge-eating disorder is listed as item "6" in this last category and is described as "recurrent episodes of binge eating in the absence of the regular use of compensatory behaviors characteristic of Bulimia Nervosa." In the section entitled "Criteria Sets and Axes Provided for Further Study," the following research criteria for binge-eating disorder are suggested:

> A. Recurrent episodes of binge eating. An episode of binge eating is characterized by both of the following: (1) eating in a discrete period of time (e.g., within any 2-hour period), an amount of food that is definitely larger than most people would eat in a similar period of time under similar circumstances; (2) a sense of lack of control over eating during the episode (e.g., a feeling that one cannot stop eating or control what or how much one is eating).
> B. The binge-eating episodes are associated with three (or more) of the following: (1) eating much more rapidly than normal; (2) eating until feeling uncomfortably full; (3) eating large amounts of food when not physically hungry; (4) eating alone because of being embarrassed by how much one is eating; (5) feeling disgusted with oneself, depressed, or very guilty after overeating.
> C. Marked distress regarding binge eating is present.
> D. The binge eating occurs, on average, at least 2 days a week for 6 months. Note: . . . future research should address whether the preferred method of setting a frequency threshold is counting the number of days on which binges occur or counting the number of episodes of binge eating.
> E. The binge eating is not associated with regular use of inappropriate compensatory behaviors (e.g., purging, fasting, excessive exercise) and does not occur exclusively during Anorexia Nervosa or Bulimia Nervosa.[25]

The Associated Features and Disorders section of the DSM-IV-TR, states the following:

> Some individuals report that the binge eating is triggered by dysphoric moods, such as depression and anxiety. Others are unable to identify specific precipitants but many report a nonspecific feeling of tension that is relieved by the binge eating. Some individuals describe a dissociative quality

to the binge episodes (feeling "numb" or "spaced out"). Many individuals eat throughout the day with no planned mealtimes. Individuals with this eating pattern seen in clinical settings have varying degrees of obesity. . . . In weight-control clinics, individuals with this eating pattern are, on the average, more obese and have a history of more marked weight fluctuations than individuals without this pattern. . . . Individuals with this eating pattern may report that their eating or weight interferes with their relationships with other people, with their work, and with their ability to feel good about themselves. In comparison with individuals of equal weight without this pattern of eating, they report higher rates of self-loathing, disgust about body size, depression, anxiety, somatic concern, and interpersonal sensitivity. There may be a higher lifetime prevalence of Major Depressive Disorder, Substance-Related Disorders, and Personality Disorders. In samples drawn from weight-control programs, the overall prevalence varies from approximately 15 to 50% (with a mean of 30%), with females approximately 1.5 times more likely to have this pattern than males. In nonpatient community samples, a prevalence rate of 0.7 to 4.0% has been reported. The onset of binge eating typically is in late adolescence or in the early 20's, often coming soon after significant weight loss from dieting. Among individuals presenting for treatment, the course appears to be chronic.[26]

While there are many obese patients who are not binge eaters according to the above criteria, there is significant disagreement in the field with regard to what constitutes a binge. For example, Nash does not limit binge eating to a discrete time limit as suggested in the DSM-IV-TR (i.e., 2 hours) and considers the following patterns also to be binges: grazing, or eating throughout the day without structured eating times; excessive amounts of food consumed "unconsciously" while watching television, reading, or working; eating excessively for pleasure because one's weight diminishes or precludes the enjoyment of other activities; eating a large amount when the opportunity of being alone near a plentiful food supply exists; and, finally, the "vengeful binge" which is used to either express or dampen hostility.[27] Most obese patients have disordered eating habits, but may not meet criteria for an eating disorder. Some eating disorders specialists feel that the DSM-IV-TR criteria for eating disorders may be too restrictive.

In 1998, C. Everett Koop's Shape Up America! reported that 35% of women and 31% of men age 20 years and older are overweight, as are approximately 25% of children and adolescents ages 6 to 17 years. More recent reports indicate that more than 50% of American adults are overweight, up to 30% meet criteria for obesity as calculated by the body mass index and 25% meet criteria to be labeled morbidly obese.[28]

The mental health of our obese patients clearly falls along a continuum. We have seen morbidly obese patients who have no diagnosable psychiatric disorder. At this end of the continuum, we have treated extremely high-functioning obese professionals, who have intact loving and supportive families, and who report many satisfying interests. At the other end of the continuum, we have patients who are severely disabled by the combination of obesity and serious mental illness. Patients in this group often spend most days sleeping, watching television, and eating. Many have completely given up on sex, either because they are so ashamed of their appearance, or find it too difficult physically, or both. Some of our more impaired patients have little contact with the outside world.

The somatic health of our morbidly obese patients also falls along a continuum. At one end are those who have none of the serious comorbid conditions such as heart disease, diabetes, sleep apnea, or degenerative joint conditions. Many of this subgroup travel, dance, exercise, and do what most people do. At the other end of the continuum we have patients who are disabled. Some of these patients have such poor respiratory function that they can walk only a few feet before they must stop and rest. Others are wheelchair bound as a consequence of orthopedic conditions, and cannot have orthopedic surgery until they lose a significant amount of weight. There are very few forms of exercise that are possible for these patients, and they find themselves in a prison of their own creation.

In the end, it may be most useful to view morbid obesity as a spectrum disorder having many etiologies and comorbidities. Future research will need to develop sturdy empirically based subgroups, and then study them with the newly developed daily process and microanalytic experimental designs. Then, in close collaboration with clinicians, empirically based treatment protocols can be developed which best fit the range of problems and needs of the morbidly obese.

PSYCHODYNAMICS

Family Dynamics

Family dynamics are influenced by cultural factors such as race, ethnicity, religion, and geographic region. Given the limited scope of this chapter, it is not possible to review the clinical and research findings germane to the development of obesity in all of the major cultural subgroups residing in the United States. Instead, a brief review of general family dynamics related to the development of obesity is presented. It is a given that most people expect to have certain needs fulfilled in life. Maslow developed a hierarchy of needs, depicted as a pyramid, that form the core bases of human motivation.[29] In ascending order these are *physiological needs* (e.g., food, water, oxygen); *safety needs* (e.g., comfort, security, freedom from fear); *belonging and love needs* (e.g., affiliation, acceptance, intimacy); *esteem needs* (e.g., competence, approval, recognition); *cognitive needs* (e.g., knowledge, understanding, novelty); *esthetic needs* (e.g., symmetry, order, beauty); *self-actualization* (e.g., problem solving, creativity, appreciation of life, commitment to personal growth); and *peak experiences* (e.g., ecstasy, transcendence). Family members have competing needs. No person gets his/her needs met all of the time. How each family member shares in the pursuit of both need gratifications and delays, while at the same time showing respect for the unique personality of each family member, determines to a large degree whether a family is healthy or dysfunctional. Nash found that healthy families discuss differences and resolve them through negotiation.[27] This process contributes to greater trust and lower anxiety. People vary a great deal in their ability to tolerate frustration. As suggested under "Individual Dynamics" (below), in addition to constitutional factors, people who frequently rely on food to deal with frustrated needs are at risk of becoming obese.

Bruch described the dynamics surrounding childbirth that contribute to obesity in one or both marital partners.[30] Some women have children based on the fantasy that a child will bring an unending supply of unconditional love into their lives. They are often unaware of the huge degree of responsibility, the amount of self-sacrifice, and the magnitude of stress that comes with caring for a helpless infant. These mothers have a rude awakening as the sleepless nights, diaper changes, and periods of inconsolable crying start to add up. Other women may have children in order to fill the emptiness created by an unhappy marriage. A husband's envy of the intense mother–infant bond and the care that the child gets can lead to his overeating and weight gain. Some women feel empty after childbirth and overeat to fill themselves up. Another group of women eat excessively in reaction to postpartum anxiety or depression.

Bruch stated that, "mothers who are insecure in their fundamental attitude toward the child tend to compensate for this by excessive feeding and overprotective measures."[30] Excessive feeding may give food an exaggerated value which can contribute to obesity. Overprotection is detrimental to development because it makes normal efforts at separation from the mother, playing with others, and exploration seem too dangerous for the child. Eating may substitute for these normal confidence-building behaviors, and thus contribute to poor social adjustment and emotional immaturity. Bruch also found that a fat child's development is often adversely affected if one or both parents react with contempt or embarrassment toward the child's obesity.[30] These attitudes, or outright denial that the child is obese, can contribute to later identity problems.

Some families are overcontrolled (i.e., rigid, repressive, lacking spontaneity), some are undercontrolled (i.e., lacking structure, organization, and predictability), and others have an adaptive level of control. Siegel et al. described the importance of a structured, but flexible, family system as follows, "family rules should flexibly shift in response to the changes in ages, needs, and capabilities. Parents of young children are watchful and protective. Parents of adolescents should decrease their previous levels of watchfulness and protectiveness. Families with rigid and fixed rules do not allow for independent behavior. Some adolescents turn to drugs, alcohol, or disordered eating behaviors when they feel helpless and controlled."[31] Siegel et al. also described three dysfunctional family patterns associated with the development of eating disorders: "overcontrolled"; "chaotic"; and "violent."[31] Healthy families have flexible rules that allow the members to express intimacy, disagree, and express needs. Siegel et al. emphasize that the direct experience and expression of intense feelings such as anger, resentment, disappointment, jealousy, sadness, and loss are necessary for healthy functioning. They explain further that children need ways to disagree and to be different in order to value and trust their subjective experiences.[31] Overcontrolled families inhibit the expression of these subjective experiences and set the children up to develop unhealthy ways of dealing with emotions, such as eating disorders. Overcontrolled families also tend to be overinvested in appearance. The insecurity that drives this orientation is passed on to the children, who may never feel good about their appearance or personal sense of taste.

Chaotic families do not have consistent family rules, and lack the necessary structure for normal development. When a chaotic family is headed by parents who abuse drugs or alcohol, life becomes even more confusing and unpredictable for the children.[31] Additionally, children may learn that the use of substances to cope with life is acceptable behavior. Violent families cross personal boundaries in pathological ways. Excessive physical punishment, verbal abuse, and sexual abuse derail development for most children and are high-risk factors for the development of eating disorders, substance abuse, and personality disorders. Zerbe reviewed the literature on sexual abuse and found that between four and sixty-five percent of eating disordered patients had been abused.[32] Nash found childhood sexual abuse to be associated with various forms of psychopathology, and greater levels of comorbidity in eating disordered individuals.[27] When a child's body has not been safe from intrusion, the child may not learn how to regulate it. Eating disorders and addictions are often described as problems of self-regulation. Physical, emotional, and sexual abuse can derail development and interfere with healthy self-regulation. Children need a sense of privacy, separateness, independence, and control as they develop. After repeated abuse, food may become the only domain that they feel they can control.

Some form of psychotherapy is almost always essential for sexual abuse victims to get back on track developmentally, and to give up their maladaptive form(s) of self-regulation. Some of these patients present as angry and rebellious, while others appear detached or without emotion. Others never reveal their experiences of abuse to others. Sexual abuse contributes to many forms of psychiatric disturbance, but it is difficult to research since many victims and their families prefer to keep it secret in order to prevent embarrassment and further emotional pain.

During interviews at our weight-management clinic, a number of patients have disclosed abuse histories that had not been revealed to anyone previously.

Individual Dynamics

People either overcontrol, undercontrol, or adaptively control their thoughts, feelings, and behaviors. Psychologists are particularly interested in the conditions under which a given person behaves in these three modes. Thoughts, feelings, and behaviors are organized in putative structures within our minds. Contemporary dynamic theories call them "self-other-affect units," or "internalized object relations," whereas cognitive theories refer to them as "schemas." Horowitz integrates the cognitive and psychodynamic models and refers to states of mind he calls "self-schemas."[33] Most people experience "superior," "inferior," and "realistic" self-schemas, and shift between them. Although thought to be mostly unconscious, they become available to the conscious mind at times.

After a significant achievement we may feel superior to others. When entering a group of unfamiliar people, or after an embarrassing moment we may feel inferior. At times of clear self-reflection we may see that we have strengths and weaknesses, that we will be liked by some and not by others, and that we are basically good enough people. The realistic state of mind is more integrated and has a better sense of balance. Patients who spend too much time in the "superior" or "inferior" states tend to have more problems in living. Simply put, some forms of psychotherapy aim at helping a person spend more time in the "realistic" state of mind, and to think, feel, and behave more adaptively.

Many of our obese patients spend too much time in the "inferior" state of mind. Bruch, however, emphasized that, "the psychiatric problems of obese people are far from uniform. It is not possible to speak of the dynamics of one basic personality type as characteristic for all obese people. Obesity may be associated with every conceivable psychiatric disorder."[30] Rather than focus on psychiatric disorders, other investigators prefer to study critical periods of development in their effort to identify risk factors contributing to disordered eating. For example, Siegel et al. observed that during times of transition such as entering adolescence, going to college, or getting married, people often experience considerable anxiety.[31] Young adults who are not prepared to make the adjustments that these role transitions require may turn to food in unhealthy ways.

Bruch found that eating-disordered patients ". . . misuse the eating function in their efforts to camouflage or solve problems in living."[30] The many meanings and uses of food for a given individual can be contradictory and confusing to both the patient and the clinician. As Bruch pointed out, excessive eating can reflect dependency and the rejection of adult responsibilities.[30] Conversely, overeating can be used to detach from others, as if to say, "I don't need anybody." Clinically, it is quite common for patients to shift from one state of mind to another (e.g., dependent to autonomous, acquiescent to rebellious) and vice versa. This makes sense of the fact that some obese patients ask for help and direction but then do not comply with the treatment. Similarly, some come to the clinic for help and then bristle when told what to do or what they cannot have.

Bruch differentiates between "developmental obesity" and "reactive obesity."[30] The former starts at a young age and is woven into the adult's whole development. Identity is shaped, in part, by their obesity. When asked when they began to have problems with their weight, these patients often say things such as "birth," or "as far back as I can remember." The other form, reactive obesity, is preceded by a traumatic event or major life change (e.g., postinjury, leaving home for college, spousal infidelity, childbirth, empty nest syndrome). Patients with reactive obesity often report that they do not feel like themselves, and are uncomfortable with their appearance. One such patient, who became obese after a work-related accident, exclaimed, "I am *not* this fat person!"

According to Bruch, unrealistic expectations of greatness and success underlie the dynamics of some obese patients.[30] They may feel that they always need to be viewed by others as special, or the "best." They may feel that the usual laws of nature do not apply to them. For example, they may believe that they can eat what they want without negative consequences, or that they will achieve great things without discipline, persistence, and a great deal of personal sacrifice. As life fails to meet their unrealistic expectations, they resort to food even more for solace. Obese patients may develop the capacity to deny certain realities. As hard as it is to believe, some obese patients are not consciously aware of the severity of their problem. Many obese patients have reported their horror at seeing a family photo (or videotape) and not initially recognizing the obese person in it, only to discover it was him or her. Some of our patients eventually reveal that they avoided full-length mirrors so they wouldn't have to acknowledge their girth, or wore loose fitting dresses or workout clothes for the same purpose.

As part of a quality-of-life assessment at our weight-management center, we have all of our patients use a 10-point (i.e., 1 = worst, 10 = best) scale to rate the quality of their marriage (or other partnership), family life, work (or school), health, finances, spirituality, and recreation. The number of patients weighing in excess of 300 to 500 pounds who rate their health as being an 8, 9, or 10 (at least 10%) truly astounds us every time it occurs. Wurmser has described "addictive behaviors" that serve to relieve pressure from a punitive conscience, or as a way to liberate one's identity from guilt.[34] Sometimes the denial seen in obese patients reflects the effort to avoid condemnation from one's own perfectionistic conscience. Other theorists view denial as an aspect of grandiosity. People who bend reality too much may do so in order to feel omniscient or omnipotent.

A major problem with excessive perfectionism is that it usually leads to excessive frustration and anger. Bruch noted the unrealistic perfectionism that torments a subgroup of obese patients.[30] Kohut and Wolf refer to addictive behaviors as "narcissistic behavior disorders."[35] These patients overvalue or idealize themselves and others in order to make up for internal deficiencies. When they perceive flaws in themselves or idealized others, they feel shattered, and may pursue an "addictive search" for something to glue them back together. The feelings of helplessness and powerlessness are to be avoided at all costs. Dodes emphasized the rage that many addicts experience.[36] He has found that rage is subjectively experienced as "taking back control." Likewise, Stolorow stated that, ". . . rage and vengefulness serve the purpose of revitalizing a crumbling but urgently needed sense of power."[37]

Anyone who has worked extensively with morbidly obese patients has sensed their feelings of helplessness vis-à-vis weight management. A subgroup of obese patients become very angry and difficult to deal with at times. Some report overeating when angry or after having an argument with someone. Donovan and O'Leary view the addiction as an attempt to control areas of physical, emotional, or behavioral function that are otherwise felt to be uncontrollable.[38] Nash found "shame" to be a central experience for many eating-disordered patients.[27] These patients feel that they are fundamentally flawed, bad, or unlovable, and food is used to deal with these feelings. For some adult-onset obese patients, overeating progressed from being an occasional coping strategy (among other ones) to that of the primary one. As the disordered eating progresses, obese patients may shift from "choosing" to eat to "having" to eat.

They lose control of their eating behavior. They may lose control over the amount of food eaten, the choice of foods eaten, the times that foods are ingested, or various combinations of these.

There is disagreement in the literature about the most fitting conceptualization for this process of losing control. Some prefer "compulsive overeating," while others prefer "food addiction" or "substance abuse." For binge eaters, there is a cognitive process called "abstinence violation syndrome"[39] that kicks in after a person experiences a minor deviation from the diet they were following at the time. This subgroup of binge eaters sees even minor slips as evidence that they are "weak" or "bad" people. They feel condemned, react with a "what-the-hell" attitude, and go on to eat enormous quantities of food. Gormally et al. found that obese patients who do not binge were more likely to report that they overeat because they "enjoy eating," whereas moderate bingers reported episodic periods of poor control, and severe bingers reported a complete lack of control and a "constant struggle to avoid a binge."[40] Regardless of the term, the notion that the person has lost control remains central to most cases of morbid and superobesity. For some obese patients, food was initially used to relieve states of emotional turmoil, but later becomes a source of emotional anguish. Patients with compulsive behaviors and addictions continue to perform the behavior despite its negative impact on emotional well-being, health, career, or relationships.

The "paradox of control" has been described in the addiction literature,[41] as well as in the compulsion literature.[42] The behavior that provides a psychological sense of control becomes ungovernable or out of control. Several theorists believe that addictions begin a pursuit of pleasure, whereas compulsions occur to limit the unpleasant feeling of anxiety. Compulsive behaviors (e.g., washing one's hands 100 times per day, or checking to see that the gas heater is turned off 20 times before going to bed) may provide some relief, but are not inherently pleasurable. Also, compulsive behaviors do not typically involve the "craving" seen in addictions.

People crave chocolate, cigarettes, and alcohol. People with compulsive behaviors usually wish they did not have them. While addictions are often initially motivated by pleasure, many patients report that they began drinking alcohol or smoking cannabis to deal with social anxiety, so that they can fit in comfortably with others. When someone exclaims, "I *need* a drink," this may have more to do with the need to get rid of a dysphoric feeling than an immediate desire for pleasure. In support groups, some of our patients feel that the term "food addict" accurately describes their plight. Other patients are quick to point out, however, that one can abstain from alcohol or street drugs, but no one can abstain from food.

Siegel et al. refer to the excessive use of food to relieve inner distress as a form of "substance abuse."[31] It becomes clear that the terms "compulsion" and "addiction" have been used to mean different things by different researchers, and it is not within the scope of this chapter to attempt to resolve the confusion among these concepts. It is important, however, to recognize that most morbidly obese patients feel that they have lost control, and are unable to self-regulate under certain conditions. This dysregulation can have external origins, internal dynamic ones, or most commonly, some combination of both.

In our support groups, we include preoperative and postoperative patients together. It is beneficial to have the postoperative patients explain to the preoperative patients how their attitudes towards food change after their surgical procedures. It is obviously important to have a trained mental health professional as the group leader, who can help group members obtain insight into their changing behaviors and needs (i.e., the surgeon should not attempt this without help).

Dynamics Between Couples

Some couples simply enjoy having good food and wine after a long day of hard work. It is their reward, and it provides a period of quality time that they both value and enjoy. Over time, however, the effects of consuming a highly caloric meal before retiring for the evening will require an important decision—live with excess weight or change the lifestyle. For other couples, however, the problem of weight gain is not so simple. Smith described a dynamic he termed the "golden fantasy."[43] This fantasy reflects the wish to have all of one's needs met in a "perfect relationship." Smith pointed out that some patients go from relationship to relationship in search of the perfect one. Others will use denial to keep them in an imperfect relationship, but develop a deep form of resentment that is highly resistant to treatment. The patient does not want to be seen as "greedy" or "infantile," but refuses to give up the insatiable wish for complete gratification. Patients expect to be rejected if their hidden desires are revealed. Smith goes on to say that patients plagued by the "golden fantasy" may not make good use of real loving relationships around them during their quest for a totally fulfilling one.[43]

A "perfect meal" is more obtainable than the perfect person, and some of our patients with "golden fantasies" become obese, either because they are disappointed in their choice of a partner or because the search for the perfect person has been replaced by the consumption of great food. Stuart and Jacobson have studied weight gain after marriage extensively.[44] The popular belief is that most couples gain weight because they are happy, or because they no longer have to compete in the singles market. In order to uncover other reasons for weight gain, these researchers collected more than 9000 surveys that assessed marital life and eating behavior. They found that the women in the happiest marriages gained an average of 18.4 pounds in 13 years, while those in the unhappiest gained an average of 42.6 pounds. The men in the happiest marriages gained an average of 19 pounds in the same amount of time, compared to the unhappiest ones who gained an average of 38 pounds.

Importantly, a significant number of respondents expected the day-to-day aspects of marriage to reflect the joys of the courtship and were disappointed. After marriage, people may discover that a spouse has certain habits that are disagreeable, and that the compromises necessary to sustain a marriage require much more work than was anticipated. When a spouse gets depressed, or becomes bereaved after the death of a relative, or becomes preoccupied with work, the other partner often feels abandoned. To deal with the lonely feelings of abandonment, some turn to food.

Couples may find that after marriage, a mismatch develops in terms of what each partner finds to be the optimal frequency of sex. A partner might find that his or her eye begins to wander, and may unconsciously eat excessively to gain weight in an effort to protect the marriage from infidelity. Some people simply substitute the pleasure of food for sex. This may be especially so when a faithful spouse discovers the infidelity of his or her partner, or when emotional or physical abuse occur within the marriage. With the stress of earning a living and adjusting to demands of being a responsible adult, some men become less affectionate and unavailable emotionally. Stuart and Jacobson found that ". . . disagreement about what intimacy means and how it is expressed is the greatest wedge between men and woman."[44]

Some women feel deceived when the tenderness and loving words of courtship begin to disappear. The authors discovered that for some people, emotional and physical deprivation become confused with hunger. Food is something they can get whenever they want it, unlike the affection of another person. When one spouse abuses alcohol or drugs, the other may turn to compulsive overeating. Once the overeating leads to obesity, some partners are so ashamed of their bodies that they will not let their spouse see them in the nude or refuse to have sex altogether. With another group of couples, the thinner partner will criticize the obese one's weight and refuse to have sex with her or him.

Interestingly, Stuart and Jacobson also found that some marital partners prefer their spouse to be obese for defensive purposes.[44] Nash also described individuals who need their partner to have some kind of behavioral disorder in order to feel stable because they cannot tolerate a relationship between equals.[27] Some feel that when their loved one is obese, it lowers the probability that they will be left for another person. At our clinic, we have had several instances of spousal jealousy increasing after the obese partner had gastric bypass surgery. Stuart and Jacobson found that couples who are frequently engaged in battles for control increase the risk of weight gain in one or both partners.[49] Some partners in the study consciously gained weight in order to thwart the other partner's efforts to keep them fit. Many eating-disorder specialists agree that the surest way to keep a spouse (or any other family member for that matter) from losing weight is to demand that they do.[31]

Stuart and Jacobson also described the double binds that one partner may place the other partner in.[44] They gave the example of a man who encouraged his wife to exercise, but then complained about the expense of her gym membership. Another example was of a partner who wanted the other to lose weight but frequently brought home fattening treats. Another complained of feeling lonely whenever their spouse was getting ready to exercise. There are many possible motivations for sabotaging the weight loss efforts of a spouse: to feel superior to the spouse; a disinclination to deal with one's own weight problem; the fear that spousal weight loss will make one look bad in comparison; refusal to give up one's own bad habits such as gambling or drinking; or feeling that the spouse is less demanding when heavy. When these types of problems are evident presurgically, we recommend that the couple receive marital therapy and/or attend our support group together.

CONDITIONS THAT MUST BE TREATED PREOPERATIVELY

Epidemiology of Psychiatric Disorders

Much more research on the incidence of the co-occurring psychiatric disorders in morbidly obese patients of various socioeconomic status, ethnicity, cultural groups, and comorbid medical conditions needs to be conducted. Because there are no epidemiological studies of obese patients that are even close to the magnitude of the National Comorbidity Study conducted by Kessler and colleagues, their findings will be briefly reviewed even though they did not address obesity in this survey. In one of the largest and best epidemiological studies of mental illness in the United States, Kessler et al. found that 48% of the people aged 15 to 54 years reported a lifetime history of at least one Composite International Diagnostic Interview or DSM-III disorder.[45] Substance abuse or dependence had a 35.4% lifetime prevalence rate in men, and a 17.9% rate in women. Anxiety had a 30.5% lifetime prevalence rate in women, and a 19.2% rate in men. Major depression had a lifetime prevalence rate of approximately 21.3% in women and 12.7% in men. Popular literature often states that about 1 in 5 American adults will have a depressive episode during their lifetime, and that virtually every American family will have at least one member who becomes clinically depressed.

Kessler et al. found that 10.4% of women and 5% of men had a lifetime prevalence of posttraumatic stress disorder (PTSD).[46] The traumas most commonly associated with women were rape and sexual molestation, whereas men were more likely to have PTSD associated with combat exposure and witnessing violent acts. Patients with PTSD have a high rate of comorbid psychiatric disorders (i.e., 88.3% of the men have a lifetime comorbidity, whereas women have a 79% rate of comorbidity). Both men and women with PTSD have a high rate of major depressive disorder, 47.9% and 48.5%, respectively. Men have a higher addiction rate, with 51.9% having alcohol abuse/dependence and 34.5% having drug abuse/dependence. Women had a comorbid alcohol abuse/dependence rate of 27.9% and a drug abuse/dependence rate of 26.9%. Kessler's group did not look at the co-occurrence of obesity in the PTSD group, but in our practice we have seen many patients with PTSD who have attempted to self-regulate with food instead of drugs or alcohol.

Problems in the Assessment of Psychological Conditions

Patients who come to our weight-management clinic wanting bariatric surgery have to jump through many hoops before they are cleared to receive the procedure. They have a nursing assessment, an internal medicine evaluation, a preoperative meeting with a surgeon, many labs, usually a sleep study, a psychosocial evaluation with a social worker, and an interview with a psychologist. In addition, they must complete a battery of tests including a Beck Depression

Index, an Eating Disorder Scale, a quality-of-life scale, and open-ended questions such as, "I get angry when _____." Response bias is a considerable challenge for us. Many patients believe that the presence of a psychiatric or emotional disorder will bar them from receiving the surgery, or slow the pace of their progression toward it. Others, because of their denial, dissociation, or lack of insight, are unaware of their emotional condition. Also (and unfortunately) some patients resist the diagnosis and treatment of psychiatric conditions in order to avoid the stigma associated with mental disorders of any kind. These three groups of patients minimize their problems on scales and oftentimes during interviews. Conversely, a small minority of patients believe that if they appear to be as polysymptomatic as possible, then they will surely get the surgery. Because some insurers only approve bariatric surgery when a potentially life-threatening comorbid medical condition exists, the exaggeration bias some patients show has some basis in reality.

We have found that interviewing patients after they have completed the scales (e.g., depression, anxiety, emotional eating) is necessary to reduce both the false-positive and false-negative diagnostic conclusions. When contradictions between the test data and a patient's presentation during the interview are explored, often a clearer sense of the patient's clinical condition emerges. As mentioned earlier, a patient may tell one clinician one thing, and then say the opposite to another. When this occurs, it is necessary to explore the discrepancy with the patient. Also, we have a daily support group which combines pre- and postsurgery patients. The group has multiple purposes: *educational* (presents potential complications and what to do about them; discussion of pre- and postoperative protocols), *therapeutic* (suggestions for lifestyle changes are made; stress management techniques are discussed), *supportive* (the climate is noncritical and accepting, and deviations from the protocols are met with kindness and encouragement), and *diagnostic* (the group therapist takes note of exacerbations of previously identified symptoms, or discrepancies between their behavior during group and their behavior during the evaluation phase, and then brings these observations to the attention of the treatment team).

Efforts to Reduce Postoperative Regression

A major reason that we treat psychological disorders preoperatively is to increase the probability that a patient will do well postoperatively. Patients without psychological disorders experience some regression after major surgery. It is normal for them to be frightened, needy, irritable, demanding, or unreasonable when they return to consciousness. When a patient wakes up with tubes going into his or her nose and/or throat, and finding his or her arms attached to intravenous lines and legs hooked to a pump on the floor, they may panic. These states of perturbation can last for hours or, in some cases, days. A more protracted state of distress may occur when a patient has not had a prior surgery of any kind, or one of the magnitude of bariatric surgery.

A subgroup of patients experience personality changes related to anesthesia which complicate postoperative care. Another group of patients cannot adjust well to the degree of discomfort and dependency that is part of the first few postoperative days. Some are so uncomfortable that they refuse to cooperate with the breathing treatments or the walking regimen. Other patients are unable to clean themselves after defecating, and find it extremely embarrassing to require assistance with this bodily function.

"Buyer's remorse" is expressed by many patients. This is especially so when a given patient had no acute life-threatening condition presurgically. After being weighed at the hospital, some patients become enraged when they discover that they gained weight after the surgery. Usually, these patients were unaware of the fact that postsurgical edema usually increases weight temporarily. After returning home, some patients find that they look worse as they lose weight. Their faces may be more wrinkled, or they notice much more loose skin hanging from various parts of their bodies, sometimes in places that they never imagined finding it. After 3 months, however, most of our bariatric surgery patients are pleased with the results, and say that they would do it again if given the choice.

It is important to give an accurate picture of the first postoperative year. Holtzclaw stated that "anxiety can actually cause an increase in poor eating behavior preoperatively and postoperatively," and that it causes patients to "ignore logic or more complex thought processes."[47] When patients are well-informed about bariatric surgery, some of them will be less anxious perioperatively. In the daily support group at our clinic, we discuss possible complications and the fact that patients are likely to feel worse before they feel better postoperatively. We also address the challenges ahead of them during the first postoperative year. It is important to note that attendance at the support group does not guarantee that patients will register, accept, or retain the information. We continue to have postoperative patients who report that they expected to "look and feel better much quicker!" The more out of line a given patient's expectations are, the more likely there will be problems in the patient's adjustment to postoperative life. Also, some patients who have been fat since early childhood experience an identity crisis when they approach normal weight. They may require therapy to help them adjust to the new demands placed on them from within and without. These latter demands may involve more attention from the opposite sex, increased jealousy from a spouse or obese friends, and possibly more interference in the patient's life and relationships from the patient's own family members.

Other processes that may contribute to postoperative regression are the changes that the patient's personality, appearance, and behavior have on others. Andrews addressed the increase in assertiveness that many bariatric surgery patients show postoperatively.[48] This can be related to increased self-esteem after weight loss, or anger for past mistreatment, and/or defensive aggressiveness in anticipation of more abuse. Andrews has observed the following negative interpersonal aspects of weight loss from bariatric surgery: some friends become envious of the patient's increased confidence; some are put off by the patient's new degree of assertiveness; and overweight friends may feel threatened or become more self-conscious because of the patient's weight loss. Some patients become vulnerable to depression from rejection, loss, and other changes in their relationships, and require ongoing support from the staff at the weight-management program. At times, this support prevents the development of a full-blown depressive episode.

It is important to mention, however, that surgeons may play a role in the postoperative regression seen in some patients. Preoperatively, most surgeons are attentive, optimistic, and supportive. After surgery, however, some become more interested in their next surgeries than in the patients who have already had it. Some surgeons react with impatience, or even annoyance, when faced with the relentless concerns and complaints from their postoperative patients. Some patients feel misled or betrayed when their postoperative years are filled with challenges, plateaus, and hard work. Obesity is a chronic illness. Surgeons and patients need to view their relationship as a long-term commitment requiring ongoing communication and collaboration. A surgeon who has rarely seen a patient more than 60 days after surgery, unless a new surgical problem has developed, is usually not prepared for the ongoing relationship that a bariatric patient requires in order to be successful in his or her first two postoperative years. Before surgeons develop a bariatric practice, they need to understand what will be required to ensure that their outcomes meet national standards.

Conditions that must be treated to the point of complete remission preoperatively include the following:

- Binge-eating disorder
- Bulimia
- Current physical abuse
- Current sexual abuse
- Current substance abuse/dependence
- Mania
- Psychosis
- Suicidality

There are many forms of psychosis. The types that we have seen at our weight-management clinic are schizophrenia, psychotic depression, and manic psychosis. We have found that it is best to have a psychiatrist treat these conditions with medications until the psychosis clears, and then have the psychiatrist agree to follow the patient pre- and postoperatively. We reassess the patient, and determine whether they have the personal strengths and social support to do well postsurgically.

When patients present with both suicidal ideation and a plan to carry it out, they must have a combination of brief psychiatric hospitalization, medication, and crisis intervention psychotherapy until the suicidality fully remits. They must also be followed pre- and postoperatively by their psychiatrist and psychotherapist.

When patients are actively bulimic, they must enter therapy (if they are not in it) and must be symptom free for 6 months. When severe, they may require inpatient treatment at an eating disorders unit to become stable. Once symptom free, they must retake our psychological tests in order to be cleared for surgery. This process is the same for binge-eating disorder.

The old psychiatric view of bariatric surgery maintained that unless an obese person has years of therapy ("which gets at the root of the problem") the patient will develop symptom substitution and become addicted to something else. We have not found this to be the case for obese patients in general. However, in the cases where we have discovered that a patient deceived us about the presence of an active addiction to alcohol, pain medications, or street drugs, the patient has been difficult to treat for our team and the addiction specialist who sees them postoperatively. Patients with histories of addiction need to enter an ongoing Alcoholics Anonymous (AA) or a Narcotics Anonymous (NA) group if they are not in one at the time of their initial evaluation for surgery. Also, we have had patients who did not follow our suggestions to develop healthier ways of dealing with stress and painful emotions. Some of them did well postoperatively until they experienced a death in the family, a break-up of a relationship, or some other significant stressor and then began drinking excessively or engaging in some other self-destructive behavior.

Current physical or sexual abuse may require that we report the abuse to the authorities, get the patient into individual therapy and/or a support group, and in some cases a shelter program. We reassess the patient and do not proceed with the preoperative phase until we feel that they are physically safe, psychiatrically stable, and emotionally prepared to undertake surgery.

Disorders that must be treated to the point of partial remission preoperatively include the following:

- Anxiety
- Depression
- Dysfunctional marriage and/or family
- Personality disorders
- Posttraumatic stress disorder

Depression is the most common psychiatric disorder that we treat at our clinic. As was indicated earlier, depression is often associated with chronic stress, sleep disorders, pain disorders, other somatic diseases, interpersonal problems, disability, losses, and the state of being obese. Sometimes, depression does not fully remit until a patient receives treatment for the problems in living and/or the somatic disorders contributing to the depression. Postsurgical depression is known to occur with any procedure that causes significant pain, discomfort, and/or immobility, or when a long period of time is needed for recovery. We use a standard depression scale to assess and monitor the course of depression. There are many good empirically based depression screens. We use the Beck Depression Index (BDI). It is norm referenced, and is widely used in both clinical practice and research. The interpretation of BDI scores is as follows: 0–9 "normal"; 10–18 "mild–moderate"; 19–29 "moderate–severe"; and 30–63 "severe–extremely severe." We usually recommend medication for patients with scores above 20. If during the clinical interview we feel that the patient minimized her or his symptoms during the test, we recommend treatment in spite of a subclinical score. We know that brain serotonin levels fall when intake is reduced, and also that many patients become more depressed in the postoperative period as a consequence of an increase in pain levels and fear of complications developing. Antidepressant therapy gives you a margin of safety when these natural destabilizing events occur postoperatively. Also, when patients endorse suicidality, hopelessness, and pessimism, we will treat them even when their scores are below 20.

When patients score in the "severe" to "extremely severe" ranges, we retest them after about 6 weeks (or whenever the medication is known to reach a good clinical level) and only clear them for surgery once they have improved significantly. While most depressed patients could benefit from concurrent cognitive behavioral or interpersonal therapies, many cannot afford it, and a significant subgroup of obese patients are unwilling to enter therapy. Some of this latter group state things such as, "My only problem is the weight. Once it is gone I will feel better." When a patient's depression is related to abuse, neglect, or other longstanding issues based in childhood, we are more likely to require the combination of therapy and medication. Finally, in cases of recent onset depression which parallels the increase in weight, we often try them first on medication, and later add a therapy recommendation if the severity of the depression persists.

Many of our patients are in treatment for depression by a primary care physician or a psychiatrist when they come to us. In these cases, we obtain a release of information from the patient, report our findings to the clinician and discuss the need for an increase or change in medication when indicated. In patients with chronic depression, who will need maintenance treatment for a long time, we discuss the need for a weight-neutral medication. The term *weight neutral* indicates that a drug has not been associated with weight gain even after years of use. There are many reports of weight gain associated with long-term use of some of the selective serotonin reuptake inhibitors (SSRIs). It is important to mention, however, that if a patient is doing very well on a maintenance antidepressant, we do not recommend a change to a weight-neutral drug preoperatively. We will develop a good line of communication with the patient's treating physician, and then revisit the issue should the patient experience an unusually long plateau in his or her weight loss, or begin to regain weight postsurgically.

Some of our patients report anxiety. Our physicians usually try them on an SSRI, BuSpar, or other medication that has good anxiolytic properties. Our clinic rarely starts patients on benzodiazepines because of their abuse and addiction potential.

In cases where trauma, physical abuse, or sexual abuse led to the development of anxiety, we recommend concurrent psychotherapy if a patient has not had a previous therapy experience. If a patient has had psychotherapy, but continues to experience flashbacks, intrusive thoughts, night terrors, avoidance behavior, and the like, we refer the patient to a PTSD specialist.

We recommend marital or family therapy for patients in emotionally destructive marriages or families. In both cases, we get a release of information in order to obtain input from the therapist about when the therapist feels that the interpersonal situation is stable enough for the patient to proceed with bariatric surgery.

Surprisingly, most of our patients presenting with personality disorders have done well with bariatric surgery. This could be for several reasons. First, if they are not in psychotherapy, we strongly suggest that they enter it before surgery. We also have the patient fill out a release form, and then request that the therapist inform us when the patient is relatively stable. Also, it is important to keep in mind that patients who are medically ill often appear more self-centered and demanding than they would ordinarily be when well. When they feel better, many of our patients behave better. This is not to say that we have not encountered patients who were difficult preoperatively, postoperatively, and for years into their follow-up treatments. Thankfully, they are rare in our experience.

We approach all our patients with a kind but firm approach and they seem to respond well to it. Many morbidly obese patients have been treated unkindly by doctors, family members, and other people who were supposed to be of help to them. When this mistreatment is added to the discrimination that they face on a day to day basis from employers, strangers, and even little children, it is no wonder why some obese patients are difficult to work with initially. When you show them some understanding, kindness, and sensitivity to their unique needs, you have over half the battle won! Finally, the fact that most of our patients do well and go on to improve their lives in remarkable ways makes working with the morbidly obese an extremely rewarding endeavor.

REFERENCES

1. Kesten D. The enlightened diet. *Spirituality and Health* Winter 2003:29–40.
2. Hobfoll SE, Schwarzer R, Chon KK. Disentangling the stress labyrinth: interpreting the meaning of the term stress as it is studied in health context. *Anxiety Stress Coping* 1998;11:181–212.
3. Swindle R, Heller K, Pescosolido B, et al. Responses to nervous breakdowns in America over a 40-year period. *Am Psychol* 2000;55:740–749.
4. Selye H. *Stress.* Montreal, Canada: Acta Medical Publisher, 1950.
5. Roy-Byrne PP, Uhde TW, Post RM, et al. The CRH stimulation testing patients with panic disorder. *Am J Psychiatry* 1986;143:396–399.
6. Gold PW, Pigott TA, Kling MK, et al. Basic and clinical studies with corticotropin releasing hormone: implications for a possible role in panic disorder. *Psychiatric Clinics of North America* 1988;11:153–160.
7. Insel TR, Kalin NH, Guttmacher LG, et al. The dexamethasone suppression test in obsessive-compulsive disorder. *Psychiatric Res* 1982;5:153–160.
8. Wand GS, Dobs AS. Alterations in the hypothalamic–pituitary axis in actively drinking alcoholics. *J Clin Endocrinol Metab* 1991;72:1290–1295.
9. Tennen H, Affleck G, Armeli S, et al. A daily process approach to coping. *Am Psychol* 2000;55:626–636.
10. Lazarus RS. Coping theory and research: past, present, and future. *Psychosom Med* 1993;55:234–237.
11. Martinez-Gonzalez D, Obermeyer WH, Benca RM. Comorbidity of insomnia with medical and psychiatric disorders. *Prim Psychiatry* 2002;9(8):37–49.
12. Quan SF. Sleep disorders centers: function, structure, and economics. *Prim Psychiatry* 2002;9(8):25–29.
13. Soldatos CR. Insomnia in relation to depression and anxiety: epidemiologic considerations. *J Psychosom Res* 1994;38(Suppl 1):3–8.

14. Ford DE, Kamerow DB: Epidemiologic study of sleep disturbance and psychiatric disorders: an opportunity for prevention? *JAMA* 1989;262:1479–1484.

15. Barnes RG, Deacon SJ, Forbes MJ, et al. Adaptation of the 6-sulphatoxymelatonin rhythm in shiftworkers on offshore oil installations during a two-week 12-hour night shift. *Neurosci Lett* 1998;241:9–12.

16. Roth T. Treating insomnia in the depressed patient: practical considerations. *Hosp Med* 1999;23–28.

17. Rosenthal NE, Sack DA, Gillin JC, et al. Seasonal affective disorder: a description of the syndrome and preliminary findings with light therapy. *Arch Gen Psychiatry* 1984;41:72–80.

18. Schenck CH, Hurwitx TD, Bundlie SR, et al. Sleep-related eating disorders: polysomnographic correlates of a heterogeneous syndrome distinct from daytime eating disorders. *Sleep* 1991;14:419–431.

19. Stunkard AJ, Grace WJ, Wolff HG. The night eating syndrome: a pattern of food intake among certain obese patients. *Am J Med* 1955;19:78–86.

20. Friedman S, Even C, Dardennes R, et al. Light therapy, obesity, and night eating syndrome. *Am J Psychiatry* 2002;259:875–876.

21. Taylor CB, Sallis JF, Needle R. The relation of physical activity and exercise to mental health. *Public Health Rep* 1985;100(2):195–202.

22. Willis JD, Campbell LF. *Exercise Psychology*. Champagne, IL: Human Kinetics Publishers, 1992.

23. Ray AL. Pain perception in the older patient. *Geriatrics* 2002;57(12):22–26.

24. American Psychiatric Association. *Diagnostic and Statistical Manuel of Mental Disorders,* 4th ed. Text Revision. Washington, DC: American Psychiatric Association, 2000.

25. American Psychiatric Association. *Diagnostic and Statistical Manuel of Mental Disorders,* 4th ed. Text Revision. Washington, DC: American Psychiatric Association, 2000:787.

26. American Psychiatric Association. *Diagnostic and Statistical Manuel of Mental Disorders,* 4th ed. Text Revision. Washington, DC: American Psychiatric Association, 2000:786–787.

27. Nash, JD: *Binge No More: A Practical Guide to Overcoming Disordered Eating.* Oakland, CA: New Harbinger Press, 1999.

28. Mokdad AH, Ford ES, Bowman BA, et al. Prevalence of obesity, diabetes, and obesity-related health risk factors, 2001. *JAMA* 2003;289:76–79.

29. Maslow AH. The instinctoid nature of basic needs. *J Pers* 1954;22:326–347.

30. Bruch H. *Eating Disorders: Obesity, Anorexia Nervosa, and the Person Within.* New York: Basic Books, 1973.

31. Siegel M, Brisman J, Weinshel M. *Surviving an Eating Disorder: Strategies for Family and Friends.* New York: Harper/Perennial, 1997.

32. Zerbe KJ. The Body Betrayed: A Deeper Understanding of Women, Eating Disorders, and Treatment. Washington, DC: American Psychiatric Press, 1993.

33. Horowitz MJ. *Introduction of Psychodynamics: A New Synthesis.* New York: Basic Books, 1988.

34. Wurmser L. The role of superego conflicts in substance abuse and their treatment. *Int J Psychoanal* 1984;10:227–258.

35. Kohut H, Wolf ES. The disorders of the self and their treatment: an outline. *Int J Psychoanal* 1978;59:413–425.

36. Dodes LM. Addiction, helplessness, and rage. *Psychoanal Q* 1990;LIX:398–419.

37. Stolorow RD. Critical reflections on the theory of self-psychology: an inside view. *Psychoanal Q* 1986;6:387–402.

38. Donovan DM, O'Leary MR. Control orientation, drinking behavior, and alcoholism. In: Lefcourt HM, ed. *Research with Locus of Control Construct.* Vol. 2: *Developmental and Social Problems.* New York: Academic Press, 1983:107–153.

39. Marlatt GA. A cognitive-behavioral model of the relapse process. In: Krasnegor NA, ed. *Behavioral Analysis and Treatment of Substance Abuse.* Washington, DC: Department of Health, Education, and Welfare, 1979. NIDI Research Monograph No. 25.

40. Gormally J, Black S, Daston S, et al. The assessment of binge eating severity among obese persons. *Addict Behav* 1982;7:47–55.

41. Marlatt GA, Gordon JR, eds. *Relapse Prevention: Maintenance Strategies in the Treatment of Addictive Behaviors.* New York: Guilford, 1995.

42. Salzman L. *The Obsessive Personality: Origins, Dynamics, and Therapy.* New York: Science House, 1968.

43. Smith S. The golden fantasy: A regressive reaction to separation anxiety. *The International Journal of Psycho-Analysis.* 1977;58(part 3):311–324.

44. Stuart RB, Jacobson B. *Weight, Sex, & Marriage: A Delicate Balance.* New York: WW Norton, 1987.

45. Kessler RC, McGonagle KA, Zhao S, et al. Lifetime and 12-month prevalence of DSM-III-R psychiatric disorders in the United States. *Arch Gen Psychiatry* 1994;51:8–19.

46. Kessler RC, Sonnega S, Bromet E, et al. Posttraumatic stress disorder in the national comorbidity study. *Arch Gen Psychiatry* 1995;52:1048–1060.

47. Holtzclaw TK. Understanding how anxiety affects eating behavior—part II. Beyond change: information regarding obesity and obesity surgery. December, 2002.

48. Andrews G. Changes. Psychologically speaking. Beyond change: information regarding obesity and obesity surgery. September, 2002.

PREOPERATIVE EVALUATION AND PREPARATION OF BARIATRIC SURGERY CANDIDATES

PETER BENOTTI / LOUIS MARTIN

Surgery is rapidly emerging as the treatment of choice for morbidly obese patients, especially as newer, less-invasive procedures allow people to return to work and full activities in weeks rather than months. The growing awareness of the vital role of surgery in the multidisciplinary management of morbid obesity is resulting in increasing numbers of patients being referred for surgical treatment. Independent market research suggests that more than 55,000 operations for morbid obesity were performed in 2002, and this number will rise to 100,000 by 2006. Operations designed to help the morbidly obese lose weight are labeled bariatric operations, or bariatric surgery, and this field of medicine is called bariatrics.

Bariatric surgery is unique among gastrointestinal operations. It is not considered an emergency procedure like an appendectomy, and is much more involved than a cholecystectomy because you are not just removing a dysfunctional organ, you are performing behavior-modification surgery. Many of the patients have illnesses that are undertreated and many have bad habits that must be addressed. The preoperative and postoperative periods are unique in that they demand full patient participation in the life change process as a prerequisite for long-term success. The necessity for complete patient understanding and full participation in the postoperative weight loss and weight maintenance process necessitates a more prolonged and labor-intensive preoperative evaluation and preparation. The long list of comorbid diseases associated with obesity and the increased mortality associated with all operations performed in the morbidly obese also necessitates careful documentation of which comorbid diseases are present and a major push to decrease the risk of surgery through positive interventions to improve the preoperative treatment of each condition. Therefore, the focus during this period is multidirectional and involves concomitant patient education, including establishing the informed consent process, medical evaluation for risk assessment, and initiation of strategies for risk reduction. It is somewhat similar to preparing a patient for organ transplantation.

PATIENT EDUCATION/INFORMED CONSENT

Surgical treatment for obesity is indicated for patients who are 45.4 kg (100 lb) overweight, or twice the desirable body weight, or who have a body mass index (BMI) of 40 kg/m^2 or more. Individuals with a body mass index of 35 to 40 kg/m^2 who have high-risk comorbidities (i.e., sleep apnea or diabetes), or who have major physical problems adversely affecting lifestyle, including their employment, mobility, or family role functions, are also candidates for surgical treatment.[1] Patients who are eligible for surgical treatment will have demonstrated failure of conservative weight-reduction programs (i.e., either failure to be able to lose weight by restricting calories or types of food, or failure to maintain weight lost on a diet by regaining all the weight lost, usually in less than a year's time). Only patients who are an acceptable operative risk should be considered for surgery. Psychosis, substance and alcohol abuse, and major organ failure are usually contradictions to surgery. The goal is to have a mortality rate of less than 1% for this elective operation in the vast majority of patients.

Patients should be made aware of the rationale for surgical treatment of obesity. This should include information about the health risks and medical hazards associated with severe obesity.[2] Discussion of health risks should also involve quality of life issues (also see Chapter 4).[3] The low probability of long-term weight control with dietary or other nonsurgical weight-control programs should be discussed. The weight-loss results of surgery should be reviewed, including failure rates of the different types of operations. The impact of weight loss on health and quality of life should be emphasized and balanced against the possible complications associated with the various bariatric procedures, including the problems that will develop from lack of compliance with the lifestyle changes each procedure necessitates.[4,5]

Prospective patients should be made aware of the mechanisms for weight loss, including gastric restriction and malabsorption. The concepts of energy balance including calories ingested versus calories consumed as mechanisms for weight gain and weight loss should be reviewed. It is especially necessary to tell patients that a high alcohol intake will prevent weight loss with any bariatric procedure.

Surgical candidates should be made aware of the available and accepted operations for obesity treatment, the results of open and minimally invasive operations, the advantages and disadvantages of the different procedures, and the operative risks. Late complications of surgical treatment (greater than 30 days to several years postoperatively) and nutritional issues from decreased food intake should also be reviewed with emphasis on the necessity for long-term follow-up by the operating surgeon. Although the mortality rate for most people considering this surgery will be less than 1%, there is a group of superobese people (those who weigh 200% above ideal body weight or who have a BMI

>60 kg/m^2) with severe medical problems such as sleep apnea, hypoventilation syndrome of obesity, and heart disease, which may be considered for surgery but will have a mortality rate of 2 to 6%.[6,7]

MEDICAL EVALUATION FOR OPERATIVE RISK ASSESSMENT

The importance of a detailed health history and examination by the bariatric surgeon and the multidisciplinary team is a critical part of the preparation for surgery. Many severely obese patients have had poor medical care because of their reluctance to deal with unsympathetic or poorly informed physicians. For this reason, many medical problems may be diagnosed at the time of the pre-operative evaluation. Collaboration with various specialists is often necessary for optimum preoperative management. Patients who are active and produc-tive, with no impairment of physical performance status despite their severe obesity, are usually good operative risks and probably will need limited study in preparation for surgery (i.e., those that can walk at least a mile on a tread-mill in under 30 minutes). At the other extreme, the patient who can barely per-form 4 metabolic equivalents of work (i.e., climb one flight of stairs) without severe dyspnea, and others who can do even less, will be at much greater risk.

Preoperative pulmonary function studies should be obtained for patients with respiratory illness (i.e., asthma or sleep apnea), and those whose perfor-mance status is limited by significant exertional dyspnea. The rationale for de-termining preoperative pulmonary function in patients with clinical pulmonary impairment, involves the awareness of the postoperative reduction in pul-monary function that invariably accompanies upper abdominal surgery.[8] Changes in pulmonary function associated with obesity include a reduction in lung and chest wall compliance, an increase in respiratory system resistance, reduced lung volumes, and an increased work of breathing.[9] Severely obese pa-tients with impaired lung function are at risk for pulmonary complications dur-ing the first 72 hours postoperation, when pulmonary function may be severely impaired. These patients need to be encouraged to lose weight preoperatively to provide the intraabdominal cavity with more room needed to compensate for the swelling caused by third space accumulation of fluid. Also a preopera-tive exercise program specifically developed for those with impaired lung func-tion can preoperatively improve pulmonary function. Treatment of reactive air-way disease, when reservable, is necessary. Obtaining arterial blood gases is important to know what, if any values are compromised, and to judge how much improvement has occurred with preoperative treatment. It also provides the treatment team with the patient's values to aim for in the postoperative period (i.e., if the arterial oxygenation level is less than 80 mm Hg preoperatively, that is as high as it can get postoperatively).

A detailed history looking for symptoms of sleep apnea is an important aspect of preoperative preparation. The presence of sleep apnea poses addi-tional risks of hypoxemia during sleep and requires special attention to nar-cotic and airway management by the anesthesiologist and other physicians.[10]

Patients suspected of having sleep apnea should be referred for sleep study and continuous positive airway pressure (CPAP) titration pre operatively. More than 80% of men and at least 10 to 15% of women with weights greater than 160 kg (352.4 lb) will have sleep apnea.[11] The preoperative use of nasal CPAP will reduce severe hypoxemia and associated pulmonary vasoconstriction, resulting in improved right ventricular function.[10] A 1-month period of adjustment is necessary for most patients to get accustomed to their CPAP apparatus and to use it successfully. Patients should bring their own equipment to the hospital to use postoperatively. If patients with severe sleep apnea cannot adjust to using CPAP, then a tracheostomy must be considered for use in the perioperative period.

Preoperative anesthesia consultation is indicated for patients with severe obstructive sleep apnea, superobese males with thick necks, anyone with major restriction of mobility of the neck, and patients with major reduction in lung volumes documented in preoperative pulmonary function testing. For these patients, airway control may be more difficult, and a reduced functional residual capacity is associated with an increased risk of severe hypoxia during endotracheal intubation at induction of anesthesia. Often a bronchoscope may be necessary for a safe intubation and the patient may need to be prepared to have an awake intubation to protect his or her airway. Postoperatively, if the patient has sleep apnea or obesity–hypoventilation syndrome, a 1 to 4-day period of mechanical ventilation may be necessary until postoperative edema has decreased and the need for intravenous pain medication has resolved.

Because cardiac dysfunction of varying degrees is not uncommon in long-standing morbid obesity, certain patients will require preoperative cardiac evaluation. Those patients with limited performance status, those with superobesity complicated by hypertension, those with sleep apnea and/or hypoxia in association with pulmonary hypertension, and those with fluid retention complicating their morbid obesity should have cardiac ultrasonography to evaluate systolic and diastolic function of their ventricles. Cardiovascular changes associated with morbid obesity include arrhythmias, especially atrial fibrillation, cardiac hypertrophy, increased preload, diastolic dysfunction, and, rarely, frank systolic dysfunction in association with cardiomyopathy.[12,13] The authors have found transesophageal ultrasonography and diagnostic right-heart catheterization helpful in the preoperative preparation of selected high-risk patients. Detailed preoperative assessment of cardiac function is extremely helpful for anesthetic management, planning perioperative monitoring, and for perioperative fluid management. Patients who cannot walk even one-tenth of a mile on a treadmill and/or who cannot complete a Bruce Stress Test may need a drug-stimulated radionucleotide stress test to evaluate for ischemia.

PREVENTION OF THROMBOEMBOLISM

Morbid obesity is associated with an increased risk of post operative thromboembolism.[14] In the authors personal experiences, the incidence of thromboembolism complicating bariatric surgery is 1 to 2% for postoperative deep venous thrombosis and 0.5% for pulmonary embolism. It has been the number one cause of mortality for the authors combined experience of more than 40 years of bariatric surgery, especially once experience is gained so that post-operative anastomotic leak rate and staple-line failures are minimized. A careful preoperative history looking for previous episodes of thromboembolism and a family history will uncover a small number of patients with hypercoagulable states.[15] Patients with hypoxia that cannot tolerate even a small decease in oxygen saturation and those with severe venous stasis associated with brawny skin changes of their lower extremities or a history of ulceration, or patients with a history of deep venous thrombosis should be considered for preoperative placement of a Greenfield filter in their inferior vena cava below the renal veins and preoperative weight loss using a high-protein, low-calorie liquid diet (see "Immediate Preoperative Dietary Changes for All Patients" and "Dietary Intervention," below).[14]

The authors have found over a 10-year experience that twice-daily injections of low-molecular-weight heparin together with sequential leg or foot compression and ambulation on the first postoperative day are the best prophylaxis for postoperative thromboembolism. The dose for morbidly obese patients should be calculated based on their BMI rather than their weight or by an attempt to estimate lean body mass. We suggest that enoxaparin (Lovenox) be given subcutaneously in a milligram dose that matches the closest multiple of 10 that is similar to the patients BMI, twice a day, starting 6–12 hours preoperatively, using the closest smaller milligram dose. This is continued until the patient is ambulating without assistance and drinking at least 3 L of water and liquid protein supplements a day, even if it must continue after discharge. This means a patient with a BMI that equals 62 kg/m^2 would receive 60 mg subcutaneously every 12 hours for 4–10 days. This suggestion is not supported yet by evidence-based medicine, but there are few tragedies worse than working with a morbidly obese patient for 4–6 months to prepare them for surgery and then learn that they have died 2 days after discharge, seconds after a bowel movement in their bathroom, from a sudden collapse. Several of these episodes experienced by the authors are the reason that most of our patients with a BMI >70 kg/m^2, or with a history of a prior thrombosis, get preoperative Greenfield filters, and all patients receive prophylaxis using enoxaparin in the manner described. We think it is important to give the preoperative dose at least 6 hours before surgery. This means that a patient can take his or her own dose at home the night before surgery or that the patient can be admitted to the hospital to be given the medication. Our hospital is convinced of the importance of starting the Lovenox preoperatively and has made arrangements for our patients to be admitted at midnight rather than at 6 A.M. on the day of surgery. This way, the Lovenox is given in the hospital, and we are able to start our first operative case each morning before other operative teams because our patients have had a longer time with the nursing staff and everything is ready for a 6:30 A.M. trip to the operating room.

We adjust the dose of enoxaparin within a range of multiples of 10, adjusting downward for lower-risk patients and upward for higher-risk patients.

A working, healthy executive with a BMI of 46 kg/m^2 will usually get a 40-mg dose every 12 hours, while an older patient who has to use a cane to walk would get a dose of 45 or 50 mg every 12 hours. If intraoperative hemorrhage or oozing is above our average, then we usually do not start the enoxaparin until 8 or 10 hours after surgery, rather than our usual 6 hours. Occasionally, we will also decrease the dose by 5 or 10 mg also. A randomized, placebo-controlled study is needed to validate this treatment model.

PREVENTION OF HYPERGLYCEMIA

Approximately 15% of morbidly obese undergoing surgery have type 2 diabetes. Glucose control in these patients is an important area of necessary preoperative attention. The association between diabetes and postoperative infections is well known. Hyperglycemia ($\geq$220 mg%) inhibits many important functions of polymorphonuclear leukocytes. Recent evidence indicates that aggressive control of hyperglycemia during the perioperative period will reduce this infection risk.[16] Preoperative patients should be made aware of the importance of proper glucose control as a preoperative requirement. If glucose levels are difficult to control with adjustments in medications, a preoperative reduction in carbohydrate intake may be necessary to bring sugars below the 200–220 mg% range. Diabetics who can spend at least 1 week on a high-protein, low-calorie liquid diet of less than 1200 kcal will decrease their medication needs by at least 50%. Patients who cannot do this as an outpatient should be considered for inpatient management of this regimen, as it becomes easier by the third day, once ketogenesis is initiated and hunger decreases. Importantly, the patient's stimulated ketogenesis mechanisms will produce the enzymes necessary for homeostasis on a liquid diet before the trauma of surgery, which will also require generation of cytokines and stress hormone responses that would compete with ketogenesis enzyme generation. Separating out these two necessary adaptations for postoperative recovery increases new protein generation in the immediate postoperative period in wound chambers placed in morbidly obese patients undergoing gastric bypass.[17] The authors insist on adequate preoperative glucose control and use a sliding scale or an intravenous insulin infusion to prevent hyperglycemia during the first 48–72 hours postoperatively, if necessary.

PREVENTION OF POSTOPERATIVE INFECTIONS

Morbidly obese patients develop more nosocomial infections during the perioperative period than do other patients.[18] Many antibiotics need to be given in higher doses to morbidly obese patients to obtain adequate serum and tissue levels. Redundant skin folds and irritation from tissue rubbing in active areas increases the percentage of morbidly obese patients who have hidradenitis, intertrigo, and frequent boils or other types of skin infections. We ask all our patients to shower at least twice a day for at least three preoperative days with antibacterial soaps such as Dial, Betadine, or Hibecleanze. We also have patients scrub their abdominal and perineal areas with Betadine scrub solution for 10 to 15 minutes, after being admitted preoperatively. We do not shave patients, however, as this increases wound infection rates.

We have also used a 3-day oral preoperative antibiotic regimen of Levaquin 500 mg once a day, Diflucan 200 mg once a day, and Flagyl 500 mg three times a day, unless allergies prevent this. With this regimen, we have not had a wound infection in more than 1000 consecutive laparoscopic gastric bypasses. The pharmaceutical companies have not examined the special needs of the morbidly obese so that very few prospective studies on such patients are available for any class of drugs, including antibiotics. Our suggestion is not based on a prospective, controlled trial, just our attempt to find a way to decrease our postoperative infection rate. A wound infection after an open procedure in a morbidly obese patient can require months to heal if the wound has to be completely opened for daily dressing changes until it granulates closed by secondary intention.

We use the same antibiotic regimen that we use preoperatively in the perioperative period, switching from oral to parenteral administration. We also think it is important to maximize oxygen saturations postoperatively, which also decreases postoperative infection rates.

MIDNIGHT ADMISSION

Another mechanism we have developed with the cooperation of our hospital is to better prepare our preoperative patients is to admit them at 12 A.M. on the day of surgery rather than at 6 A.M. Almost all medical insurance companies deny preoperative days for all but the most critically ill patients. The postoperative complication rate for bariatric surgery, however, is higher than for all other commonly performed gastrointestinal procedures. Many insurance companies reimburse hospitals at fixed rates based on the operative procedure and medical diagnoses without compensation for perioperative complications. This encourages the hospital to help the surgeon control the rate of perioperative complications for high-risk procedures. Although a midnight admission adds extra work for nursing night shifts that are often managed with skeleton crews, if it only involves two to four patients that all have common orders, it has not proved to overburden our nursing staff. It allows us to initiate deep venous thrombosis prophylaxis 6 hours before surgical procedures, helping to prevent thrombosis while decreasing the risk of perioperative bleeding. It provides time to rehydrate patients with intravenous fluids who have been on our liquid diet for 3 to more than 30 days. It places the patient in a less-stressful environment in the immediate preoperative period because the patient and the patient's family and/or friends are not fighting traffic or competing against all the other preoperative patients to get in line for the admission process. Our operating room schedule routinely starts on time and there are fewer medical errors committed because there is more time to check that all routine orders have been completed. If a patient with sleep apnea has forgotten his CPAP machine or needs special medication, there is more time to retrieve such items before the operation has been completed.

Additionally, as mentioned in Chapter 8, it is important to have pre-arranged standards and care plans for bariatric patients that are specialized for the type of operation they receive. Once the volume of bariatric patients is sufficient, it is helpful to have a specialized postoperative area to care for them the first night or two, which is not usually at an intensive care unit (ICU) level but more like a cardiac step-down unit except equipment and care plans are designed for bariatric, rather than cardiac patients. As an example, we try not to operate on patients who are not still ambulatory. We want all patients to ambulate within 24 hours of their procedure. This is not typical of patients who are admitted to most ICUs but important for bariatric patients. The nurses in our step-down unit follow bariatric care plans more routinely than the ICU nurses do because it is a specialized unit. Nurses need to be attuned to the discrimination issues bariatric patients face and to their special hygiene needs (e.g., heavier patients after open procedures often cannot reach their perineal area). Not all nurses enjoy working with bariatric patients. This is a specialty practice like many other patient areas (e.g., neonatal units, cardiac units, the various types of intensive care units) where nurses need to develop a comfort level with the types of patients they will care for so that they do not appear anxious or misinformed. Our patients feel more confident having an operation scheduled in a hospital that has a special care unit devoted to their needs. This enhances our practice and the hospital's reputation.

IMMEDIATE PREOPERATIVE DIETARY CHANGES FOR ALL PATIENTS

In addition to asking most of our diabetic patients to start on a high-protein, low-calorie liquid diet preoperatively for the reasons outlined above, we ask all of our patients to start this diet for at least 3 days preoperatively or for as long as their preoperative instruction period (usually 2–3 months). Diabetic patients and all those with central (android) obesity have enlarged livers from steatosis. An enlarged liver can make it impossible to complete a laparoscopic procedure if the liver is so thick that a space is not available underneath it to visualize the stomach adequately. Because the gut and the liver have all nutrients pass through their domain before being transported to the rest of the body, the liver stores glycogen (like the muscles) that is released immediately once semistarvation is initiated. The gut fat (visceral adipose tissue) in the mesentery and omentum also appears to undergo lipolysis quicker than subcutaneous adipose stores.[19] Glycogen release from the liver will be complete in 3 days of semistarvation but the longer a patient remains on a low-calorie liquid diet, the smaller the liver becomes, especially the left lobe of the liver. We documented this in 1987,[17] and it was more definitively documented in 2002.[19] This regimen decreases intraabdominal fat more than subcutaneous fat for at least the 2 months of use,[19] further increasing operative access to the abdomen and helping to prevent the development of postoperative intraabdominal compartment syndrome with decreased pulmonary function from postoperative edema and traumatic swelling.[20]

Patients that are on this regimen also have a general diuresis and remain relatively underhydrated with lower blood pressures (see Chapter 3 for the physiology of this response). The anesthesia team needs to be aware of this especially if intravenous fluids are not initiated before the patient enters the preoperatively holding area because at least 1 L of normal saline should be infused before induction of anesthesia.

EVALUATION OF GASTROINTESTINAL SYMPTOMS

A careful gastrointestinal history is important in order to assess upper gastrointestinal symptoms. Significant symptoms of gastroesophageal reflux on a patient who has not been previously evaluated is an indication for gastrointestinal evaluation with endoscopy or a barium swallow to determine if a significant hiatal hernia is present and if it is fixed in the mediastinum. It is important to look for any esophageal dysmotility disorders as gastrorestrictive operations may be counterindicated.[21] Occasional cases of Barrett esophagus will be diagnosed. Documentation of the presence of a significant hiatus hernia will allow better planning of the operation. If *Helicobacter pylori* infection is found, it should be treated preoperatively. Although, physicians have worried that bariatric operations that use an excluded section of the gastrointestinal tract to produce malabsorption exclude these areas from further diagnostic exams, few problems occur. Bariatric operations will correct reflux disease in a much higher percentage of morbidly obese patients than will a Nissan fundoplication because acid and bile will no longer be in contact with the esophagus (the acid-producing cells are below the proximal gastric pouch), and as important, the patient will lose weight and decrease intraabdominal pressure, greatly decreasing pressure differences between the intraabdominal and pleural cavities which contribute to the production of reflux in most obese patients.

PSYCHOSOCIAL EVALUATION

Preoperative psychiatric consultation is indicated for patients receiving active psychiatric care, those taking major psychotropic drugs, and those with a history of major mental illness. All patients should be screened by obtaining a psychosocial interview by someone trained to be able to elicit a history of sexual abuse, poor social support, bulimia, or other eating disorders, undiagnosed depression and/or anxiety, and for thought disorders. Standard tests like the Beck Depression Index,[22] the Eating Inventory,[23] the SF-36,[24] or other quality-of-life scales are very useful in documenting the degree of preoperative impairment. A psychologist or psychiatrist (psychotherapist or therapist) should be consulted if problems are identified by these screening tests. These consultants need to independently judge the patient's interest and knowledge of bariatric surgery, and provide opinions regarding the impact of surgery, the impact of the major weight loss caused by the surgery and the constraints on eating behavior on the patient's future mental health. It should not be the therapist's role to approve or disapprove the patient for a bariatric, that is the surgeon's responsibility. The therapist should be helping the surgeon prepare the patient for surgery by identifying what supportive strategies might be helpful.

A supportive home environment is an important prerequisite for surgical success. Therefore, family conflicts which may add to perioperative stress should be addressed before surgery. Starting antidepressants on patients with depression without current treatment or increasing the dose of those inadequately treated deceases the chances of the patients developing severe depression postoperatively when they cannot use overeating or emotional eating to treat themselves, especially if complications develop. It is best to have a licensed psychotherapist who is willing to work with you regularly as part of your multidisciplinary team, both preoperatively and postoperatively.

When a psychiatrist refers a patient and supports the patient in the patient's efforts to have bariatric surgery, we ask them to apply for temporary privileges at our hospital so that they can participate in postoperative care as needed. When patients who are under a psychiatrist's care, are traveling from outside their immediate area to receive surgical therapy to us, we want them evaluated preoperatively by our team's psychotherapist just like one would have a patient with brittle diabetes evaluated by your team's endocrinologist. Your psychotherapist, who helps you when postoperative problems develop, needs the opportunity to interview and examine the patient preoperatively before the operative stress and possible complications develop, have the opportunity to get old records and discuss the patient's treatments with the long-term psychotherapist, and decide if additional preoperative interventions are necessary or desirable to better prepare the patient for the procedure. This information needs to be communicated to you and the risks discussed before you agree to proceed with operating on such a patient.

SUPPORT GROUPS

We also have our psychologist direct our perioperative support groups. All of our patients are encouraged to attend these support groups both preoperatively and postoperatively which are conducted weekly at several different scheduled times. In these sessions, postoperative patients discuss how they perceived the operative experience and how they are adjusting to the postoperative dietary and behavioral changes we suggest are necessary for success (i.e., smaller portion sizes, increased time spent chewing of food, slower intake of food, elimination of high fat and concentrated sweets, etc.). The group members discuss whether our preoperative teaching is accurate and helpful, their feelings throughout the process, the reactions of their family and friends and a great deal more. Not all patients are candidates to participate in group and the psychologist screens all patients as part of their evaluation. Patients must be respectful of group rules (only one person talks at a time, no one is allowed to dominate conversation, confidentiality of all statements in group must be respected, and the group leader's role respected) and have adequate social skills to participate.

Preoperative patients often learn more from group discussions than they do from the other teaching we provide because it comes from the people who have "walked the walk" already, so they are more willing to listen to them. Often similar types of patients pair up as "buddies," helping and supporting each other through surgery. This is especially important if the patient has limited social support or has friends or family members who are resisting their attempts to proceed with surgery. We find that the number of sessions a patient attends correlates with the percentage of excess weight they lose postoperatively, with the patients who attend the most groups losing the highest percentage of excess weight. This is somewhat expected, however, because the patients who are attending group are usually the most motivated, have good social skills, and are taking the time and energy to really try to change their behavior.

When a new bariatric practice is started, the volume of patients, especially the volume of patients who have had surgery, may not be enough to sustain one or more weekly group therapy sessions. Ideally, a group session should have 4 or more patients, but not more than 12, so that all members have a chance to talk and interact with each other. When this is not possible, another approach is to have monthly support meetings run by the surgeon and other members of the multidisciplinary team (dietician, exercise specialist, nurse, psychotherapist) and invite not only your own patients but everyone in the area who has had bariatric surgery. Many patients of other surgeons from other areas are still very willing to help morbidly obese people decide whether a surgical treatment is right for them. Advertisements in the papers are usually enough incentive to gather a group.

Groups that meet monthly or less often may not provide enough support for preoperative patients who are trying to make a decision whether or not to have surgery in a timely fashion. We have had some preoperative patients, especially men, attend more than 50 group meetings before deciding that surgery is appropriate. They had to meet enough successful people and make sure all the people they were interacting with who were like them successfully lost weight after surgery. This monthly approach to group meetings, however, can provide support for many postoperative patients who will need to make incremental behavioral changes for at least the next year to be maximally successful and do not feel comfortable intermittently attending weekly group sessions where they can feel like an outsider.

A new bariatric surgeon who is developing a practice can also help some patients obtain the support they need from other weight-loss support groups such as Weight Watchers or TOPS. Bariatric surgery practices and patients have also developed chat rooms on the internet and web sites that share information, although, as with any unregulated site, not all the information provided on these sites is factually correct. A list of these sites now includes:

www.spotlighthealth.com/morbid_obesity/mo/mo.htm
www.endosec.com/pated/edtgs22.htm

www.mynewtritionist.com
www.007secrets@egroups.com
www.dietwatch.com
www.vitalady.com
www.obesityhelp.com
www.yahoogroups.com/community/OSSG
www.duodenalswitch.com
www.beyondchange-obesity.com
www.office@obesity-online.com
www.obesity-online.com

These sites constantly evolve and search engines will undoubtedly include additional ones if one periodically searches the Internet for this type of activity.

Nonprofit organizations, such as the Shape Up America! Foundation, the American Diabetes Association, the American Dietetic Association, the American Obesity Association, and major companies involved in selling bariatric products, such as Ethicon EndoSurgery, a division of the Johnson & Johnson Company, and Inamed Corporation, have web sites that are designed to help people lose weight or find resources to help them lose weight.

DIETARY INTERVENTION

Every preoperative patient should be interviewed and helped preoperatively and postoperative by a dietician who is a member of the bariatric surgeon's multidisciplinary team. A surgeon can ask to use a hospital's dietician for the patients using a given hospital, but each dietician who participates in such an endeavor needs to know how the surgeon plans to use diets both preoperatively and postoperatively. A dietician needs to take a food history, finding out food preferences, who prepares the patient's meals, and who purchases food, and how many meals are consumed at home versus at restaurants and fast food outlets. Does the patient feel they overeat regularly (a big meal eater), eat the wrong foods (a "sweets" eater or one who has fat cravings), or do they graze all day or night, eating small to large amounts of certain foods? How many empty calories are consumed as sugared beverages or nonnutritional foods per day? The dietician has to determine whether the patient understands the food pyramid, how to count calories consumed, grams of protein consumed, how to read food labels in stores, and how to measure portion sizes. The dietician will need to teach these skills to patients who do not know these skills and/or to family members or friends who will help the patients.

Either the dietician or the psychosocial interviewer needs to determine how the patient uses food. Is the patient an emotional eater and what emotions lead to food consumption? Depression, anger, boredom, loneliness, confusion? What else triggers eating other than hunger and emotions? How often does the patient overeat and to what level of discomfort? Does this cause guilt? Does the patient purge, binge, and how often or how long ago in the past? Does the patient secretly eat (usually at night), hide or horde food, especially nonnutritional food such as candy? The answers to these questions will help the dietician and psychotherapist develop a care plan for this patient and help the patient create a list of habits that need to be changed to enhance successful postoperative weight loss.

Most practices prepare very specific food lists that patient's progress through each week and teach patients how to count grams of protein consumed per day to help them in the postoperative period. The dietician needs to interview most patients on each postoperative visit to help then relearn how to eat and reinforce their good habits while discouraging their bad habits.

EXERCISE EVALUATION AND INTERVENTIONS

Each patient should also be seen by an exercise specialist. Most morbidly obese people have to work hard just to walk and perform activities of daily living. The average normal weight individual could not tolerate completing his or her average daily activities if required to wear a hundred-pound backpack everywhere. Morbidly obese patients, who are still active, usually have good cardiopulmonary function. We evaluate everyone by asking them to try to walk a mile, or as close to it as they can, on a heavy duty, industrial treadmill that can work at very slow speeds on a level track. It is extremely rare for anyone who can walk a mile to have a postoperative complication that is not technically related. People who cannot walk at least a quarter mile need to either lose weight preoperatively or to begin an exercise program to prepare them for the additional perioperative stress that their cardiopulmonary system will experience. As mentioned, pulmonary reserve is already compromised in most morbidly obese patients. Patients who cannot walk a tenth of a mile have problems breathing after postoperative swelling occurs. The cardiovascular system will still need to be functional with the heart working at a rate 10 to 25% above resting without the development of atrial fibrillation or other problems. Exercise programs can improve cardiopulmonary status to levels which allow these patients to function even if a complication occurs such as a small pulmonary embolus or sepsis which will further stress these systems.

Additionally, patients need to use pedometers to know how active they are. Most morbidly obese patients take fewer than 2000 steps a day. We encourage patients to increase activity to 10,000 steps a day. This level of activity usually requires a walking program or extra activities. Walking, pool aerobics, or low-impact activities such as biking are preferred activities in a population that usually has osteoarthritis or increased joint stresses. Periodically retesting patients on the treadmill where they can see improvement in the distance they can walk, or how fast they can walk a distance, encourages additional activities.

A patient's sense of improvement in their physical condition can be supported by body composition measurements. Determining their total fat mass and muscle mass initially and then every few months postoperatively allows each patient to see his or her fat mass decrease. More importantly, it allows the physician to make sure the patient does not lose muscle mass while losing weight and allows the physician and the patient to evaluate whether his or her physical activity program is successfully improving his or her muscle mass.

CONCLUSIONS

Not all surgeons will be comfortable accommodating their practices to the special needs of bariatric patients. It must be remembered that this is behavior-modification surgery in a group of patients who often have several associated serious comorbid medical problems that contribute to higher rates of morbidity and mortality than most other patients, except for the geriatric population, on whom general surgeons perform electric operations. It is very hard to provide the level of perioperative support a bariatric patient needs if you and your staff are not treating at least five patients per month. A surgeon has to perform at least 25 or more bariatric procedures a year to make it feasible for the associated hospital to have the special equipment and care plans in place to treat these patients. At rates lower than these, you are not improving protocols with practice but relearning the special needs of the obese with each patient. You will also not have the volume of patients necessary to recruit consultants to work with you to help these challenging patients. Most consultants will initially be afraid of morbidly obese patients.

Once your practice is adjusted to helping bariatric patients, you will see that the revenue generated from these elective surgical patients helps you and your consultants develop more economic stability. Although the multidisciplinary team approach used for the bariatric surgical patient most resembles the organ transplant team approach, with bariatric patients you do not have to wait for an organ to become available. Those of us who have chosen to dedicate our practice to bariatrics like the challenges these patients present and enjoy watching people receive immense benefits from their surgical procedures. We also enjoy the long-term relationships we develop with these patients. We are rewarded by the major reversals that occur in their disease burden and the improvement that occurs in their quality of life. It is a difficult type of practice to establish because it contains many parts. If you decide that this type of practice might be of interest to you, we would encourage you to visit an established bariatric surgeon's practice. The American Society for Bariatric Surgery (www.asbs.org) has a list of members and their practice locations, as well as a list of surgeons who are willing to serve as preceptors for surgeons interested in starting such a practice. The American Society for Bariatric Surgery also has biyearly courses to help surgeons learn more about this field. You will find that most bariatric surgeons are willing to help other surgeons initiate such a practice if they ask for help because the reputation of all of us who perform these types of procedures depends on each having the best possible results.

REFERENCES

1. Consensus Development Conference Panel. Gastrointestinal surgery for severe obesity. *Ann Intern Med.* 1991;115: 956–960.

2. Pi-Sunyer FX. Medical hazards of obesity. *Ann Intern Med.* 1993;119:655–660.

3. Deitel M, Camilleri A. Overlooked problems in morbidly obese patients [abstract 4]. *Obes Surg.* 2000;10:125.

4. Mason E, Amaral J, Cowan G, et al. Surgery for severe obesity: information for patients. *Obes Surg.* 1994;4:66–72.

5. Mason E, Hesson W. Informed consent for obesity surgery. *Obes Surg.* 1998;8:419–428.

6. Livingston EH, Huerta S, Arthur D, et al. Male gender as a predictor of morbidity and age as a predictor of mortality for patients undergoing gastric bypass surgery. *Ann Surg.* 2002;236:576–579.

7. Oliak D, Ballantyne G, Davies RJ, et al. Short-term results of laparoscopic gastric bypass in patients with BMI ≥60. *Obes Surg.* 2002;12:643–647.

8. Smetana GW. Preoperative pulmonary evaluation. *N Engl J Med.* 1999; 340: 937–944.

9. Koenig SM. Pulmonary complications of obesity. *Am J Med Sci.* 2001;321:249–279.

10. Benumof JL. Obstructive sleep apnea in the adult obese patient: implication for airway management. *J Clin Anesth.* 2001;13:144–156.

11. Vgontzas AN, Tan TL, Bixler EO, Martin LF, Shubert D, Kales A. Sleep apnea and sleep disruption in obese patients. *Arch Intern Med.* 1994;154:1705–1711.

12. Thakur V, Richards R, Reisin E. Obesity, hypertension, and the heart. *Am J Med Sci.* 2001;321:242–248.

13. Alpert MA. Management of obesity cardiomyopathy. *Am J Med Sci.* 2001;321:237–241.

14. Clagett G, Anderson F, Geerts W, et al. Prevention of venous thromboembolism. *Chest.* 1998; 114:531s–560s.

15. Batist G, Bothe A, Bern M, et al. Low antithrombin III in morbid obesity: return to normal with weight reduction. *JPEN J Parent Enteral Nutr.* 1983;7:447–449.

16. Van Den Berghe G. Woutern P, Weekers F, et al. Intensive insulin therapy in critically ill patients. *N Engl J Med.* 2001;345:1359–1367.

17. Martin LF, Tan TL, Holmes PA, Becker D, Horn JR, Bixler EO. Can morbidly obese patients safely lose weight preoperatively? *Am J Surg.* 1995;169:245–253.

18. Choban PS, Heckler R, Burge J, Flancbaum L. Increased incidence of nosocomial infections in obese surgical patients. *Am Surg.* 1995;11:1001–1005.

19. Busetto L, Tregnaghi A, DeMarchi F, et al. Liver volume and visceral obesity in women with hepatic steatosis undergoing gastric banding. *Obes Surg.* 2002;10:408–411.

20. Sugerman HJ, Windsor ACJ, Bessos MK, et al. Abdominal pressure, sagittal abdominal diameter and obesity co-morbidity. *J Intern Med.* 1997;241:71–79.

21. Greenstein RJ, Nissan A, Jaffin BW. Esophageal anatomy and finction in laparoscopic gastric restrictive bariatric surgery: implications for patient selection. *Obes Surg.* 1998;8:199–206.

22. Beck AT, Steer RT. *Manual for the Beck Depression Inventory (MBDI).* San Antonio, TX: Psychological Corporation, 1993.

23. Gardner DM. *Eating Disorders 2.* Odessa, FL: Psychological Assessment Resources, 1991.

24. Ware JE Jr, Sherbourne CD. The MOS 36-item short-form health survey (SF-36). I. Conceptual framework and item selection. *Med Care.* 1992;30:473–483.

SPECIAL NEEDS OF THE BARIATRIC SURGICAL OFFICE

TRACY MARTINEZ OWENS / WALTER LINDSTROM

UNDERSTANDING THE PATIENT

Obesity is a disease largely caused by a person's genetic makeup. Twin studies show that two-thirds of the variation in body weight can be attributed to genetic factors.[1] Morbid obesity is a multifactorial process characterized by an impaired satiety mechanism and a dysfunctional basal metabolic rate. Morbid obesity is manifested by an abnormal conversion of ingested calories to fat rather than their dissipation by body fat.

Those choosing to work in the field of bariatrics must be aware and sensitive to obese patients' strife with obesity, and the difficulty living in a cruel and ignorant society when dealing with morbid obesity is only the beginning. Patients often enter the bariatric practice with an enormous amount of hurt, which is sometimes displayed with behaviors such as anger, fear, anxiety, and depression. Patients' self-esteem and confidence have been compromised as a consequence of the discrimination they have experienced. An individual who has been overweight since childhood has most likely endured years of humiliation and a sense of failure, not realizing that it is not their fault. On the contrary, they have often been told that they have a lack of willpower.

As health care professionals working with this population, we must convey our understanding of the disease process to our patients, as well as the discrimination they most likely have experienced.

Many people describe the morbidly obese as lazy, less intelligent, and lacking willpower. In a study conducted on children's attitudes toward obesity in psychological aspects of human obesity, Stunkard and Waddin write, "Children no more than six years of age describe silhouettes of an obese child as 'lazy, dirty, stupid, ugly, cheats, and liars.'"[2] Black-and-white line drawings of a normal-weight child, an obese child, and children with various handicaps, including missing hands and facial disfigurements, were also shown to a variety of audiences. Both children and adults rated the obese child as less likable. This prejudice extended across races, across rural and urban dwellers, and, saddest of all, even to the obese persons themselves.[2]

Other documented psychosocial effects include impaired childhood body image, reduced acceptance to major colleges, employment discrimination, and disrespectful treatment by the medical profession. The psychological aspects of this disease are as important as more publicized major medical comorbid conditions when one considers the quality of life of the morbidly obese.[2-7]

Studies of severely overweight persons conducted before undergoing antiobesity surgery show that there is no single personality type that characterizes the severely obese. This population does not report greater levels of psychopathology than do average-weight controls.[3]

Studies conducted after surgical treatment and weight loss show that self-esteem and positive emotions increase and body image disparagement decreases. Marital satisfaction increases, but only if a measure of satisfaction existed before surgery. Eating behavior is improved dramatically. The results of surgical treatment are superior to those of dietary treatment alone. Practitioners should be aware that severely obese persons are subjected to prejudice and discrimination, and should be treated with an extreme measure of compassion and concern to help alleviate their feelings of rejection and shame.[8]

Needless to say, morbid obesity is an enormous burden. Individuals have endured unspeakable discrimination. To laugh at the obese is one of the last generally permitted prejudices of our society.[9]

Creating a practice that provides a safe and empathetic environment to help patients maximize their pre- and postoperative success potential is the obligation of the surgeon and the surgeon's staff. Life after bariatric surgery has commonalities, as well as unique experiences, for each patient. The bottom line is life will not be the same. To help prevent unnecessary stress and to maximize the individual's success potential, a dynamic, supportive, educated, and dedicated office staff is invaluable.

EDUCATION

Educating the bariatric surgical patient is the obligation of the multidisciplinary staff. The purpose of education is to maximize the patient's success potential while decreasing stress from lack of knowledge. Patient education should be a mandatory component of all bariatric programs. Many practitioners in the field describe bariatric surgery as a "tool." Teaching the patient to use his or her "tool" adequately and to his or her best advantage is the professional obligation of the multidisciplinary team. Education is a team effort. Each member of the team should be dedicated to convey his or her expertise to the bariatric patient. Each patient needs to understand that morbid obesity is a chronic disease, one for which we have no cure. Understanding that lifelong treatment and lifelong followup is required. A patient's success or failure depends on his or her acceptance of surgery as a tool, and using the tool appropriately can help them change their relationship with food, as well as with life.

Education begins with the first interaction with the prospective patient. This may occur with an inquiry telephone call. The receptionist should possess enough basic knowledge about the process a patient follows to enter into the practice.

CONSULTATION

Often this first interaction is at a consultation. This may be done one-on-one by the surgeon or in a group setting at an information lecture. Regardless of style, the informational gathering consultation should be conducted in an appropriate setting for morbidly obese individuals. A comprehensive overview of the surgical procedure performed, alternatives, lifestyle changes needed for compliance and success, risks, expected benefits, patients' responsibility, long-term consequences, and lifelong followup should be explained. Adequate time for questions should be accommodated. This is an appropriate time to introduce your staff to prospective patients.

As stated in the American Society for Bariatric Surgery (ASBS) and Society of American Gastrointestinal Endoscopic Surgeons (SAGES) *Guidelines: For Surgical Treatment—Bariatric Surgery*, published in 2000, "The multidisciplinary approach includes medical management of a comorbidities, dietary instruction, exercise training, specialized nursing care and psychological assistance as needed. Having a multidisciplinary team who can address these necessary components of bariatric patients' needs are imperative."

Education is an essential component to a comprehensive bariatric program. Often the sharing of knowledge between staff, surgeons, and patients provides a shared responsibility, a sense of teamwork, and builds a foundation that supports patients throughout their pre- and postoperative journey.

PREOPERATIVE EDUCATION

Preoperative education is extremely valuable. All the routine risks and outcomes of any abdominal surgery—risks such as infection, hemorrhage, or damage to adjacent organs and outcomes such as muscle pains, inability to continue with a routine diet due to nausea, diarrhea, or constipation—must be explained in preoperative teaching. But more importantly, educating the patient on specific aspects unique to bariatric surgery is essential. Preoperative education is the key to enabling the patient to understand what their responsibilities are to be an active participant in their operation.

Educating the patient one-on-one or in a group setting can be equally effective. Group dynamics often stimulate open conversations, questions, or patient concerns.

To insure thoroughness, consistency, and accuracy, an agreed outline and format are helpful. This outline should include all the components needed to be covered in preoperative education. Preoperative education should cover the following:

- Preadmission orders including any bowel preparation, meal restrictions; nothing by mouth (NPO) instructions
- When to arrive at the hospital and what to bring—for example, secure walking shoes that are easy to put on
- What will take place prior to surgery, that is, vital signs, consent, intravenous access, premedication
- Waking up in the postanesthesia care unit after the operation, and the importance of early ambulation to decrease risk of pulmonary embolism
- How to use the spirometer including a demonstration
- Pain management
- Introduction of fluids and diet progression
- Grocery lists for home
- Activity at home, that is, the importance of continued ambulation, fluid intake
- Followup in office

All information should be clear and in writing to reinforce instruction provided. Examples of high-quality protein foods, examples of soft foods, and advancing guidelines (a schedule of how to advance the diet from liquids to the first category of soft foods and then onto a more regular schedule of vegetables, seafood, and other solid protein sources) are helpful.

Postoperative education is an ongoing process and is provided in many forms. Postoperative education begins at discharge and continues thereafter. Postoperative instructions and education given prior to surgery may be ineffective. Often patients are so focused on the surgical experience itself that they cannot look beyond surgery. Overloading the patient with too much information preoperatively may limit, and therefore interfere with, comprehension. Pre- and postoperative education is uniquely different with separate focuses.

Postoperative education focuses on early postoperative recovery, lifestyle changes, and patient obligations for compliance and wellness, both physically and emotionally. The bariatric surgical patient needs to be educated about the following:

- Pouch size, dumping syndrome, or restrictions, depending on surgical procedure performed
- Food advancement, emphasizing protein; examples of high-protein foods and examples of advancing from fluids to soft to regular foods are helpful
- Importance of hydration
- Need for frequent ambulation to help prevent pulmonary embolism and to rebuild stamina
- Wound care—distinguishing between normal and abnormal, and instructing patient to call if any abdominal drainage, foul odor, or increased tenderness occurs
- Necessity of vitamin replacement for specific bariatric procedure
- Need to call the office. Reasons may include: increased temperature, prolonged vomiting, shortness of breath, increased pain, change in wound or drainage, diarrhea, difficulty swallowing, leg pain or

swelling, unable to pass gas, or for any other concerns. Make it clear that you are available at all times.

- Specific things to avoid such as alcohol intake, antiinflammatory medications, pregnancy in the first postoperation year
- Follow-up expectations, reinforcing that, ultimately, followup is the patient's responsibility.
- Exercise is a mandatory component for success
- Importance of followup and support group attendance.

All education should be reinforced orally by the staff, as well as in written form for reference and clarification. Always explain why the patient needs to do something. This helps to reinforce and enhance compliance.

A structured class with a systematic presentation outline helps to ensure thoroughness by the presenter. Offering postoperation discharge teaching in the same office setting and at times when both pre- and postoperative patients are seen by the staff decreases the potential for confusion and the possibility of patients missing this valuable opportunity. You might consider having patients sign a registration form to validate attendance. Commonly, when patients are well educated, anxiety is decreased, compliance is improved, and patients call the office less often with repetitive questions.

OFFICE FOLLOWUP

Office visits can be an excellent opportunity to continue to educate and reinforce important information to help success and to clarify misunderstanding.

Preprinted follow-up forms used in the office can help ensure completeness of various aspects you wish to cover with your patient. These forms can cover such things as vitamin supplementation, nutrition intake by asking your patient to do a 24-hour meal recall. This recall can evaluate patient's protein intake, including healthy or unhealthy habits such as snacking. Inquiring about exercise, including type and frequency, can be helpful and motivating. Special emphasis on specific needs identified in a comprehensive follow-up visit can address all aspects of a successful postoperative experience. Identifying special needs, offering education or reinforcement, as well as establishing agreed-upon goals, can facilitate achieving and maintaining a healthy weight.

The office must be equipped for the morbidly obese individual. Adequate waiting room seating that is armless or has extra width and is appropriately weight bearing is essential. Scales that can accommodate the largest patient are mandatory. Another necessity is to stock blood pressure cuffs that are varied in size so accuracy is ensured, as well as to avoid embarrassment if the cuff is too small. Patient gowns that are large and roomy for patients to change into for their history and physical are important. Wide doorways are important to have in the office. It is not uncommon to have patients who are wheelchair dependent as a consequence of their arthralgia in weight-bearing joints. Toilets that are affixed to the floor instead of the wall can prevent a potentially dangerous situation if the added weight stresses the wall fixture. Wall handrails can help a patient on and off the toilet. A rule of thumb is to walk around your office as if you are 45.4 kg (100 lb) heavier. How does your office measure up? Providing a compassionate and accepting environment puts the patient at ease, something that is not often possible in our society for a morbidly obese individual.

ONGOING EDUCATION

The bariatric surgical patient must understand that morbid obesity is a chronic disease that surgery does not cure. The patient must accept the fact that achieving and maintaining weight loss is an ongoing, lifetime effort.

Newsletters can be an effective way to offer ongoing education. Varied contributors can write articles that are specific to the bariatric patient. These articles can be creative yet informative. It is also a great way to incorporate other physicians into the program. A gynecologist can write about women's health issues or the role of calcium supplementation. The program psychologist can highlight topics such as self-esteem, body image, or even successful hints while job interviewing. The exercise coordinator can share some guidance on a certain type of exercise and fitness equipment. Program support group meetings can also be listed.

All the while your newsletter has become an extension of your educational efforts. The newsletter can reinforce the importance of a "team" approach and the need for ongoing education.

The World Wide Web has opened up an unlimited opportunity to gain information with little effort, time, and expense. Although the Internet can be detrimental when medical advice or other information given through chat rooms is inaccurate, it can also be a powerful mechanism to your patient.

Your Web site has unlimited possibilities from an educational standpoint. They range from listing frequently asked questions, postoperative instructions, copies of newsletters, current media coverage on bariatric surgery, and summaries of support group meetings, to active video teleconferencing of support group meetings.

SUPPORT GROUPS

Patients must assume responsibility for their progress postoperatively. Informing the patient of this obligation preoperatively is imperative. The patient needs to understand that obesity surgery does not cure obesity. Like any chronic disease, lifelong effort and attention is necessary for long-term weight loss maintenance. It is the multidisciplinary team's responsibility to provide ongoing education in a supportive environment. Support groups offer the education to use their tool (surgery) and to maximize success while decreasing fear and anxiety in a compassionate environment. The education offered in a support group empowers the individual to take ownership of their new lifestyle and master it. The peer support enhances an environment that facilitates success.

Preoperative patients often attend a support group because their surgeon suggested it. Often, these patients get a sense of not being alone for the first time in their lives. The sense of shame and failure is lightened. It is also a valuable way to gain knowledge about the surgical experience through other postoperative patients sharing their experience at various stages. This, in turn, helps to reduce anxiety and to establish realistic expectations. Often, physicians make preoperative attendance mandatory in order to achieve additional informed consent. Although the patient will tell you that weight loss is their lifelong dream and that obesity has caused hurt and shame and hardened them for years, weight loss itself can cause anxiety, fear, and an array of unpredictable feelings. Friendships, job responsibilities, family dynamics, spousal relationships, and coworker relations are all subject to change, as is society's response to a morbidly obese person who becomes "average" or "normal" in size.

After becoming more normal weighted, patients encounter many new experiences that evoke responses. Patients can find camaraderie, understanding, and absence of judgment, often for the first time in their lives, in a support group.

Individuals who had damaged self-esteem and limited friends often overcompensate by doing for others while negating their own needs. As self-worth increases, as is commonly seen postoperatively, patients may choose not to be the people pleaser at their own expense. When they say, "No, I can't" or "I don't want to do this or that," often for the first time in their life, relationships are changed—sometimes forever, sometimes and often for the best. Giving a safe and supportive environment to share these experiences is invaluable.

Numerous and wide-ranging topics of discussion and concern arise at support group meetings. Many times questions about diabetes, hypertension, and the need for continuous positive airway pressure (CPAP) are resolved. "Fitting in" to society is experienced when patients share the experience of no longer needing a seatbelt extension on an airplane; of fitting into a theater seat, restaurant booth, or ride at an amusement park; or of getting promoted, getting a raise, or quitting a job one despised. Social opportunities arise. Dating for the first time in one's life is often experienced—with both excitement and fear. Abusive friendships or abusive intimate relationships are no longer tolerated as patients' self-esteem increase and patients gain enough self-confidence that being the victim is no longer acceptable.

The fear of failure or weight gain is normal. A support group can facilitate and reinforce the active role the patient must take to be successful in optimizing weight loss and resolving comorbidities.

Support group meetings should provide opportunities for the pre- and postoperative patient to learn new ways of relating to issues, rather than turning to food; to deal with body-image changes and relationship dynamics; to share successes; to reinforce nutritional and program guidelines; and to learn about self-care and nurturing. Participants share their feelings in order to get feedback and wisdom from others.

SETTING UP YOUR SUPPORT GROUP

Organizing a support group within a bariatric program requires several important factors. One of the most productive steps in the process of establishing a new support group occurs well before the group begins. There should be a support group meeting for the first patient who enters your program. One of the first things to consider when setting up your support group meeting is who will facilitate.

The unique and important role of the professional facilitator is a critical factor that sets the tone of the meetings. Facilitators should be trained to help the group establish the framework of the meeting and provide a safe, compassionate environment of people to connect to one another in productive and meaningful ways. The facilitator will share in the discussions as appropriate and share some of his or her views, feelings, and expertise. The group facilitator must be experienced at understanding how groups work effectively, as well as be knowledgeable about the aims and goals of the bariatric practice. Group facilitators should not be patients. Patients need their own recovery opportunity. Sometimes in remote areas the support group's patients facilitate the group. This is not ideal. A well-trained professional facilitator represents your practice the best by having in-depth knowledge of the procedure performed, possible complications, and common psychological issues, and is knowledgeable about group dynamics and facilitation. The facilitator must know his or her limitations and be knowledgeable enough to defer questions, to request immediate medical intervention, and to call upon an expert more qualified. The facilitator should seek to facilitate matters in five basic areas:

1. Feelings—empathy, understanding, acceptance, and self-worth
2. Communication—good listening skills, emotionally supportive discussions, and open and honest communication
3. Information—medical and health knowledge, program guidelines, successful coping strategies, options and alternatives, and the like
4. Connection—a sense of community, bonding, belonging, fellowship, "you're not alone"
5. Opportunities—personal growth (coping, adjusting, overcoming), helping others in the group, and mutual exchanges

Ideally, the support group facilitator is part of the program's multidisciplinary team.

The support group facilitators should be:

- Knowledgeable about group behaviors and leadership
- Possess a basic commitment to the self-help process
- Capable of distinguishing and controlling personal views
- Willing to work toward the group's goals
- Able to initiate activity and discussion
- Comfortable with the expression of emotion, tension, and conflict
- Committed to the welfare of the group and all its members
- Respectful of and value each member as a unique individual
- Understand that they are a representative of the surgeon and the surgeon's bariatric program

Facilitators can be registered nurses, psychologists, registered dietitians, or even the surgeon.

PLANNING THE MEETING

One thing to consider when planning your support group meetings is making concrete arrangements for a regular time and place to hold the meetings. Scheduling the meetings for the same place and time helps to build a successful group and eliminates confusion. Many hospital conference rooms, medical center education rooms, physician office buildings, churches, libraries, and community centers provide adequate space at little or no charge.

Armless and appropriate weight-bearing chairs, adequate and convenient parking, reasonable walking distance, wheelchair- and handicap-friendly restrooms are a few things to consider when selecting a location for the meeting. Decide on the frequency and time the group will meet; for example, every third Wednesday of the month from 7:00 to 9:00 P.M. This will help you to secure a meeting place. Publishing a calendar will ensure attendance by patients. Meetings should respect the multidisciplinary approach to bariatric surgery. Planning specific topics and guest speakers in advance is an important step in assuring the success of your group. Lining up guest speakers may sound like a daunting task, but it can be as easy as a phone call. Most speakers welcome the opportunity to introduce their services to a large number of possible clients. Meetings should be unbiased educational forums, not sales pitches for products or product endorsements. Remember to keep the focus of your group on proven information, support education, and wellness. This ongoing education is valuable in helping the patient achieve and maintain success. Support group meetings are an excellent opportunity for various experts in the field to share their knowledge.

Experts to include in the meetings could include dietitians, nutritionists, fashion consultants, gynecologists, plastic surgeons, massage therapists, psychologists, exercise specialists, travel consultants, yoga instructors, and make-up artists to name a few.

Support group meetings are most successful when a time structure is followed. It is important that the facilitator start and close the meeting on time, allowing time for introductions, guest speaker presentation, questions and answers, and socialization among patients.

It is helpful to record patients who sign in, date, and topic, along with the guest speaker and any handouts distributed. These records can be helpful as a resource for planning other meetings and patients' attendance.

It is important to establish ground rules for your support group meetings. These ground rules should address privacy and confidentiality. One ground rule to be addressed is whether children should be allowed. Often topics that stimulate emotional expressions, discussions of sexuality, and vulnerability are inappropriate for children. The meetings should not have to be edited for children. Toddlers and babies are often disruptive, and their attendance at support group meetings is inappropriate. Another ground rule to decide is whether your program will allow patients of other surgeons to attend. Different or conflicting postoperative instructions can be confusing to the group. Regardless of what you decide, ground rules should be printed on your support group schedule so that patients know them in advance. Confidentiality must be stated and reinforced at the beginning of each meeting.

Changes in body image, family and friend dynamics, work environment, social encounters, and food relationships will occur. The surgeon has an obligation to his or her patients to create a place where the patients can go, be understood, and not be judged.

INFORMED CONSENT

Consent is a prerequisite to medical treatment. Informed consent is a consent given by a patient only after having received detailed information regarding the proposed medical treatment. The purpose of informed consent is to:

- Maintain trust between the medical practitioner and the patient
- Enable the patient to participate in the decision-making process
- Minimize doubt and stress by maximizing information

Specialized Informed Consent

All patients undergoing any invasive procedure are required to sign an informed consent form. Because bariatric surgery is so life-changing and a change in necessary lifestyle behaviors is important for success, many practitioners require a specialized bariatric surgical consent in addition to the conventional informed consent. This "specialized consent" consists of indications for surgery, alternatives, mortality risk, results, patient obligations, and short- and long-term complications. A summation that documents understanding by signature is important. Much of this information is first provided in the consultation. Record keeping of those who attended an informational seminar can document what information a patient was provided. If the informational seminar is a PowerPoint presentation, archiving each presentation as it changes with the dates it was provided may be helpful from a legal aspect to demonstrate informed consent. Documentation of support group attendance can also demonstrate an aspect of informed consent.

True/False Exam

A true/false exam given to patients preoperatively gives the surgeon and team an opportunity to validate the patients' clear understanding of the surgical procedure to be performed, the necessary lifestyle changes, and the risks and benefits, as well as the importance of lifelong followup. This exam should be developed and customized based on the procedure performed. The following are examples of statements that might appear on a preoperation true/false exam:

You will be able to eat as much as you wish after surgery.

Reoperation is sometimes necessary for hernias, bleeding, bowel obstruction, or leakage.

Staple or suture lines never leak and never result in infection, reoperation, or death.

Lifelong followup is recommended following bariatric surgery.

I have been informed that support group attendance is recommended after surgery.

Vitamin supplementation is required after gastric bypass surgery, and if not taken, may result in deficiency and permanent nerve damage.

If a preoperative patient chooses a few incorrect answers, either the surgeon or registered nurse should explain why his or her answers are incorrect. The patient should then circle the correct answers and initial them to demonstrate understanding and clarification. If a preoperative patient misses many questions, the surgeon and the surgeon's team need to reevaluate and decide on the patient's readiness for surgery. It may be appropriate to request the patient to reread program materials or attend another informational seminar and/or support group meeting. There is nothing wrong with delaying surgery until the team thinks the patient is better educated and prepared. Retesting the patient to ensure readiness and appropriate knowledge is good practice.

EXERCISE

The importance of exercise for the long-term success of bariatric patients cannot be overemphasized. Exercise may be something very foreign and intimidating to a morbidly obese individual. Arthralgia in weight-bearing joints, as well as respiratory difficulty with any exertion, may limit a patient's ability to walk, let alone exercise. However, it is an important component in the postoperative phase of bariatric surgery. Patients early on lose a significant amount of weight. It is not uncommon for a superobese individual to lose a pound per day for several months. To help prevent muscle mass loss and to build lean muscle mass, weight-bearing exercise is important, especially during the first postoperative year. Long-term weight management is dependent on decreased or controlled caloric intake and expenditure. In other words, exercise is necessary for ideal weight loss (fat tissue loss) and weight management.

Identifying an exercise coordinator for your program is essential. This individual may be an exercise physiologist, physical therapist, or certified personal trainer. Whomever you choose, it is extremely important that the exercise coordinator have an in-depth understanding of the disease of morbid obesity and of postoperative recovery, and have empathy and understanding for the morbidly obese. The coordinator must possess the ability to teach individuals based on knowledge about exercise and to respond to individual needs and expectations, as well as to a patient's physical limitations. Motivational skills are also extremely important. The benefits of exercise must be repeatedly communicated to the patient. Educating bariatric patients preoperatively, upon discharge, and throughout followup about the benefits of exercise is valuable toward achieving short- and long-term success. Integrating your exercise coordinator into the discharge education process, as well as a frequent guest speaker, adds value to your program and enhances your patients' likely success.

During rapid weight loss, resistance training can help to minimize muscle mass loss, which may be a contributor to a lower metabolic rate, thereby making weight management more difficult. Educating patients about the benefits of resistance training, and demonstrating and mentoring them on resistance training, are important contributions to patients' recovery and long-term health.

Patients have an investment in their bariatric surgery. Exercise is an added deposit into that investment and the dividends are endlessly rewarding. Express to the patients the benefits of exercise such as increased muscle mass, which increases metabolic rate; lowers blood pressure; helps to control cholesterol; enhances self-esteem and self-concept; and reduces stress, anxiety, and maybe even depression.

Keeping an exercise journal might be something that the exercise coordinator should recommend. This can be a motivating tool, as well as an educating tool, to share with the coordinator for further instruction and feedback.

An exercise manual that explains the benefits of exercise, and that illustrates both aerobic and anaerobic exercises, will be helpful for your patients. Setting an exercise plan without guidance can be an overwhelming task that can contribute to failure. Helping patients pick an activity, guiding them through exercise equipment, and assisting them to plan a schedule are helpful activities. Encourage patients to set goals, such as, "by 1 month, I will walk 2 miles 2 days per week and weight train 2 days per week." This can help measure success and progress. Encouraging patients to reward themselves for reaching a goal helps to continue the momentum and gives them a sense of success, instead of the failure they have often experienced.

Exercise is an essential component of a comprehensive bariatric program. Exercise is mandatory to maximize postoperative success. An exercise coordinator is crucial in implementing and maintaining this important component. Ongoing education, as well as hands-on mentoring, maximizes patients' health and weight loss in both the short and long terms. Aerobic and anaerobic exercises are both beneficial. Developing a program to secure this important need is the obligation of the surgeon and the surgeon's team.

DISCHARGE CLASS

Discharge education can be provided one-on-one or in a group setting. Ideally, discharge education occurs on discharge day. The most appropriate instructor is a registered nurse (RN) who has in-depth knowledge of the bariatric surgery performed, of the surgeon's routine postoperative instructions, of common complications, and of the follow-up schedule. A significant other or an adult support person should be encouraged to attend because she or he usually is the caretaker at home.

INTERACTING WITH MEDICAL INSURANCE COMPANIES

Perhaps no other disease state receives as much scrutiny from insurance companies, both positive and negative, than does bariatric surgery. This section briefly outlines the ramifications of the insurance precertification process. Because virtually all insurance companies handling these matters now require some type of precertification (also called predetermination, preauthorization, and other similar names), it is beneficial to evaluate how to submit these cases correctly the first time for third-party payer approvals, rather than go through multiple approval processes. Typically, medical insurance companies demand that the applicant documents that bariatric surgery is medically necessary not just because he or she is morbidly obese but because he or she has expensive comorbid disease (such as diabetes, sleep apnea, or atherosclerosis) that cannot be successfully treated in the obese unless the patient loses weight or has damaged organ systems (such as the development of steatosis of the liver, oseoarthritis of the major weight-bearing joints, venous stasis ulcers in the lower legs, or brawny skin changes). Additionally, most insurance companies want documentation of multiple prior attempts to lose weight, including copies of physician records if supervised in an outpatient medical setting or commercial reciepts if one went to programs such as Weight Watchers or Jenny Craig. Other requirements specific to individual insurance plans may include a preoperative evaluation by a psychologist or psychiatrist, a letter of endorsement for surgery from the patient's primary care physician, a limitation to specific bariatric procedures based on a company's evaluation of the effectiveness of a procedure as documented by "evidence-based" medical literature, or other specific requirements (such as weight or age), which often are not revealed either to the insured member or his/her physicians until initial approval for a bariatric surgical procedure has been denied.

First consider how your office is organized to handle the insurance process. A practice can often find that transitioning from a basic general surgery practice to a bariatric orientation requires a great deal more patient contact than the office is accustomed to, and the vast majority of that patient contact is a direct consequence of the difficulty in obtaining insurance approval for the surgery. Bariatric surgery is very different from conventional surgery such as gall bladder, hernia, or cancer surgery. Consequently, you need to consider how the office should be set up and whether you will need additional billing personnel.

The office needs to be set up in a way that places your patient and your practice in the best possible position at the earliest possible time for an insurance approval. There is a substantial time delay between the time a patient first contacts a bariatric practice until that patient is scheduled for surgery. That time delay may be because of scheduling limitations within the individual practice's clinical protocol, or it may be a result of patient "shopping" practices regarding different types of bariatric procedures and the time it takes for the patient to decide which type of surgery to have. It is essential to have the patient actively involved in the insurance process, and one of the mistakes many bariatric practices make is not giving patients enough information to assist them in getting insurance approvals.

The information that a patient needs to have is relevant to two particular time frames. The first time frame is documentation for past medical treatments. Patients need to be told specifically that they should be seeking out their primary care medical records, specialty care medical records, and, most importantly, to start collecting records of their "conservative" weight-loss treatments. This documentation is necessary because insurance companies are not generally interested in weight loss; rather, they are interested in having their prerequisites met before they will approve a bariatric surgical procedure.

Your office should approach the insurance approval process as a painter would approach a blank canvas. It is up to the patient and the practice, working as a team, to create a picture that demonstrates the medical necessity for treating morbid obesity and its multiple comorbid conditions. That medical necessity can often be demonstrated through the patient's prior medical records that show long-standing treatment for comorbidities well known to be associated with morbid obesity, such as type 2 diabetes, cardiovascular disease, hypertension, obstructive sleep apnea, urinary stress incontinence, and gastroesophageal reflux disease.

Most insurance companies, if not all third-party payers have medical policy criteria that they rely upon to determine whether they will cover bariatric surgery. That medical policy criteria may vastly differ from what the practice considers medically necessary. A primary barrier that patients need to overcome to obtain coverage for bariatric surgery is full documentation of prior weight-loss efforts that have been unsuccessful over the course of several years.

While virtually every patient who approaches a bariatric surgical procedure has done "just about everything" that insurance companies require, the insurance companies routinely require standard documentation of those efforts. For instance, at the time of publication, Cigna Health Care generally required, among its other medical policy criteria, three professionally supervised weight-loss efforts of a 12-week duration, one of those efforts having been completed within the last 12 months prior to the request for bariatric surgery. Cigna would consider professional weight-loss efforts inclusive of commercial weight-loss programs such as Weight Watchers, Jenny Craig, and Take Off Pounds Sensibly (TOPS), in addition to medically supervised weight-loss efforts.

Contrast that requirement with Aetna insurance. As of January 2003, Aetna requires 6 consecutive months of medically supervised weight loss that includes regular weigh-in and legible chart notes. No nonmedical, commercial plans are acceptable. Local and regional insurance companies will likely have a variation of these types of requirements. Some insurance companies require as much as 18 to 36 consecutive months of conservative medically supervised weight-loss treatment, all the while knowing that those efforts will be unsuccessful in 98% of the population. One of their hopes is that you will change your insurance plan or job to find a way to obtain surgery sooner than they allow it.[10]

One reason why we belabor the concept of medically or professionally supervised weight-loss efforts is because many bariatric patients are not told early enough in the process that these documents may be important in getting surgical approval. If not told to obtain these immediately, these documents may be lost to the patient. The earlier the patient is made aware of this need, the more likely the patient is to get those documents and to make them available when they apply for predetermination.

In setting up your bariatric practice, it is important to have the person(s) who will have direct patient contact be empathetic and understanding of the patient's frustration with the insurance approval process system. The patient has been told time and again by various doctors that bariatric surgery is medically necessary, but the patient generally does not understand that blanket statements by their doctors are insufficient to obtain insurance coverage for the procedure. The patient often becomes frustrated, and often takes this frustration out on the person in the "front line" of the bariatric practice. A high degree of empathy, sympathy, caring, and knowledge of insurance processing will certainly serve that patient and the practice extremely well.

Once the office is set up to instruct the patient about the medical documentation needs, with an emphasis on documenting prior medically supervised weight-loss efforts, the office can then start to set up an office "template" that will act as the basis for producing "letters of medical necessities." The letter of medical necessity is the critical document because it paints a picture for each patient of the medical need and medical propriety of bariatric surgery. The letter of medical necessity has two components: (1) background information that is applicable regardless of the type of bariatric procedure being requested, and (2) patient-specific information that truly outlines the medical need for that particular patient to have bariatric surgery. We address these issues below.

We think it is important for an insurance company to be made aware that the requested procedure is approved by independent authorities that endorse bariatric surgery. Most notably, the 1991 National Institutes of Health's (NIH) Consensus Conference Statement[11] endorsed bariatric surgery for the treatment of morbid obesity, including both gastric restrictive surgery and Roux-en-Y gastric bypass (RYGB). The NIH Consensus Conference established that the body mass index (BMI) thresholds are commonly used as benchmarks for defining medical necessity conditions. The two levels of medical necessity include a BMI of 40 kg/m^2 or above, regardless of comorbid status, and 35 to 39 kg/m^2 with high-risk comorbid conditions and or interference with major life activities (see Chapter 5).

Often, these standards are similar, but not identical, to the requirements of a third-party payer, although some medical insurance companies use more restrictive limits (i.e., higher BMI before they approve coverage). A good letter of medical necessity will establish for an insurance company that the fundamental requirements set forth by the NIH are met by this particular patient. Therefore, it is important to outline these requirements as part of the body of the letter, and then add something to the template that will change for each patient, demonstrating that in your medical judgment the patient's comorbid medical conditions warrant bariatric surgery and that this is also consistent with outside authorities.

An important aspect of the bariatric practice is its multiple disciplinary nature. One of the requirements of the NIH Consensus Conference in suggesting that bariatric surgery could be medically appropriate for certain patients who are highly motivated to lose weight is the fact that it is done in a multidisciplinary team setting. If your program does offer that type of multidisciplinary approach, then it is important to let the third-party payer know that your team is in place and to give it some information about that team. Again, this is information that can be provided on a template basis, changing it only when your team or program changes markedly.

In addition to the 1991 NIH Consensus Conference, there are other guideline statements that can be reviewed by the practice and integrated into the letter of medical necessity template. The NIH's *Clinical Guidelines on the Identification, Evaluation and Treatment of Overweight and Obesity in Adults* (1998) is an example.[12] Many insurance companies rely on this document to require bariatric patients to document that they have undergone supervised weight-loss attempts, because in it, the NIH establishes conservative treatment as a precondition to documenting the medical necessity of bariatric surgery. With the exception of this precondition, these NIH guidelines are consistent with the early consensus conference statements.

Other sources of information that the practice might consider adding to its template are guidelines published in 2000 by the American Society for Bariatric Surgery (ASBS), whose administrative office is in Gainesville, FL (www.asbs.org), and the Society of American Gastrointestinal Endoscopic Surgeons (SAGES), whose administrative office is in Los Angeles, CA (www.sages.org), as well as recommendations as promulgated by the American College of Surgeons (ACS), whose administrative office is in Chicago, IL (www.facs.org). What is desirable in a letter of medical necessity is to clearly set out that the patient meets treatment guidelines as established by government bodies and medical specialty organizations and that the program meets the multidisciplinary approach set up by good medical practice, by the NIH, and by medicine's peer review system, consisting of the nationally recognized subspecialty organizations, such as the ASBS, SAGES, and ACS.

The following items can be included in the letter of medical necessity in addition to the patient-specific information:

- Name of hospital/facility where the procedure is to be performed
- Date of operation
- Expected outcome (especially if your practice has published the results of a large series of procedures performed on your patients in a peer reviewed journal)

We now turn to the patient-specific information that is contained in the letter of medical necessity. A key mistake made by practices, especially with physicians who were not trained in the United States, is to fail to outline the patient's medical problems in a way that matches them to the NIH requirements in a readily understood manner. Because there are so many nonclinicians reviewing these letters and making the initial determination within the payer community as to whether surgery is warranted, it is important to state height in feet and inches and weight in pounds. It is also necessary to correctly calculate the

BMI for the reviewer. This information should be placed in the beginning of the letter so that the reviewer can easily determine that the patient meets these NIH criteria.

After clearly stating the patient's height, weight, and BMI, it is important to outline the other comorbid conditions suffered by the patient with respect to the need for bariatric surgery. For example, many practices clearly outline each and every comorbid condition in a separate paragraph with its relevant International Classification of Diseases (ICD-9) diagnostic code.[13] It is, in our opinion, the best practice because it clearly demonstrates and documents the urgent medical need for surgery by outlining each and every comorbid condition and how surgery can be expected to improve these conditions. It is also a superior way of handling it, rather than by specifically describing the benefits of bariatric surgery for each comorbid condition, risking that the reviewer will understand how these comorbidities will be corrected. Because there are numerous references available in the literature and in this textbook to link bariatric surgery to the reversal or correction of a specific disease, whether it be by gastric bypass, biliopancreatic diversion (with or without) duodenal switch, or BioEnteric's gastric LAP-BAND system, there should be linkage to each procedure and whether it corrects each particular comorbid condition that the patient has. While it may not be necessary to physically attach those references, abstracts, or citations for the benefit of any medical director or clinical personnel reviewing this at the third-party payer's office, it will certainly assist them in their understanding of the benefits of bariatric gastric surgery for the patient with respect to the patient's comorbid conditions.

In summary, a good letter of medical necessity is not necessarily a short letter of medical necessity. We have seen numerous letters in our law practice that are of the fill-in-the-blank style and that neither demonstrate a medical urgency nor clearly document the compelling needs of the particular patient.[11] That does a disservice to the patient, as well as to the practice, and often creates unnecessary denials.

Bariatric surgery practices must confirm the specific medical policy requirements of each payer. For instance, as stated earlier, many payers have requirements for bariatric surgery that are different from the NIH Consensus Conference suggestions or the surgeon's clinical judgment. Many payers require specific documentation to be provided with the letter of medical necessity (e.g., chart notes or a letter of support from the patient's primary physician) while other payers simply want to see a comprehensive letter of medical necessity that meets their requirements for demonstrating that the patient meets the payer's medical policy requirements. It is important to develop a cooperative relationship with the payer and an understanding of what the payer is requiring in order to facilitate approval for your patients. Many good practices spend time meeting with the medical directors of their major payers to educate them about their bariatric practice and to let the payers specify their requirements in order to maximize approval for their patients. A cooperative relationship between practice and payer often leads to accelerated appeals that can be done either with a quick letter or by telephone because the level of cooperation and trust between the practice and the payer is high. While this may sound unusual to practices that routinely fight with insurance payers, it is often the norm for many practices that have taken the time to develop those relationships over the long term.

One important aspect of the letter of medical necessity that should be separately addressed is the question of CPT (current procedure terminology) coding. CPT codes are required by the insurance industry to link the treatment provided to the diseases presented by the patient.[13] While bariatric surgery has a slate of codes for procedures done by an open laparotomy, it becomes more difficult to address coding issues when the procedure is to be completed laparoscopically (Table 6–1).

There is a series of codes for gastric restrictive procedures such as vertical-banded gastroplasty (VBG) and non–vertical-banded gastroplasty, as well as proximal and distal RYGB. There is no specific code for the biliopancreatic diversion with or without the duodenal switch.

When it comes to laparoscopic procedures, until there is a slate of codes available for those procedures, which is a time-consuming and burdensome process for the specialty medical society and practitioners to create, "unlisted" codes such as CPT43659 (unlisted laparoscopic stomach) and CPT43999 or CPT49320 (if the procedure is started laparoscopically and then converted to an open operation) changed as of January 1, 2003, and are viable options for the various procedures done laparoscopically.

Coding with an unlisted code is generally a burdensome process that requires hand processing, rather than computer processing, and is often interpreted by an insurance carrier as a coding error. This is, again, an opportunity to deal with the executives of your third-party payers to develop a payment strategy and protocol for the payment for laparoscopic procedures. Until there is an agreement between the practice and the third-party payer to use a "code" for a laparoscopic bariatric procedure, the unlisted codes referenced in Table 6–1 are the only available codes. However, so long as there is an appropriately documented agreement between the practice and the third-party payer, there should be no issues of fraud or improper coding when using the open code. Issues of fraud, however, would arise if a practice chose to code a particular procedure for purposes of obtaining payment that is otherwise not entitled for such reimbursement.

With respect to the ICD-9 coding for the diseases implicated, in addition to the comorbid conditions referenced earlier, it is critical that the practice always properly code the disease of morbid obesity, which bears ICD-9 code

TABLE 6–1. CURRENT PROCEDURE TERMINOLOGY (CPT) CODES FOR BARIATRIC PROCEDURES	
CPT #	DESCRIPTION
43633	Gastrectomy with Roux-en-Y reconstruction
43842	Vertical-band gastroplasty
43843	LAP-BAND ® or other adjustable gastric band
43848	Revision of gastric procedure—restrictive
43860	Revision gastrojejunal anastomosis

278.01.[12] There are other codes for "obesity" that are not relevant to a person suffering from the disease of morbid obesity.

Once a letter of medical necessity has exited your office and gone to the third-party payer, your office insurance protocol must include a system to track the third-party payer's response. Because of their anxieties, bariatric patients will often be very persistent in contacting the practice about insurance approval; letting them know what the specific time frame is (and following that time frame) will reduce the number of redundant phone calls that a bariatric practice must endure.

The response by the insurance company usually comes in one of three forms: an approval for surgery; a denial for surgery; or a request for more information. Obviously, if there is a request for more information, the practice must ascertain specifically what information is needed and endeavor to provide it.

DEALING WITH APPROVAL AND DENIALS

In this era of managed care, one mistake that is occasionally made by some bariatric practices is believing that a certification of the "medical necessity" of the procedure acts as an approval for coverage. While this may sometimes be the case, it is not always the case, and this is where knowledge of the third-party payer is important. Some businesses, especially those that have their own self-insurance plans, hire a third-party administrator that only acts to certify medical necessity for a particular procedure based on whether there is documentation using appropriate diagnoses and other criteria in the letter of medical necessity. Often those letters of "approval" contain a proviso that the letter is not a guarantee of payment but rather payment is subject to the terms and conditions of the policy. That "certification of medical necessity" is meaningless when you try to obtain reimbursement of a procedure for the patient if the plan itself excludes coverage. Therefore, for those payers, where it is a two-step process, it is important for the practice to know its payer system and to obtain all necessary approvals, not just the certification for medical necessity.

A significant portion of the time of a person whose assignment is to obtain insurance approvals in a bariatric practice will be spent addressing the denials of requested procedures. These denials can occur for a number of reasons. Each reason should be treated a bit differently by the practice.

Bariatric procedures are generally denied because the medical necessity criteria is not met, or because there is an exclusion of coverage of some sort in the certificate of coverage. With respect to denial for medical necessity, this is often the result of a disconnect between what the office provides and what the insurance carrier thinks it needs in order to approve the surgery. Again, direct prompt communication between the office and the insurance company prior to submitting these letters will help to eliminate many of these types of denials. Alternatively, your practice may chose to appeal the denial depending on the particular basis stated by the insurance company as its reason for the denial. Most state laws require that an insurance company clearly define and specify why a matter is being denied and a practice or patient must take whatever steps are necessary in order to provide that information.

It is important to know that a right to appeal is generally the patient's right to appeal. Therefore, it would be a better practice for the bariatric surgeon's office to ensure that there is a written authorization from the patient to the practice to appeal a denial of coverage. Because every insurance company has a limited number of appeals and a specific appeal or grievance process that must be followed, a bariatric practice can "use up" appeals that the patient may want to reserve for other advocates to advance their position. Although the bariatric practice may feel that it is serving the patient by aggressively appealing these matters, if it is not meeting a specific request for more information or specific issues that have resulted in the denial, it may be simply exhausting an appeal that the patient could use more productively through other means.

An exclusive coverage actually takes on multiple meaning depending on the nature of the exclusion and the procedure being sought. We address these in turn. There are some insurance companies that very specifically exclude bariatric surgery. They may use formulation such as, "We do not cover the surgical treatment of morbid obesity regardless of the associated medical conditions, whether psychological, emotional, or physical."

This is a very specific policy formulation that addresses the disease ("morbid obesity"), the comorbidities ("associated illnesses"), and the nature of the treatment ("surgery"). Other policy formulations may address specific procedures, such as gastric bypass, gastric banding, and gastric balloons, as procedures they do not cover. Other companies may reference the diseases by using the terms overweight, obesity, and morbid obesity as diseases for which they do not provide treatment. In fact, there are virtually hundreds, if not thousands, of ways insurance companies attempt to exclude bariatric procedures or treatments. Some of these exclusions are well constructed and not generally subject to attack: other exclusions relied upon by insurance companies are poorly drafted and so ambiguous that they are subject to challenge or can be challenged by both practice or other appropriate patient advocate.

Another type of exclusion may exist that may be related to the procedure performed by the bariatric surgeon. Quite frequently, insurance companies are denying certain types of procedures on the basis that they are either "experimental" or "investigational." These procedures include distal RYGB, biliopancreatic diversion with or without duodenal switch, and adjustable gastric-banding procedures. The general position taken by many insurance companies is that the more extensive malabsorptive procedures do not provide enough additional weight loss or additional comorbidity resolution to justify the potential metabolic sequelae that are inherent in an extensive malabsorptive procedure. While this may be a debate that should be reserved for clinicians, the company can state the position of the insurance industry because many members of the insurance industry do not provide coverage for these malabsorptive procedures.

With respect to adjustable laparoscopic gastric banding, the Food and Drug Administration (FDA) approved the INAMED Health (Santa Barbara,

CA) Lap Band System on June 5, 2001. Some insurance companies approve the use of the device and procedure, while others are taking a more conservative approach and seeking additional data to support the safety and advocacy of this device and technology as a treatment for morbid obesity. Often, however, even though a company refuses to provide coverage for malabsorptive procedures or adjustable gastric-banding technology, it does cover bariatric procedures such as the more "conventional" treatments of vertical-banding gastroplasty and RYGB.

If a bariatric practice chooses to become involved with the appeal process, it is important that the practice understands a few fundamentals. Policy language in a certificate of coverage is generally construed in the favor of the policyholder. This is less true in cases where the insurance policy is governed by the federal Employee Retirement Income Security Act of 1974 (ERISA), which gives a great deal of deference to the plan. That deference, however, can be used both ways. A plan can be amended to cover bariatric surgery once the company is confronted with the data and evidence demonstrating that the plan as a whole may benefit from providing coverage for bariatric surgery in appropriate clinical incidences.

A bariatric practice can and must, if it's going to be involved in the insurance appeal process, address the basis for denial in each individual case. This can be time-consuming and the practice must be aware of time constraints to initiate appeals, which can range from 30 to 180 days. Again, it is important to have the patient consent to the practice being involved with bariatric surgery appeals.

In the instance of denials based on experimental or investigative treatments, many state statutes provide for separate external review processes. It would be beneficial for the practice to be aware of those opportunities to accelerate the appeal process and to determine whether or not these processes may be in the patient's best interest.

Although it is beyond the scope of this chapter to address the entire claims process (the process that occurs after the surgical procedure has been performed), we offer a few principles that will assist you in maximizing your reimbursement. A good preauthorization process will assist in maximizing reimbursements. By submitting accurate claims, the practice or the billing service working with the claims form will be able to improve reimbursements. It is important for bariatric surgeons to communicate directly with the billings/coding staff so that the staff may be aware of anatomical nuances and operative procedure issues that might be the difference between payment and nonpayment for a particular procedure. This is particularly true when dealing with issues related to operations that are not routinely performed by the practice and whenever a revision of a previous operation is performed. Revisions or unusual procedures must be preauthorized in a manner that does not allow the insurance company to claim they were deceived or misinformed. Submission of a "clean claim" often generates an insurance company's obligation under state "prompt pay" laws, while confusion generated by an inaccurate preauthorization letter or a poorly dictated operative note that does not match the claim form can result in the claim being denied payment, which results in a lot of extra work and explanation before the practice can be reimbursed. The practice can also lose the opportunity to obtain any reimbursement, which may also affect the hospital's ability to get paid but still means the practice and the hospital can be sued for a bad outcome.

REFERENCES

1. Stunkard AJ, Foch TT, Hrubec Z. A twin study of human obesity. *JAMA* 1986;256:51–54.
2. Stunkard AJ, Wadden T. Psychological aspects of human obesity. *Human Obesity: General Aspects* 1992;352–358.
3. Stunkard AJ, Wadden TA. Psychological aspects of severe obesity. *Am J Clin Nutr* 1992;55:5224s–5232s.
4. Staffieri JR. A study of social stereotype of body image in children. *J Pers Soc Psychol* 1967;7:101–104.
5. Canning H, Mayer J. Obesity—its possible effects on college admissions. *N Engl J Med* 1966; 275:1172–1174.
6. Larkin JE, Pines HA. No fat person need apply. *Soc Work Occup* 1979;6:312–327.
7. Rand CSW, Macgriegor AMC. Successful weight loss following obesity surgery and the perceived liability of morbid obesity. *Int J Obes* 1991;15:577–579.
8. Valles JM, Ross MA. The role of psychologic factors in bariatric surgery for morbid obesity: identification psychologic predictors of success obesity surgery. *Obes Surg* 1993;4:346–359.
9. Coloman JA. Discrimination at large. *Newsweek* 1993;1:9.
10. Lindstrom W Jr. Believe it or not, sometimes lawyers are the good guys. *Obes Surg* 1996;6:371–376.
11. NIH Conference. Gastrointestinal surgery for severe obesity. Consensus Development Conference Panel. *Ann Intern Med* 1991;115:956–961.
12. National Institutes of Health. Clinical guidelines on the identification, evaluation, and treatment of overweight and obesity in adults—the evidence report. *Obes Res* 1998;6(Suppl 2):51S–209S.
13. Martin LF, White S, Lindstrom W Jr. Cost-benefit analysis for the treatment of severe obesity. *World J Surg.* 1998;22:1008–1017.

POSTOPERATIVE MEDICAL MANAGEMENT OF BARIATRIC PATIENTS

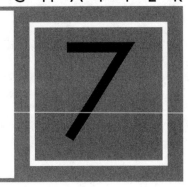

WILLIAM J. RAUM

This chapter addresses a variety of issues that are commonly encountered in the postoperative medical management of patients who have undergone procedures like the LAP-BAND (LB), gastric bypass (GB), or biliopancreatic diversion. A few of the more rarely observed problems are touched upon to instill the notion that the unexpected can, and often does, occur. Experience and coordinated interaction with a team of nurses, internists, surgeons, dietitians, psychosocial counselors, and exercise physiologists who are all following the same management plan allows for the best results for the patient physically and psychologically, with the least number of complications.

MANAGEMENT OF PRIOR MEDICAL CONDITIONS

Obstructive Sleep Apnea

Preoperative diagnosis and treatment is essential to prevent postoperative complications related to this potentially catastrophic disease (see Chapter 5). Obstructive sleep apnea is a primary cause of sudden death in the morbid obesity[1] and nearly all patients are completely cured by the level of weight loss produced by bariatric surgery.[2] However, until enough weight is lost, continuous positive airway pressure (CPAP) treatment must be initiated preoperatively until the patient is accustomed to sleeping with the mask on, and it must be maintained postoperatively in the hospital and at home afterwards. When the patient reaches a weight where he or she has stopped snoring, another sleep study can be performed to confirm that the obstruction has been resolved.

Other Pulmonary Disorders

Asthma (especially when secondary to reflux), chronic obstructive airway disease, obesity-hypoventilation syndrome, and hypoxia from shunting are completely reversed or markedly improved by weight loss. Patients are given an incentive spirometer and flutter valve during their hospitalization and taught how to use the devices by respiratory therapists. They should be encouraged to continue to use these and, if indicated, bronchodilators and inhalable steroids for several weeks postoperatively, even if asymptomatic. Most patients develop some significant degree of atelectasis postoperatively. Occasionally, even more severe atelectasis results from a left-sided pleural effusion. Continuing an aggressive pulmonary toilet during this early postoperative period reduces the chance of developing more severe problems, such as pneumonia, bronchiectasis, or empyema. Interestingly, chronic, mild to severe asthma and sinus symptoms are cured or markedly reduced by weight loss. The improvement may be the result of a reduction in food allergies that exacerbate allergic reactions in respiratory tract. The diet is drastically changed and some foods that caused unrecognized allergic reactions may have been eliminated from the diet. In addition, fat tissue in the head and neck are lost rapidly, increasing the diameter of respiratory passages, which may reduce the severity of symptoms from milder episodes of mucosal swelling and inflammation. Also, reflux of acid washing over into the trachea is usually eliminated by LB and always by GB.

Hypertension

No antihypertensive treatment is usually required after discharge unless the patient was hypersensitive before they became obese. Decreased caloric intake, particularly sugar or sucrose, causes a marked decreased in blood pressure. The effect occurs within 1 week, well ahead of any significant weight loss. The few patients who have primary hypertension, not hypertension secondary to obesity, may require some therapy, but usually at a reduced dosage. Thiazide and loop (furosemide) diuretics should be avoided. Volume depletion is the norm rather than volume overload at this time, thus diuretics are not indicated. Prerenal azotemia, hyperuricemia, hypercalciuria, renal stones, hypokalemia, and hypomagnesemia are other undesirable side effects. Some increased extracellular fluid may be present with pitting edema, but this should simply be treated with a low-salt diet and elevation of legs when at rest. If blood pressure is still a concern at discharge, calcium channel blockers, angiotensin-converting enzyme inhibitors, or clonidine by transdermal delivery are usually effective and well tolerated. Beta-blockers may cause some significant muscle weakness and hypoglycemia and should be avoided if not essential for other indications. Antihypertensive therapy must be reevaluated frequently to avoid hypotension and syncope. The latter is much more likely at this time than a hypertensive crisis.

Adult-Onset Diabetes Mellitus (Type 2 Diabetes)

Insulin resistance and glucose levels fall rapidly during the first week and month after surgery,[3] regardless of the procedure used, and usually occurs with rapid weight loss induced by nonsurgical methods. Like hypertension, this decrease precedes a significant decrease in weight and is caused by the decrease in calorie intake. Tight control of blood sugar during this time is not desirable and can be detrimental. Caloric intake can be erratic and physical activity generally increases after discharge. Hypoglycemia and the effects of neuroglycopenia with syncope and coma are a much greater risk at this time with certain diabetic agents than with others. Unless unavoidable for special circumstances, intermediate-acting and even short-acting insulin should be avoided. Not only can this therapy induce rapid and prolonged hypoglycemia, high insulin levels are a primary cause of obesity. The deposition of fat and hyperphagia caused by excess insulin should be eliminated as quickly as feasible. Metformin is commonly used preoperatively. It does not stimulate insulin levels and it does little to induce hypoglycemia. The "glitazones" can be used alone or with metformin. Sulfonylureas and their combinations with other agents should be avoided because of the risk of hypoglycemia. Blood sugars less than 180 mg% before meals is considered reasonable control at this time. It would be unusual if insulin or oral agents were needed to attain this level of control. However, if needed, ensure that the patient will perform home glucose monitoring. Provide the patient with a schedule to reduce the dose and number of medications taken to avoid hypoglycemia. Blood sugar that increases suddenly and persistently above 200 mg% usually has one or two potential causes: consumed sugar or stress caused by infection or psychosocial problems. The likely infections as this point include wound abscess, infected seroma, respiratory tract, or urinary tract. Dietary intake should be reviewed and the onset of family or other social stressors should be addressed. Blood sugar levels do need to be treated to reduce levels to below 180 mg%. Once the cause is treated, blood sugar will continue its descent.

Reflux Disease and Gastritis

After gastric bypass, proton pump inhibitors, H_2 blockers, and antacids may all be discontinued. Because acid from the stomach can no longer reach the proximal stomach pouch or esophagus, there is no more reflux disease. The LAP-BAND may also markedly reduce the ability of acid to reflux proximal to the band or reach the esophagus as long as the LAP-BAND outlet remains small and abdominal girth decreases from weight loss. Marginal ulcers at the gastrojejunal anastomosis may occur with the biliopancreatic diversion (BPD), and for this reason, antacid therapy is usually maintained for months to years after this procedure.

Arthritis and Back Disease

Nonsteroidal antiinflammatory drugs (NSAIDs), glucocorticoids, and cyclooxygenase (COX)-2 inhibitors used to treat the pain and inflammation possess a number of side effects that range from theoretical to life-threatening. All of these agents result in the breakdown of gastric mucus and the mucosa that can affect the pouch or distal stomach in all three procedures, and result in nausea, abdominal pain, and gastric bleeding that could be catastrophic. Glucocorticoids also cause the loss of lean body mass, exacerbate diabetes, increase risk of infection, impede the loss of fat mass, and contribute to the development of osteoporosis. For these reasons, the use of these agents should be avoided whenever possible. If essential to treat severe rheumatoid disease or debilitating pain, and no other substitutes are effective, then the stomach should be protected with proton pump inhibitors or H_2 blockers. Oral intake should be in liquid form and/or with food to reduce contact with the gastric mucosa and taken in the smallest effective dose.

Acetaminophen and narcotic analgesics are given for the first 4 to 8 weeks to treat pain; this is sufficient for most patients. Except for the most severely debilitated, joint and back pain are completely relieved or markedly reduced within the first 2 months after the procedures, and continue to resolve with time. Severe degenerative joint disease, inflammatory joint disease, and degenerative disk disease generally require antiinflammatory agents. Having a pain specialist who is aware of the special requirements of the bariatric surgery patient is essential, allowing the design of a therapeutic regimen that avoids NSAIDs with morphine or Marcaine pumps, transcutaneous electrical nerve stimulation (TENS), biofeedback, or Botox, to name a few agents that are useful. It is essential that pain be relieved in order to be able to perform some exercises and to allow patients to increase their physical activity.

Urinary Incontinence

Urinary incontinence not caused by autonomic neuropathy responds very quickly to weight loss. First, this is a result of a decrease in the volume of liquid that can be consumed. Second, there is a decrease in intraabdominal pressure from the decrease in bulk food consumed and a reduction in abdominal fat. Thus, there is less pressure on the urethral sphincter and it is less likely to become incompetent. As abdominal weight continues to decrease, the incidence of incontinence diminishes. Most women who require anticholinergics before surgery do not require them at discharge. Only those with other structural abnormalities that require surgical procedures need drug treatment beyond the first postoperative month.

Dependent Edema

Increased levels of intraabdominal pressure adversely affect venous return from the lower extremities leading to edema of the legs in most morbidly obese patients. The edema generally decreases overnight and recurs by evening. With time, varicose veins may develop, skin darkens as a consequence of pigments causing brawny changes, and the skin thickens. Recurrent episodes of cellulitis develop and skin ulcers, deep vein thrombosis, and even pulmonary embolus can occur. Diuretics, usually furosemide, are used to treat these conditions, but treatment is rarely successful. For dependent edema from congestive heart failure, diuretics may be indicated, but in obesity, the treatment is weight loss. Following surgery, some edema may be present from intravenous fluids collecting as part of the third space accumulation of fluid caused by the injury response, but it will resolve quickly. Postoperatively, the diet is very low in sodium, fluid intake is low, and some level of volume depletion develops in most patients. Rarely should patients be discharged from the hospital on diuretics, and even more rarely should diuretics be used during postoperative weight loss. The mild and diminishing edema postoperatively poses no threat, whereas the side effects of diuretic therapy, including prerenal azotemia, electrolyte imbalance, hyperuricemia, and nephrolithiasis are to be avoided.

Menstrual Disorders and Estrogens

Delay restarting estrogens or progestogens postoperatively for as long as feasible. These hormones increase fat deposition (mostly subcutaneous),[4] increase risk of the development of deep vein thrombosis,[5] and potentially pulmonary embolus. Examine the reasons for the treatment preoperatively, evaluate the actual benefit in light of the risks outlined above, and determine if alternative treatment is available. Usually, no treatment is needed. Some women have been placed on estrogens for hot flashes, or just because they are postmenopausal (surgical or natural), for the potential development of osteoporosis, for birth control, to regulate abnormal menses, or for mood disorders. All women will have been off these hormones for a month or two at this time to reduce the incidence of postoperative deep vein thrombosis. If they are no longer having hot flashes, major mood swings, abnormal menses, or other minimal indications, then there is no reason to restart these medications and it is probably better to wait for a clear indication. It is unlikely that a morbidly obese woman will develop osteoporosis in the immediate postoperative period. The mechanical stress of carrying an extra 45.4 kg (100 lb) or more is an excellent stimulus for maintaining strong and well-mineralized bones. There are alternate therapies for most of the conditions listed above so that restarting estrogens during this rapid-weight-loss phase can be avoided. Clonidine delivered by transdermal patch may reduce hot flashes. Moods swings can be treated with antidepressants. There are many other methods of birth control that do not involve estrogens or progesterone, including condoms, spermicides, diaphragms, or intrauterine devices. Calcitonin may be used to treat documented osteoporosis.

Thyroid Disorders

Generally, only hypothyroid disorders should be present postoperatively. Patients with hyperthyroidism do not become candidates for treatment of morbid obesity until those disorders are treated and cured, or they are in remission. Hyperthyroidism caused by intrinsic disease, excessive replacement, either intentional (for treatment of thyroid cancer) or unintentional, carries a high risk for arrhythmias during anesthesia induction, and postoperatively leads to excessive loss of lean body mass especially the heart with the development of cardiomyopathy, and loss of bone leading to osteoporosis. The management of hypothyroidism should be done with levothyroxine (T_4) only and without mixed preparations that contain triiodothyronine (T_3). Doses should be adjusted to keep thyroid-stimulating hormone (TSH) in the mid-normal or high-normal range, and avoid excessive thyroid hormone to avoid loss of lean body mass. Absorption of thyroxin may be somewhat erratic and can vary significantly from the preoperative dose. Taking thyroxin before bed, with no other medications or food tends to reduce some of the variability encountered.

Hyperlipidemias

Most secondary hyperlipidemias are resolved by weight loss over time. Unless total cholesterol was above 350 or triglycerides were greater than 750, antilipidemic agents need not be restarted immediately. The diet and weight loss should be given 4 to 6 months to have an effect on lipid metabolism and then a fasting lipid panel should be obtained. The results usually confirm that the secondary hyperlipidemia has been cured. If primary disease is present, then lipid levels will not have returned to normal and it is unlikely that they ever will without pharmacologic treatment. Restarting antilipid agents in the 4- to 6-month postoperative period is more readily tolerated by liver and muscle than in the immediate postoperative period, and it will be clear then that treatment will be needed regardless of the patient's final weight.

Depression

Postoperative depression layered on existing depression can overwhelm preoperative treatment regimens. Psychological and psychosocial evaluation pre- and postoperatively is essential to ensure treatment is adequate to meet the additional challenges of this period. Tricyclic antidepressants (amitriptyline, desipramine, imipramine) are to be avoided. Many times they are prescribed for insomnia or as adjuncts to pain therapy. These agents, however, are potent appetite stimulators[6] and may be a cause of obesity, as well contribute to the failure of methods to treat obesity, including surgical procedures. Antiserotonergic agents (e.g., Prozac [fluoxetine], Paxil [paroxetine], and Zoloft [sertraline]) can increase appetite in some patients. If this effect is suspected, changing to agents such as Wellbutrin (bupropion) may reduce appetite. A number of these agents are available in liquid form, and are preferred in the first month after surgery to avoid obstructing the gastric outlet.

MANAGEMENT OF NEW PROBLEMS AT 4 WEEKS POSTOPERATIVELY

Volume Depletion

Patients must be encouraged to consume adequate fluids to prevent urinary tract infections, kidney stones, hyperuricemia, constipation, and hypotension. Men, and some women, tend to swallow large volumes too quickly and overfill their 2- or 3-ounce gastric pouch. Vomiting or severe substernal and epigastric pain from spasms of the esophagus or gastric pouch ensue, which result in a further decrease in volume intake. Patients must be taught and reminded to sip small quantities of liquid on a regular basis to avoid the consequences of volume depletion. Patients should be advised to avoid situations that cause excessive sweating or situations where access to fluids is limited. Urine specific gravity is a reasonably good indicator of fluid balance and patients can be taught to use dipsticks. Fortunately, this problem is usually resolved by the second postoperative month.

Gas

There are four primary reasons for problems with gas after bariatric surgery. Most gas in the gastrointestinal tract comes from swallowed air. Air is introduced in the following manner: Chewing gum puts bubbles in saliva that is swallowed; a long period of conversation puts bubbles in saliva that is swallowed; carbonated beverages, beer, and soda, have gas; blended protein supplements can contain a lot of air. First look to these and other foods that may contain carbonation or air and eliminate them. Swallowed gas is usually dissolved into the liquid contained in the stomach. Because the stomach size has been reduced at operation and liquid consumption is low, more gas enters the intestine, producing gas pains and excessive flatus. Treatment of gas, other than treatment to reduce swallowed air, can be accomplished by using products containing *simethicone* as chewable tablets or liquid.

Although most adults already know when they have a lactase deficiency because they have problems digesting milk, others only develop symptoms when taking larger quantities than they were accustomed to preoperatively. After surgery, some patients develop a mild deficiency that usually resolves over time. Milk and dairy products are usually an essential part of the recommended postoperative nutritional plan because they contain large amounts of protein. To reduce the symptoms, lactose-free milk and other lactose-free dairy products may be used. There are tablets containing the enzyme lactase that can be chewed before eating or drinking dairy products. Also, soy liquid products can be substituted for dairy products.

Certain vegetables can cause gas because of the lack of the intestinal enzyme α-galactosidase. Some drugs can inhibit the enzymes and surgery can cause a relative deficiency. If it is difficult to avoid foods that cause gas, or if the foods cannot be identified, then an enzyme supplement, such as Beano, may be used, by simply putting a few drops of this preparation right on vegetable being consumed.

The last likely cause for excessive gas may be the overgrowth of the fungus *Candida,*[7] or of anaerobic bacteria, which produces gas. If none of the solutions above reduce the problem, then a serology test can be obtained to detect excessive titers of *Candida* antibody, or a stool culture may be obtained to identify an infection, or overgrowth of intestinal *Candida*. Antibiotics used during and after surgery may eliminate the normal intestinal flora that prevents fungus from growing. The fungus or yeast produces gas in the intestine. DiFlucan (fluconazole) may be used to eliminate the fungus. Flagyl (metronidazole) can be used to decrease anaerobic bacteria levels.

Nausea and Vomiting

Not chewing food completely, or eating or drinking too fast are the most common reasons for nausea or vomiting, regardless of the bariatric procedure performed. Treating nausea with antiemetics can prolong this behavior and increases the risk of inadequate long-term weight loss. Patients need to clearly understand the consequences of eating or drinking too fast. They may develop either structural defects in their new anatomy, or tachyphylaxis of the noxious hormonal feedback that limits food intake. Some of the structural defects that can occur from overeating include dilatation of the esophagus with LAP-BAND (Figure 7–1); GB, or BPD, dilation of the gastric pouch with LAP-BAND, GB, and BPD, dilation of the gastric outlet with GB, slippage or erosion of the LAP-BAND, dilatation of the alimentary limb of the GB, or dilation of the blind end of the biliopancreatic limb. By repeatedly overstimulating gastrointestinal hormones that decrease food intake, such as gastric inhibitory peptide, glucagon-like peptide-1, and enterostatin (see Chapter 3), they will no longer inhibit appetite and weight loss will not occur.

Alternatively, nausea and vomiting can occur if a stricture develops at the gastric outlet stoma of a LB, GB, or BPD, or if a small-bowel obstruction occurs. Radiographs of the abdomen can be essential in determining whether these structural defects have occurred.

Constipation and Diarrhea

Patients must understand what constipation means. It is not infrequent bowel movements; rather, it is dry, hard stools. The two most common causes for constipation are the lack of fiber in the diet and volume depletion. Very-low-calorie liquid diets (formula) and most postoperative gastric bypass diets have very little fiber in them. Some of this is designed intentionally, some unintentionally. After bariatric surgery, fluid intake is usually low. Therefore, the first goal is to increase the water content of the stool by using either a stool softener, such as docusate sodium, and/or by encouraging fluid intake as tolerated. When

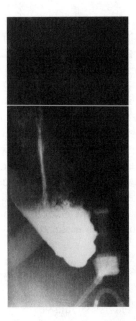

FIGURE 7–1   Radiograph with dilation of the esophagus with LAP-BAND, GB, or BPD.

someone presents with painful constipation, adding a stimulant (laxative) such as Peri-Colace (docusate sodium and casanthranol) may be more effective. If no results are obtained from taking two doses of Peri-Colace 6 to 12 hours apart, then an enema is indicated to physically break up the stool. Sometimes it is necessary to digitally break up a large circumference piece of stool. To do this comfortably for the patient, it is often necessary to paralyze the rectal sphincter muscles by injecting 1% lidocaine. Then, with the addition of one or two mineral oil or phosphosoda enemas, results are usually obtained. The enemas should be followed with an oral laxative, phosphosoda (oral liquid), magnesium citrate oral solution, or bisacodyl tablets or suppositories. Severe constipation may require several treatments with the enemas and oral laxatives to clear out the colon. Once accomplished, docusate sodium or docusate casanthranol should be taken daily and the fiber content of the diet increased compatible with the current stage of their LB, GB, or BPD diet.

Clostridium difficile, an opportunistic organism whose growth is favored by loss of normal enteric flora induced by antibiotics, can cause diarrhea. The disease caused by this organism, pseudomembranous colitis, may be lethal if not diagnosed and treated appropriately. It occurs most commonly days to weeks after discharge from the hospital and cessation of prophylactic antibiotics. Using Flagyl as one of the prophylactic antibiotics reduces, but does not eliminate the risk of pseudomembranous colitis. The characteristic diarrhea is unrelated to food intake, occurs around the clock, and continues to produce very frequent, watery stools even when fasting. If a patient presents with this symptom complex, a stool titer for *C. difficile* should be obtained, and either oral vancomycin or Flagyl should be given. Antidiarrheals, Lomotil (diphenoxylate and atropine), or kaolin, pectin, and Imodium (loperamide) are ineffective in reducing the diarrhea, but the antibiotics are usually effective in 24 to 48 hours.

Diarrhea caused by excessive fat intake is most severe in the BPD, but may be moderately severe after GB and generally does not occur in the LB. Diarrhea, abdominal cramping, and gas usually occur within 20 minutes to several hours after consuming foods high in fat content.[8] The treatment is to stop eating the offending high-fat foods. Although antidiarrheals will help to reduce symptoms, they will also prolong the time for patients to modify their behavior to avoid fat intake. Like nausea and vomiting, the more times inappropriate foods are taken, the less potent the noxious stimuli, and the less likely that dysfunctional food behavior will be modified.

Nutrition: Macro- and Micronutrients

Protein is the primary nutrient that should be the center point of every weight-loss diet, whether surgical, medical, or behavioral. For it is not, precisely, weight loss that we wish to achieve, but loss of excess body fat and retention of lean body mass (protein). Because the body tends to break down protein and convert it to sugar in times of semi-starvation, the preferred source of energy production, protein must be replenished and protected in all weight-loss diets. As a reasonable estimate, patients are encouraged to consume a certain amount of protein in grams per day based on a calculation where they multiply their body weight in pounds times 0.3 to obtain the total grams of protein they need to consume a day. Thus, a patient weighing 250 pounds should consume 75 grams of protein per day ($0.3 \times 250 = 75$). A patient weighing 400 pounds would consume 120 grams of protein per day ($0.3 \times 400 = 120$). The result of the patient's protein intake is assessed by measurement of serum prealbumin and changes in body composition (see Review Resting Energy Expediture and Body Composition Trends, below). Protein consumption must be high quality; that is, it must contain all of the essential amino acids. Products or protein supplements made from gelatin or collagen are not high quality and will not protect the endogenous protein stores of the heart, the liver, the skin, and the muscle. Sources of high-quality protein include milk, cheese, whey, soy, eggs, fish, and meat. All must be low fat or fat free.

Vitamin B_{12} deficiency occurs when a portion of the stomach is removed or separated from ingested food (GB or BPD). A protein is made in the stomach (intrinsic factor) that binds to B_{12} and allows it to be absorbed in the intestine. To prevent vitamin B_{12} deficiency after GB or BPD, one strategy is to give high doses of B_{12} orally and hope that enough of the binding protein will eventually reach the B_{12}, enabling it to be absorbed in the intestine and into the blood stream. Injections of B_{12} into the muscle will go into the bloodstream and do not need the binding protein. Pills that contain both vitamin B_{12} and the binding protein, intrinsic factor, are available. Chewable multivitamins that come in both children's and adult formulations contain a form of vitamin B_{12} that can be absorbed into the bloodstream through the oral mucosa. Sublingual tablets that contain only B_{12} are also available. Adult or children's chewable multivitamins supply most of the vitamins needed and are inexpensive. Vitamin B_{12} levels can be measured while taking the chewable vitamins and produce normal level in more than 95% of patients. The remaining 5% of patients can be treated with sublingual B_{12}. Because chewable and sublingual forms of B_{12} are now readily available and very inexpensive, it is very rare for a patient to require monthly parenteral injections of B_{12}.

Other vitamins and minerals can be deficient in the diet or not absorbed as well after surgery. Fat-soluble vitamins A and D usually must be supplemented in BPD, and occasionally in GB, if a patient is unable to curb fat intake and the patient has significant diarrhea. Magnesium or zinc may be in deficient in any of the procedures because of decreased intake and increased loss by the kidneys. Generally, it is best to measure these vitamin and minerals because excessive replacement can lead to diarrhea and other effects, resulting in additional risks and no added benefits. Additionally, taking a host of vitamins and minerals will reduce the capacity to take the large quantities of protein that are clearly essential.

Anemia

Patients are frequently anemic in this early postoperative period, especially menstruating women. Iron-deficiency anemia is the usual type. The causes of iron-deficiency anemia include some operative blood loss, reduced intake of iron as a consequence of necessary dietary restrictions, decreased absorption of iron from lack of gastric acidity (GB only), and continued losses in menstruating women. Other causes include new or continuing blood loss from the gastrointestinal tract that usually occurs at the anastomoses. Although macrocytic anemia occurs with vitamin B_{12} deficiency, it is unlikely to occur this early. Deficiency in iron stems from gastric surgery and from dieting alone. The deficiency can be very severe and can lead to significant anemia and fatigue. Unfortunately, taking iron orally causes constipation and often causes nausea, too. Iron injections are painful, expensive, and difficult to administer. All oral preparations are expensive and there is little difference in the cost. Liquid forms stain the teeth and are very expensive. Branded names of ferrous sulfate or ferrous fumarate cost more than generic brands or contain less elemental iron. Measure several serum iron levels, blood counts, and reticulocyte counts. If the patient is gradually improving it may be prudent to not give an iron supplement. If significant anemia persists, then pick some preparation of iron to administer. Consider giving epoetin alfa to stimulate red cell production, and have the patient take a stool softener and mild laxative to avoid constipation. Iron tablets should be taken with either chewable ascorbic acid or citrus juice (2 oz of orange or grapefruit juice) to increase ionization of iron and thus absorption. Iron tablets are better tolerated when taken immediately after a meal is consumed.

The intensity of the treatment should be matched to the severity of the anemia. Clearly, issues that must be addressed directly include loses from the gastrointestinal tract with endoscopy, or excessive menses with gynecologic consultation. Anemia may also occur or fail to correct rapidly from moderate to severe protein-calorie malnutrition, but usually shows indices of a normochromic, normocytic anemia. Resolution results from continued improvement in protein intake and nutritional balance over time. Monitoring blood count and indices, reticulocyte count, serum iron, and vitamin B_{12} levels, and protein balance will usually provide a guide to the appropriate treatment.

Activity

Regular exercise helps to maintain lean body mass or protein balance.[9] Some tissues and organs that rely on protein for proper function include skeletal muscle, heart, hair, skin, nails, and liver, to name a few. Exercise reduces appetite and increases sense of well-being through the secretion of endorphins during the activity.[10] Moderate exercise increases basal metabolic rate, prevents fatigue, increases stamina, and enhances weight loss, especially fat loss.[9] In the absence of regular graded exercise activities, there is a risk of losing too much lean body mass resulting in excessive hair loss, dry skin, easy bruising, broken finger nails, reduced resistance to infection, increased risk of blood clots, less overall weight loss, increased risk of regaining fat, and poor cardiovascular fitness.

Note that this section is labeled "activity," not "exercise," or "aerobics." For the morbidly obesity, the latter terms may have a negative connotation. Many have severe arthritis, back disease, and pulmonary and cardiac disease that can limit the type and activity that they can perform. Exercises performed in a swimming pool are probably the best that could be accomplished by everyone, but access to pools is very limited. Walking is the next best activity that almost everyone can complete.

Walking exercises most of the major muscle groups in the body and does not require special facilities, equipment or trainers. Walking is just a series of steps and every step counts, whether the steps are to answer the telephone, clean the garage, put away files, shop at the mall, or steps taken on a treadmill or in the park. We recommend that patients use a device such as a step meter or pedometer. The device is worn on a belt or waistband and counts steps. Patients are instructed to put the meter on their waistband first thing in the morning, record their steps at the end of the day when they go to bed, and reset the number so that it will be zero for the next day. For the first week, they are to simply record the number of steps completed each day. The next week, they are encouraged to maintain the same number of steps each day and eliminate any wide fluctuations from day to day by monitoring their step total at several time points per day. Beginning with the third week, they are to increase their steps by 250 to 500 per day each week. For example, if they are taking an average of 2000 steps per day, the next week they should increase by 500 steps to 2500 steps per day. Each subsequent week, they should increase their steps per day until they reach 10,000 steps per day.

Attempting to initiate a strenuous exercise program while losing weight on a very-low-calorie diet can lead to excessive loss of lean body mass, and an undesirable result. Sugar, specifically glucose, is needed for intense exercise. Low-calorie diets do not provide a sufficient supply of sugar, and the body's supply of glycogen is used up in the first week of dieting so that muscle (body protein) is broken down to amino acids and converted to glucose for these high-energy requirements of a strenuous exercise program if one is on a low-calorie diet. Fat and its breakdown products, glycerol and free fatty acids, cannot be converted to glucose to meet the high-energy demands of strenuous exercise. In many ways, too much exercise can be worse than too little. While metabolic studies can be done to determine how much exercise each patient can perform without reaching detrimental levels, the tests are expensive and complicated. Some advice on limits can be provided to prevent excessive loss of lean body mass to exercise. The exercise program is too intense if more than mild dyspnea is produced or if heavy perspiration is produced. If muscles burn or feel weak or rubbery immediately after exercise, or certain muscle groups are sore or stiff the next day, then the exercises were too intense. We recommend that patients avoid these symptoms, by starting slow, using light weights or low levels of resistance. Rest between activities on each muscle group. Perform the exercise for short periods several times per day rather than all at one time.

Postoperatively, walking is the only recommended activity. The type and intensity of activity in the months to come are best guided by a physical therapist or exercise physiologist who understands the physiology described above, the limitations of the patient's musculoskeletal and cardiopulmonary system, and can provide a variety of convenient and interesting activities to keep the patient motivated and aware of the benefits of their activities.[11]

Cholelithiasis Prophylaxis

Gall stones occur in approximately 30% of patients who undergo significant weight loss regardless of the method used to lose weight, medical or surgical.[12,13] Ursodiol increases the solubility of bile salts and reduces the risk of developing gallstones to approximately 2% if taken at the rate of 300 mg four times per day. Once-per-day dosing reduces the risk of developing gallstones to 50%, two times a day to 25%, and three times a day to 12 to 13%. Ursodiol is given for 6 months or for as long as the patient is losing a significant amount of weight (more than 3% of body weight per month). There are no other medications, changes in diet, or lifestyle that will prevent the development of gallstones to the same magnitude as ursodiol. The medication comes as a rather large pill and is fairly expensive. Both of these features limit the number of patients who can follow this recommendation.

Expected Weight Changes

Although fat loss is the primary goal, weight loss and hip and waist circumference are easy to measure and help the patient see how rapidly they are improving their health. The difference between calories consumed and burned will be the major contributor to weight loss, if the patient was not severely edematous prior to surgery. During the first month, 5 to 15% of total body weight loss can be expected with GB and BPD; losses with the LB are usually half that. The more the patient walks and the more carefully they follow their new dietary guidelines, the faster they will lose weight.

Review Medications

Many medications will have been discontinued at hospital discharge, including antacids, antidiabetics, antihypertensives, NSAIDs, estrogens and birth control, other over-the-counter herbs, vitamins and minerals, and antihyperlipidemics. If patients do not need these medications, ensure that they have not restarted them because of some miscommunication at each of the first four postoperative visits. Review their discharge medications to ensure that they still need them, or if they can or should be altered. Ensure that they are taking some form of chewable multivitamin, antidepressant (if indicated) and chronic medications such as thyroxin, and none of the medications that previously were mentioned to avoid if possible. Reduce the medications to the least number possible to allow room for protein and fluid intake.

Diagnostic Studies to be Ordered

The tests obtained to monitor changes that occur in the first few postoperative weeks are those that are used to monitor a very-low-calorie intake, low urine output, and those needed to monitor the changes in multiple medications. Table 7–1 lists frequently ordered tests, as well as other tests that may be indicated for the usual bariatric operations. Of course, the physician should obtain all those that are medically justified, and eliminate all those that are not. Resting energy expenditure by indirect calorimetry and body composition analysis by body impedance analysis should be obtained preoperatively and just prior to the first postoperative visit, usually within 1 month. The results of the blood tests should be reviewed as soon as available and the patient contacted to make changes in their medications, nutrition, or activity to address any abnormalities. The metabolic rate and body composition tests should be obtained every 2 to 3 months after the first postoperative month to compare to preoperative tests and to examine current trends.

TABLE 7–1. ROUTINE DIAGNOSTIC STUDIES AT FIRST POSTOPERATIVE VISITS	
TEST	PROCEDURE
Albumin	LB, GB, BPD
Body composition by BIA	LB, GB, BPD
CBC (complete blood count)	LB, GB, BPD
Electrolytes	LB, GB, BPD
Mid-stream urinalysis	LB, GB, BPD
Prealbumin	LB, GB, BPD
Resting energy expenditure	LB, GB, BPD
Serum iron	GB, BPD
Uric acid	LB, GB, BPD
Vitamin A	BPD
Vitamin B_{12}	GB, BPD
Vitamin D_{25}	BPD

Consider these optional tests to monitor presurgical problems:
   Glycated hemoglobin
   Lipid panel
   Liver panel
   Thyroid panel

Consider optional tests to monitor perioperative problems
   Abdominal/wound ultrasonography
   Chest radiograph
   Magnesium
   Phosphorus

Abbreviations: BIA = body impedance analysis; BPD = biliopancreatic diversion; GB = gastric bypass; LB = lap-band.

MANAGEMENT AT 2 TO 5 MONTHS POSTOPERATIVELY

Nutritional Review of Macro- and Micronutrients

Before each physician visit, patients should be seen by the dietitian to briefly review their progress in following instructions, including estimated protein intake in grams, estimated calorie intake, problems with intake of various food types, compliance with dietary instructions given previously, and liquid intake. The dietitian should then determine the need for further discussion that day or another day, or tell the physician that the patient is well informed and educated. The physician should be alerted to any significant deficiencies, or problems the patient is having adapting to their procedure.

   Instructions are reinforced concerning the types of foods, and volume that should be consumed, and which foods and behaviors that should be avoided. Reinforcing by providing brief written instructions should accompany the discussion to ensure there are no misunderstandings.

Recommendations for Physical Activity

The exercise physiologist should review compliance with activity recommendations, average number of steps taken daily and methods to achieve the current level of activity. The exercise specialist should provide instructions for the addition of weights, more aerobic activities, and stretch exercises for patients who are at least 2 months past their procedure. For patients with serious disability, it is important for the office to know facilities that have activities that meet the patients' capabilities and encourage the patients to become engaged in those activities. The physician should be alerted to problems with motivation and too little or too much activity.

For the average patient, upper body weights at 1 to 2.3 kg (2 to 5 lb) per arm (or the equivalent in resistance equipment) are added with recommendations for the amount of time and number of repetitions that should be done daily. It is important for patients to build some muscle in their arms to prevent loose skin from forming a "bat wing" effect that makes them self-conscious.

Review of Diagnostic Studies

Laboratory results should be reviewed with the patient along with their current list of medications. This helps to ensure that the patient is in compliance with treatment recommendations and helps them see how their activities are reflected in their studies.

If there is no significant progress in the resolution of anemia in menstruating women, review the status of their menstrual cycle and refer them to a gynecologist if heavy menses is occurring monthly. If there is no evidence of blood loss and serum iron is low, increase the intensity of iron therapy as described in the previous section.

Normal vitamin B_{12} levels are the usual result when patients are taking chewable multivitamins. If there is a desire to change to multivitamins to a pill format, obtain another measurement 1 month after the change has occurred. Low vitamin B_{12} levels with oral intake of a pill-type multivitamin after normal levels with chewable multivitamins should initiate the addition of 1 mg of sublingual B_{12} taken weekly, or sometimes daily.[14] Laboratory levels should be taken just before the next dose of B_{12} is taken to ensure that the lowest possible levels are being measured.

Elevated levels of uric acid occur because of the breakdown of lean body mass to provide energy during the period when the patient is on a low-calorie diet and from the conversion of nuclear purines to uric acid. The higher the breakdown of lean body mass, the higher the level of uric acid being generated. Uric acid is excreted by the kidney and tends to accumulate because fluid intake and urine output tend to be low at this point following surgery.[15] Additionally, uric acid shares an active transport system with ketones for urinary excretion.[16] Ketone production from the breakdown of fat is also high at this time. The primary risk of elevated uric acid is not gout (unless genetic predisposition exists), but uric acid renal stones, which can lead to uric acid nephropathy if not treated appropriately.[17] The treatment is to encourage fluid intake to increase urine volume and to give allopurinol to block the production of uric acid. The decision to give allopurinol and the dose depends on the severity of the problem and likelihood of resolution by fluid intake alone. Additional treatment includes methods to reduce losses of endogenous protein with increased activity and increased intake of protein.

Prealbumin is the best marker of nutritional status and of protein intake and balance.[18] The half-life if prealbumin is approximately 48 hours, thus it is sensitive to rapid changes in protein intake and is unaffected by hydration status. If levels are low, the patient is not taking in adequate protein. With proper consumption, levels can increase at the rate of 2 mg%/d and should reach normal levels (greater than 20 mg%) in a week. In addition to the intake of high-quality protein, prealbumin may be affected by excessive loss of lean body mass and low activity levels. To correct low prealbumin, patients need to increase the intake of high-quality protein and decrease the loss of lean body mass by following the postoperative exercise recommendations.

Review Resting Energy Expenditure and Body Composition Trends

Calorimetry is a measure of the amount of energy being used or generated. The precise definition is the amount of heat (measured in kilocalories) that is generated by a process, chemical reaction, or a person over some time period such as seconds, minutes, hours, or days. For chemical reactions, special chambers will measure the heat exchanged. For people, special rooms can measure all the heat produced by an individual. For chemical reactions, chambers are fine, but for people, the chambers are very expensive to build and impractical to use unless a small number of people are being measured as part of a scientific study. Indirect methods have been developed that measure exhaled gases to determine the volume of oxygen extracted and the volume of carbon dioxide generated to calculate energy expenditure.

The calorie content of most foods is known and is usually printed on the food packaging. The caloric content of foods is also published in lists and tables in many books and pamphlets. Body weight is determined by the number of food calories consumed and the number of calories burned for energy. It is possible to keep careful track of the amount and calorie content of food consumed to calculate precisely how many calories are consumed. However, determining the number of calories burned is more difficult. If it is not measured, as it is done for food, then only an estimation can be made. There are hundreds of formulas and permutations published to calculate energy expenditure under a variety of conditions, including disease states, such as obesity, and others.[19] The

Harris-Benedict equations[20] are probably the most commonly used. The estimation makes many assumptions about an individual's metabolic rate and efficiency. Some of these assumptions may not be valid and the estimated energy expenditure for an individual varies greatly from the actual measurement when validated methodology is used to accurately measure energy expenditure. The best way to know how much energy is being used is to measure it. Indirect calorimetry can be used to calculate the current metabolic rate. The measurement, taken while the patient is resting, is labeled the resting energy expenditure (REE). REE is expressed in kilocalories per day, and is derived from the Weir equation.[21] An average measurement is approximately 2000 kcal/d. The range could be 10,000 to 600 kcal/d or less.

The respiratory quotient (RQ) is obtained during the indirect calorimetry measurements as carbon dioxide output in mL/min divided by oxygen uptake (mL/min). This value is a measure of the current primary source of energy in the diet, which will be fat, protein, or carbohydrate. How well dietary regimens are being followed may be deduced from this measurement.[19,21]

Review of the REE measurement is compared to the estimate obtained from the Harris-Benedict equation or some other equation that attempts to predict the REE for the patient and is usually expressed as a percent of normal. After some weight loss or several weight-loss cycles, some people complain that their metabolism is very low. They eat almost nothing and yet cannot lose weight. If this is true, a measurement of their REE will show a very low rate, perhaps only 900 kcal/d, while their predicted rate maybe 2000 kcal/d based on their weight and some assumption of their activity level. The percent of normal would be 900/2000, which equals 45%. To lose weight, caloric intake must be decreased to less than 600 to 700 calories per day. Alternatively, REE may increase. Some patients with similar symptoms and complaints, however, may have a measured REE of 3000 kcal/d, or 150% of predicted value, and a very active metabolism. A careful analysis of their caloric intake must be made and those calories decreased.

For a low REE, exercise is the best way to increase metabolic rate. Exercise is to be done at a low to moderate level. If there are no physical limitations, walking at 3 to 4 miles per hour for 15 to 20 minutes per day is a good form of exercise at this point for the bariatric patient. The activity should be repeated every day to have the best effect on increasing basal metabolic rate. To get the most activity out of the widest range of patients, a step meter or pedometer to measure the number of steps taken each day should be used. If the patient still does not have their step meter, encourage them to get it now. They need to record their average number of daily steps over a week, and then increase their daily steps by 500 each week until they reach 10,000 steps per day. This method takes into account all activity because every step counts toward maintaining or increasing their metabolic rate and lean body mass. The REE should be measured at 3-month intervals to ensure that normal levels are maintained and that low levels are identified and interventions are initiated to increase the level to "normal".

The metabolic rate of some patients may not increase significantly with the maximum activity level they can perform. Physical disability may limit the type and amount of activity they can perform. Some have such a low metabolism that they complain that they do not have the "energy" to exercise. In selected patients, ephedrine has been used to increase metabolic rate, enhance weight loss, and provide the impetus to exercise.

Ephedrine stimulates the β_3 receptor to increase thermogenesis, and thus metabolic rate.[22] Fat becomes the preferred source for metabolic fuel,[23] metabolism becomes less efficient, metabolic rate increases producing more heat, and more energy becomes available for exercise. Ephedrine also stimulates β_1 receptors that increase the heart rate and cause palpitations, and β_2 receptors that cause tremor, anxiety, and insomnia. Fortunately, tachyphylaxis develops for these undesirable effects and they dissipate with time.[24–26]

Even better, the beneficial effects on fat metabolism actually increase over time.[23] To overcome some of the unwanted effects of ephedrine, the dose is gradually increased over a prolonged period. The goal is to take 25 mg of ephedrine three times per day. This can be accomplished by starting with ephedrine 25 mg daily for several days, then twice a day, and later three times per day. The dose is only increased after the unwanted side effects dissipate. It is important to increase activity while taking this medication. The goal is to be able to maintain a higher metabolism with exercise and not with medications.

Some patients are not candidates for this treatment. Difficult to control hypertension, coronary artery disease, panic attacks and tachyarrhythmias are a few conditions that may make administration unwise. Some higher risk patients may still be candidates. High-risk patients need to start on even smaller doses (12.5 mg) taken with food to slow absorption. They need frequent monitoring of their response. For most patients, these doses of ephedrine possess far less adrenergic stimulation than do medications that they took before they had surgery, including phentermine, albuterol, Adderall (amphetamine mixed salts), pseudoephedrine, sibutramine, Elavil (amitriptyline), and Desyrel (trazodone). Postoperative patients are also in better medical condition than when they took these other medications in the preoperative period.

Body composition measurement by body impedance analysis (BIA) is essential to ensure that fat is being lost and lean body mass preserved following surgery. The most sensitive and accurate method to obtain this measurement is underwater weighing. Another method that is far more convenient is the measurement by BIA. This measures the conductivity of the body and estimates fat and body mass in percent and pounds. Drinking a lot of fluid, exercising, or eating within a few hours of the test can significantly affect this measurement. While not perfect, serial measurements taken with the proper preparation provide far more accurate estimates of body composition than skin fold thickness and hip and waist measurements.

Important values to track are the percent of lean body mass and percent of fat mass. These should be approximately 75% or more and 25% or less, respectively. Many patients start with only 55 to 65% lean body mass and 35 to 45% fat. Lack of proper protein intake and a RQ of <0.7 for a prolonged period can lead to a marked loss of lean body mass and preservation of fat. The result is a body with a low metabolic rate, poor muscle tone, lack of energy, poor wound healing, increased susceptibility to infectious diseases, weight gain with minimal increase in caloric intake, and feeling cold when everyone else is warm. This condition should be avoided and is never considered a successful result regardless of the number of pounds registered on the scale.

Body composition results are best used by tracking changes over time. Measurements should have been taken before surgery and at this point one can subtract current lean body mass in pounds from that present before surgery. Likewise, current fat mass can be subtracted from fat mass before surgery. The loss of fat should be greater than the loss of lean by a ratio of 2:1 or more. A table can be made for each patient to record their preoperative body composition from some estimate of ideal. We use a BMI of 25 and lean body mass of 75% for women and 80% for men. Because patients begin with a wide variation of lean body mass, the amount of lean mass that can be lost safely varies for each. For example, a 167.6-cm (66-inch) woman might start with a total body weight of 136.1 kg (300lb) (BMI 48) of which 50% is lean (68 kg [150 lb]) and 50% is fat (68 kg [150 lb]). Her goal is to obtain a BMI of 25 (70.3 kg [155 lb]) of which 75% would be lean (52.6 kg (116 lb]) and 25% would be fat (17.7 kg (39 lb]). She loses 22.3 kg (50 lb) in the first 2 months after surgery and she is now 54% lean (61.2 kg [135 lb]) and 46% fat (52.2 kg [115 lb]). For her 22.3-kg (50-lb) weight loss, she lost 6.8 kg (15 lb) of lean mass and 15.9 kg (35 lb) of fat, a better than 2:1 ratio. If she, however continues this rate over the next 45.4 kg (100 lb) (29.9 kg [66 lb] of fat and 15 kg [33 lb] of lean), when she reaches a BMI near 25 she will have only 46.3 kg (102 lb) of lean (67%) and still 22.2 kg (49 lb) of fat (33%). Her lean mass is a negative 6.4 kg (14 lb) and she still has 4.5 kg (10 lb) of excess fat. This will be a difficult situation to reverse, adding lean body weight. It is best to avoid this by working to retain her lean mass while it is in excess, rather than trying to add it later. Some patients lose at the rate of 1:1 or worse. Tracking the loss of lean and fat mass and making corrections early provides far more optimal results in the end.

If lean body mass is being lost at a high rate and intake of high-quality protein and exercise is ineffective in modifying the trend, then ephedrine can be used to achieve the desired results. While ephedrine increases metabolic rate it does it by enhancing the loss of fat mass and protecting lean body mass.[27]

If adequate results are not obtained with ephedrine alone, caffeine or theophylline may be added to prolong and enhance its effects on metabolic rate and enhanced fat metabolism.[28]

Review Problem List

Sleep apnea may be resolved by this time. If the patient is no longer snoring, it is unlikely that they have sleep apnea. It is recommended that a sleep study with titration of their CPAP be performed to document that sleep apnea has been resolved rather just reduced in severity at this time. As weight loss continues, sleep apnea will almost certainly be cured.

Hypertension has already been resolved or should be by this time. If not, it is likely that the patient does not have hypertension secondary to obesity, but has a primary cause. While the number and dose of antihypertensive will probably be less, they may require continued treatment regardless of how much further weight loss is obtained. If treatment is required, avoid diuretics for the reasons given previously.[29] Beta-blockers tend to cause muscle weakness and is not advisable at a time when activity is being encouraged to maintain lean body mass.

Nausea and vomiting, if acute and severe, could always be signs of gastric outlet obstruction, or small-bowel obstruction. A barium swallow or upper endoscopy may be indicated. Food could be lodged in the gastric outlet at a stricture or inflammation could be the cause of obstruction. Endoscopy may be used to remove the foreign body, and balloon dilation to open the gastric outlet. Small-bowel obstructions may occur at any time, but those caused by adhesions seem to be most prevalent and usually occur before 6 months postoperatively. If the nausea and vomiting is a result of continued inappropriate eating behavior or food selection, intensive dietary and psychological support needs to be instituted before permanent structural damage occurs and the procedure becomes incompetent to modify food intake.

Dyspnea on exertion is either markedly improved or resolved at this time. If not, then this may be an indication that other cardiopulmonary problems are present. This could be related to surgery, increasing pleural effusion from infection or severe malnutrition, or unrelated new or advancing disease.

Diabetes mellitus is usually cured at this point. Patients with supermorbid obesity and diabetes may take a few more months to resolve their insulin resistance. If diabetes has suddenly gotten worse, there is a risk that some major new stress has occurred. The stress could be psychosocial, but is usually due to infection, wound, pulmonary, or urinary tract as the most likely candidates.

Arthritis symptoms and low back pain usually are significantly improved. Less weight bearing is the primary cause for improvement as well as an improvement in mood that likely minimizes pain. Some patients have some increase in pain especially knees and hips where they require replacement. The increased activity, that they feel so much better in performing, increases pain in their most debilitated joints.

Antidepressants may be discontinued at this time if prescribed for a reversible chemical imbalance, or a situation that has resolved. Patients with long histories preoperatively may require treatment indefinitely or for extended periods. Psychological reassessment can aid in arriving at a decision in any situations that are questionable.

Diagnostic Studies to be Ordered

Laboratory tests based on any ongoing problems or adjustment in medications may be obtained, such as thyroid functions, vitamin levels, or glycated hemoglobin, but the usual tests that are needed at this time to ensure that common problems are resolved include blood count, basic metabolic panel, prealbumin, and uric acid. Lipid panel may be ordered before the next visit. If the hyperlipidemia was likely to be secondary to obesity, wait for 5 to 6 months postopoperatively before ordering the lipid panel to allow sufficient time for a cure. If patient was likely to have a primary cause of hyperlipidemia, then obtain the lipid panel before 6 months so that antilipid agents can be restarted as soon as adequate protein intake has been established.

If the patient required ephedrine treatment, the patient will return within 1 month to check vital signs and symptomatic response to the medications. REE and body composition will be obtained in 2 to 3 months from that appointment. Patients not taking ephedrine will have REE and body composition measured 3 months from the current visit.

If the patient's BMI will be near 30 by the next visit, then testing for osteoporosis should be done. A DXA (dual-energy x-ray absorption), or bone density, scan should be obtained before the next visit.[30] If the equipment is available (usually attached to the DXA scanner), then body fat analysis by DXA should also be performed at this time. A blood test for N-telopeptide index is also obtained to aid in the measurement of bone turnover should the risk for osteoporosis be detected.[31] The index may be used to measure the effect of treatment, if needed, before a second DXA scan is obtained. The evaluation for osteoporosis is usually not done before this time. Bone density is commonly very high in the morbidly obese and DXA scans reflect this state. Once significant weight has been lost, and if patients have a high risk of osteoporosis because of long-term lack of estrogen, family history, poor calcium intake history, repeated treatment with glucocorticoids for asthma, autoimmune disease, or joint disease, then the DXA scan can detect the initial signs of osteoporosis and preventative treatment can be instituted.

MANAGEMENT AT 6 TO 12 MONTHS POSTOPERATIVELY

Nutritional Review

Patients should be able to eat approximately 1 cup of food in 30 to 45 minutes, three meals per day, and a snack at this time. Protein intake should not be a problem by this time and a variety of foods should be easy to ingest to maintain protein levels, including white fish, tuna, shellfish, chicken breast, very lean ground beef, eggs, beans, low-fat cheese, and milk. Other foods that should be taken include vegetables for fiber and a limited quantity of fruit for desserts.

Physical Activity Recommendations

If weight is beginning to plateau, then activities that include more strength training and aerobic exercises are indicated. More weights and more cardiopulmonary exercises may be performed, but again at a gradually increasing intensity. Higher impact exercises should only be prescribed if the cardiovascular system can tolerate the activity and weight loss has indeed begun to plateau. If weight loss is still significant, then excessive loss of lean body mass is still a risk until caloric intake nearly matches calories burned. If the patient is taking ephedrine, then exercises are performed before the morning dose of ephedrine or at least 4 hours after the last dose to avoid excessive strain on the cardiovascular system.

Review Diagnostic Studies

Lipid panel should be normal and there will be no need to repeat this as long as patient maintains their weight loss. If it is abnormal and the patient has lost 60% or more of their excess body weight, then it is likely that the patient has a primary form of hyperlipidemia and will require pharmacologic treatment.

DXA bone density scan is usually normal, but now the test is more sensitive at detecting osteoporosis than with patients who have a BMI of 40, 50, or 60 kg/m^2. Measurements are usually taken of both hips and the lumbar spine. If there is indication of moderate risk at more than two sites, or high risk at any site, the patient should be treated. If calcium intake is, or has been relatively low, then start the patient on calcium citrate, the best absorbed of the calcium preparations available. If a patient has no contraindication to taking estrogen and has no uterus, then estrogen can be given. If a patient requires progesterone as well because of an intact uterus, then it may be better to use calcitonin to avoid side effects from the combination estrogen–progesterone therapy that includes weight gain, migraine headaches, resumption of menses, and others. Do not use alendronate because of the potential for severe reflux esophagitis. In 1 to 2 months, the *N*-telopeptide index may be obtained to see if bone turnover has been affected and to decide on further modification of treatment if indicated. A DXA scan should be repeated at about 6 months to monitor the effect of treatment and modify as appropriate.

REE and body composition should be evaluated to ensure that metabolic rate is being maintained, or responding appropriately, if ephedrine treatment was begun. Likewise, the trend in body composition analysis of lean mass and fat mass should be reevaluated. If the combination of protein intake, activity and the maximum dose of ephedrine are being taken (25 mg three times per day), then the addition of theophylline slow release at 200 to 600 mg or caffeine at up to 200 mg three times per day may be added to increase the effectiveness of ephedrine.

Cholelithiasis Prophylaxis

If weight loss has stabilized, then ursodiol may be discontinued.

Elective Procedures

If weight loss has stabilized, prealbumin levels are normal, lean body mass is 75 to 80% of total weight, then wound healing, resistance to infection, and tolerance to stress should be very good. Patients should be good candidates for elective procedures for panniculectomy, orthopedic procedures, dentures or other major dental work, or plastic surgical procedures.

MANAGEMENT AFTER 12 MONTHS POSTOPERATIVELY

At this time, the goals are to lose weight, obtain a body composition that can be maintained, and achieve resolution of most comorbid diseases.

The attempt is made for patients to reach a BMI of less than 25 but greater than 21. However, the more important measure is that of body composition. Regardless of weight, women should have a lean body mass greater than 75%, and men, greater than 80%. Any modification of body weight, once these lean body masses are achieved is considered cosmetic and no longer would have any significant impact on their medical risk factors.

If patients are still on ephedrine, then attempts should be made to wean them off while ensuring that they are maintaining a normal metabolic rate and body composition without it. This is rarely a problem, and most patients discontinue ephedrine on their own when they find they no longer need it.

All comorbid diseases that were potentially reversible should be resolved by this time.

Maintenance

Even if all comorbid disease has resolved, patients should be reevaluated at annual intervals. The long-term effects of these procedures are poorly defined. The LAP-BAND experience in the United States is limited to less than 10 years and effects or response for more than 5 years is not well known. The BPD produces a greater risk for loss of fat-soluble vitamins, osteomalacia, and protein malnutrition than other procedures and should be monitored on a regular basis. The GB effects on vitamin B_{12}, iron, protein balance, and osteoporosis should continue to be monitored on an annual basis.

Changes in lifestyle that may be detrimental to the continuing function of the bariatric procedure should be addressed aggressively by the entire treatment team to avoid either revision procedures or failure of maintenance of weight loss.

SUMMARY

Bariatric surgical procedures for weight loss are by far the most effective methods currently available to help morbidly obese people achieve a healthy weight. To maximize the benefit from these procedures and to reduce the complications, a well-organized management program is essential. The keys to this management are to concentrate on preventing problems early and to avoid trying to do everything immediately. To minimize long-term problems from protein loss, the adequate intake of protein must be stressed with adequate counseling to help the patient find a source of palatable and affordable protein. Activity that is tolerated, convenient to perform with immediate feedback provided with a step meter is crucial. Keep the number of drugs as low as possible. Do not try to treat every minor symptom or give medications that will require more medications to control side effects.

The goal of the procedure and program is to teach the patient to eat a normal healthy diet and to perform regular physical activity. It is not to test the procedure to see if it is working, or challenge it to see how long it will last. To avoid destructive approaches such as these, education is essential, with support groups and a knowledgeable staff.

The entire team needs to be consistent in following the management protocols, and the management program needs to be flexible so that new information can be incorporated and outdated notions discarded. To meet these goals, it is critical to have a quality control program in place to evaluate the protocols being followed and monitor the effects of new plans that are initiated.

After undergoing this drastic, expensive and painful procedure, it is only logical to ensure that the most healthy result is obtained, and it remains functional for as long as possible.

REFERENCES

1. Fletcher EC. Obstructive sleep apnea and cardiovascular morbidity. *Monaldi Arch Chest Dis* 1996;51(1):77–80.
2. Pekarovics S, WJ Raum, SR Klein. Vertical-banded gastroplasty versus gastric bypass: weight loss and impact on comorbid conditions. *Obes Surg* 1998;8:169.
3. Guldstand M, Ahren B, Adamson U. Improved beta-cell function after standardized weight reduction in severely obese subjects *Am J Physiol Endocrinol Metab* 2003;284(3)E557–E565.
4. Ryan AS, Nicklas BJ, Berman DM. Hormone replacement therapy, insulin sensitivity, and abdominal obesity in postmenopausal women. *Diabetes Care* 2002;25(1):127–133.
5. Ardern DW, Atkinson DR, Fenton AJ. Peri-operative use of oestrogen containing medications and deep vein thrombosis—a national survey. *N Z Med J* 2002;115(1157):U26.
6. Berken GH, Weinstein DO, Stern WC. Weight gain. A side-effect of tricyclic antidepressants. *J Affect Disord* 1984;7(2):133–138.
7. Levine J, Dykoski RK, Janoff EN. *Candida*-associated diarrhea: a syndrome in search of credibility. *Clin Infect Dis* 1995;21(4):881–886.
8. Hasler WL. Dumping syndrome. *Curr Treat Options Gastroenterol* 2002;5(2):139–145.
9. Svendsen OL, Hassager C, Christiansen C. Effect of an energy-restrictive diet, with or without exercise, on lean tissue mass, resting metabolic rate, cardiovascular risk factors and bone in overweight postmenopausal women. *Am J Med* 1993;95:131–140.

10. Dunn AL, Blain SN. Exercise prescription. In: Morgan WP, ed. *Physical Activity and Mental Health.* Washington, DC: Taylor and Francis; 1997:49–62.

11. Marcus BH, Pinto BM, Clark MM, DePue JD, Goldstein MG, Silverman LS. Physician-delivered physical activity and nutrition interventions. *Med Exerc Nutr Health* 1995;4:325–334.

12. Sugarman HJ, Brewer WH, Shiffman ML, et al. A multicenter, placebo-controlled, randomized, double-blind, prospective trial of prophylactic ursodiol for the prevention of gallstone formation following gastric-bypass-induced rapid weight loss. *Am J Surg* 1995;169(1)91–96.

13. Shiffman ML, Kaplan GD, Brinkman-Kaplan V, Vickers FF. Prophylaxis against gallstone formation with ursodeoxycholic acid in patients participating in a very-low-calorie diet program. *Ann Intern Med* 1995;122(12):899–905.

14. Delpre G, Stark P, Niv Y. Sublingual therapy for cobalamin deficiency as an alternative to oral and parenteral cobalamin supplementation. *Lancet* 1999;354(9180):740–741.

15. Gougeon R. The metabolic response to two very-low-energy diets (VLED) of differing amino acid composition during weight reduction. *Int J Obes Relat Metab Disord* 1992;16(12):1005–1012.

16. Roch-Ramel F, Werner D, Guisan B. Urate transport in brush-border membrane of human kidney. *Am J Physiol* 1994;266(5 pt 2):F797–F805.

17. Zurcher HU, Meier HR, Huber M, Lammli J, Wick A, Binswanger U. Acute kidney failure as a complication of fasting therapy. *Schweiz Med Wochenschr Suppl* 1977;107(29):1025–1028.

18. Beck FK, Rosenthal TC. Prealbumin: a marker for nutritional evaluation. *Am Fam Physician* 2002;65(8):1575–1578.

19. McClave SA, Snider HL. Use of indirect calorimetry in clinical nutrition. *Nutr Clin Prac* 1992;7:207–221.

20. Garrell DR, Jobin N, de Jonge LH. Should we still use the Harris and Benedict equations? *Nutr Clin Prac* 1996;11:99–103.

21. Feurer I, Mullen JL. Bedside measurement of resting energy expenditure and respiratory quotient via indirect calorimetry. *Nutr Clin Prac* 1986;1:43–49.

22. Astrup A. Thermogenesis in human brown adipose tissue and skeletal muscle induced by sympathomimetic stimulation. *Acta Endocrinol Suppl* 1986;278:1–32.

23. Malecka-Tendera E. Effect of ephedrine and theophylline on weight loss, resting energy expenditure and lipoprotein lipase activity in obese over-fed rats. *Int J Obes Relat Metab Disord* 1993;17(6):343–347.

24. Pasquali R, Cesari MP, Melchionda N, Stefanini C, Raitano A, Labo G. Does ephedrine promote weight loss in low-energy-adapted obese women? *Int J Obes* 1987;11(2):163–168.

25. Daly PA, Krieger DR, Dulloo AG, Young JB, Landsberg L. Ephedrine, caffeine and aspirin: safety and efficacy for treatment of human obesity. *Int J Obes Relat Metab Disord* 1993;17(Suppl 1):S73–S78.

26. Waluga M, Janusz M, Karpel E, Hartleb M, Nowak A. Cardiovascular effects of ephedrine, caffeine and yohimbine measured by thoracic electrical bioimpedance in obese women. *Clin Physiol* 1998;18(1):69–76.

27. Greenway FL. The safety and efficacy of pharmaceutical and herbal caffeine and ephedrine use as a weight loss agent. *Obes Rev* 2001;2(3):199–211.

28. Astrup A, Breum L, Toubro S, Hein P, Quaade F. The effect and safety of an ephedrine/caffeine compound compared to ephedrine, caffeine and placebo in obese subjects on an energy-restricted diet. A double-blind trial. *Int J Obes Relat Metab Disord* 1992;16(4):269–77.

29. Ogilvie RI. Diuretic treatment in essential hypertension. *Curr Med Res Opin* 1983;8(Suppl 3):53–58.
30. Blake GM, Fogelman I. Dual-energy x-ray absorptiometry and its clinical applications. *Semin Musculoskelet Radiol* 2002;6(3):207–218.
31. Demers LM. Bone markers in the management of patients with skeletal metastases. *Cancer* 2003;97(3 Suppl):874–879.

CHAPTER

PREPARING A HOSPITAL FOR BARIATRIC PATIENTS

LOUIS F. MARTIN / MERITA BURNEY / VONDA GAITOR-STAMPLEY / TERRY WHEELER / WILLIAM J. RAUM

Bariatric surgery began in the 1950s, in several hospitals, with several surgical teams attempting radically new ideas to provide operations for a very few morbid/superobese patients who presented with not only a weight above 181.4 kg (400 lb) but with life-threatening comorbid diseases such as obesity–hypoventilation syndrome (Pickwickian syndrome), recurrent cellulitis of their edematous lower legs or abdominal pannus, or uncontrollable adult-onset diabetes, where it was believed that these patients would die unless a surgical solution could be improvised (see Chapter 2). Since these early beginnings, the field of bariatric surgery has provided many patients with great hope and permanent changes in weight, associated with huge increases in quality of life. On the other hand, some of these ideas that produced weight loss initiated other problems, sometimes life-threatening, that have challenged anesthesiologists, internists, endocrinologists, pulmonologists, cardiologists, critical care specialists, and psychiatrists to rethink many axioms in their own fields that failed when they were applied to treating the morbidly obese.

ONE SIZE DOES NOT FIT ALL!

Not only have medical and surgical techniques and treatments had to change, but morbidly obese patients have shown physicians and hospital administrators that they cannot use most of the standard equipment that is purchased by physician offices and hospitals. Medical manufacturers usually design their products by applying the adage that "one size fits all," which really means only for those patients who weigh less than 136.1 kg (300 lb) or at most 158.8 kg (350 lb). A 226.8-kg (500-lb) patient will break most standard armless chairs and cannot fit inside any chair with arms. They will break wall-mounted toilets (when the toilet is bolted into the wall instead of being bolted on the floor) in hospitals rooms or lobbies or in physician offices. They need wider doors and wider hallways to move through comfortably and many will not be able to walk more than 200 to 300 feet without needing a bench to sit on and rest.

There are even bigger problems with the most expensive hospital diagnostic and supportive supplies. Initially, surgeons bolted two hospital operating room (OR) tables together and two hospital single beds to accommodate these patients who often broke single tables and single beds, just like they broke toilets off the walls in bathrooms. Bolting beds together was not a satisfactory solution, however, because patients could not be transported to other areas in the hospital in this double-wide bed because it would not fit in elevators or even through most doors or hallways. The operating room situation was even worse. Patients' intraabdominal contents that surgeons needed to reach to perform their operations were between the two tables. Reaching over both the patients' external fat and the bed and then into a deeper abdominal cavity was backbreaking work. The need for standard-width operating tables and beds that could support patients up to 294.8 kg (650 lb), or even 362.9 kg (800 lb), was quickly realized.

Although morbidly obese patients are a small percentage of the population, their health needs are probably 10 times greater than most other patient groups, especially in light of their admission rates in any given year to hospitals. This is recognized by some hospital supply companies and by medical insurance companies, who are aware of how much more medical care is needed by the morbidly obese. Medical insurance companies try to avoid covering them. When the Northern California Kaiser-Permanente insurance region reviewed all health care costs for all their members in one year, they found that the morbidly obese cost 44% more to treat per year than did the members who were not overweight or obese.[1] Hospital charges are 35% higher for morbidly obese patients who receive artificial joints than for the nonmorbidly obese, in large part because of longer lengths of hospital stay. We have previously reviewed these data.[2]

While medical insurance companies and some hospitals choose to shun the morbidly obese, other aspects of the medical industry see the market need for special products. The American Society for Bariatric Surgery (ASBS) members have worked diligently for years to convince many companies to make products that they desperately need to safely treat these patients. The ASBS web site (www.asbs.org) has a list of these products that is constantly updated with contact information for each company. Products that are now readily available include regular-size operating room tables (remember the skeleton of morbidly obese patients is not bigger than that of lighter patients) that can perform all their usual functions for weights up to 294.8 kg (650 lb) and a heavy duty model that supports up to 385.6 kg (850 lb). There are hospital beds and hospital gurneys (the stretchers on wheels) that can support similar weights. These are also extra-wide, heavy-duty wheelchairs, walkers, port-a-potties, and hospital/office chairs and sofas that support between 294.8 kg (650 lb) and 453.6+ kg (1000+ lb). Hospital gowns for patients and scrub uniforms worn by nurses and physicians (our whole population is becoming more obese yearly,[3] including hospital personnel) now come in extra-large (XL), 2X, 3X, 4X, and 5X sizes. These plus-size hospital gowns are prized even by other patients who can wrap the gowns around them at least twice, eliminating one of the more embarrassing patient problems.

Bariatric surgeons and their hospitals need extra-wide, extra-long (circumference) blood pressure cuffs; big platform scales that a patient can hold onto for balance that provide accurate weights to 362.9 kg (800 lb) to 453.6 kg (1000 lb) (these eliminate asking patients to weigh themselves on truck or laundry scales at the hospital); heavy-duty exam tables; wide doors and hallways; and bathrooms equipped with handicap rails.

Almost all the instruments routinely manufactured for abdominal operations are "standard size" and, therefore, too short to be used for patients weighing more than 158.8 kg (350 lb). To special order longer instruments significantly increases the price, but is usually possible for the instrument companies. When disposable "stapling" devices and other disposable instruments for laparoscopic and open operations were developed beginning in the 1970s, no manufacturer was willing to produce more than one size. When adjustable gastric banding procedures and gastric bypass where demonstrated to be equally safe and less disabling than open procedures to treat morbid obesity, only the lighter group of this population could be treated because, again, the instruments were not long enough to reach the intraabdominal organs after first having to transverse 12.7 cm (5 inches) or more of subcutaneous fat (see Chapter 2).

The increase in acceptance of laparoscopic bariatric operations, however, created a much greater demand for longer disposable instruments. Smaller companies were the first to respond to this market; now several *Fortune* 500 companies have convinced themselves that providing products for the morbidly obese is a profitable way to increase their market share. This competition will help to control costs. More importantly, it has added the engineering creativity and the educational resources these big companies have to the creation of better medical equipment, which should decrease morbidity rates for these patients and better educational tools to improve the patients' transition to new lifestyles.

It has taken longer to have radiology equipment manufacturers understand that they also need to make their products suitable for patients who weigh more than 136.1 kg (300 lb). More than 90% of the fluoroscopy suites in the world do not have a table to accommodate someone who weighs more than 136.1 kg (300 lb). Most computed axial tomography (CAT) scanners and magnetic resonance imaging (MRI) tables do not have a heavy-duty motor that will move patients who weigh more than 147.4 kg (325 lb) into the image-producing tunnel of these machines. Those of us who were trained before there were CAT scanners or MRI imaging devices are not as handicapped by this unavailability of diagnostic services. Physicians younger than 45 years of age, however, have always had these services available. All of their diagnostic routines to make certain diagnoses incorporate these tools, and they have had to develop the confidence to make decisions for the heavier morbidly obese patient without having had this type of information available. There are also, finally, a few manufacturers who have modified their equipment so that it can handle patients who weigh 204.1 kg (450 lb). But as our American population continues to increase yearly in weight,[3] even heavier-duty equipment needs to be manufactured.

HOW IS THIS FIELD EVOLVING?

This book, the first by a major publishing company in more than a decade, is just one example of the realization that the morbidly obese have been vastly undertreated for at least the last two decades and that there are a great many morbidly obese patients who are now seeking operative therapy. *Fortune* 500 companies are designating bariatric surgery products as a major growth industry for their business and are creating new divisions dedicated to new product lines. Although it takes years to obtain permission from the FDA to sell a new product to be used surgically, these companies know that with so few products available, everyone is at the same starting line. They also know that there are not enough trained surgeons to treat all the morbidly obese patients seeking bariatric operations at this time, so it is premature to overadvertise until more are trained to perform these procedures. The companies are trying to prepare for an expanding market.

The successful introduction of the first adjustable gastric band to treat morbid obesity in the United States and the availability of at least five other bands elsewhere in the world are another sign of both the increased acceptance of bariatric surgery (especially less-invasive laparoscopic procedures) and of the exponential market growth for new bariatric products. There are societies of bariatric surgeons in countries of all the inhabited continents and the number of general surgeons who are interested in mastering these difficult operations has also grown exponentially for at least the past 5 years.

This expansion of interest in bariatric operations and the influx of talent and energy to this field are also creating problems. First, every health insurance program—from Medicare and Medicaid to the smallest insurance companies—worries about how to pay for this backlog of morbidly obese patients who either had a clause denying coverage for any obesity treatments (often lumping bariatric procedures used to treat life-threatening disease with cosmetic procedures or liquid diets) or who did not have access to a bariatric surgical center in their locale. This discriminatory treatment of the people with morbid obesity, trying to deny that their disease was not as life-threatening as coronary artery disease or some forms of cancer, was exposed by the (NIH) National Institutes of Health's and the (WHO) World Health Organization's publication of their evidence-based reports on obesity, imploring all governments to spend more money on obesity research to look for better curative and preventative strategies and outlining for all physicians how important it is to treat obesity.[4,5]

In Louisiana, the state's Office of Group Benefits (a state-run insurance program for state employees) completed a survey of its approximately 250,000 members in 2002. This insurance program had not covered any obesity treatments for at least 10 years. The survey stated that a trial of a limited number of bariatric operations would be contracted for in 2003 and asked anyone who met the NIH criteria to be considered for bariatric surgery to send in a letter indicating their interest. The state was in the process of contracting for 40 bariatric operations, not wanting to spend over $1 million. The state received 1000 responses requesting surgery from members who met NIH criteria. State officials and the executive board were stunned. They have missed several self-created deadlines to start the contract, trying to resolve the issues involved in this overwhelming demand, including considering creating criteria different than that of the NIH so as to minimize the state's risk and make it harder to qualify for surgery.

Even though there are multiple publications suggesting that treating morbid obesity effectively in midlife should be cheaper than treating all of the consequences of the comorbid diseases caused by being morbidly obese, the insurance companies have cost analyses and data enabling them to predict expenses by using their current benefit packages. They are afraid of the unknown: What will it cost for the next several years if bariatric surgery is offered to this undertreated population? Can they stay in business long enough to benefit from the decreased costs of treating future medical problems? Executives lose jobs over quarterly income and expense reports; they do not retain their jobs based on 10-year savings.

Until 2001, fewer than 20% of academic medical centers training surgical residents had a bariatric treatment program. Now, general surgeons everywhere are interested in learning how to perform bariatric operations to increase their income. All general surgeons who had learned to perform a laparoscopic gastric bypass consider it the hardest abdominal operation to master laparoscopically of those procedures performed regularly. Academic centers who do not teach these techniques to their residents may be cited by the review organizations that monitor the quality of training programs as deficient in providing this high-level training, so now every center wants to develop a program.

PROBLEMS INITIATING A NEW PROGRAM

This rush to start new hospital programs and train all general surgeons to perform bariatric procedures worries the executive counsel of the American Society for Bariatric Surgeons (ASBS). Almost all of the 200 to 300 members of this organization in the late 1990s viewed bariatric surgery as a specialty that required a full-time and expensive support system to get the best results. While the programs in the early 1960s usually consisted of the surgeon, their office staff, and the hospital's dietician, this has changed over time. Currently, most established ASBS members' office staff is set up as outlined in Chapter 6 and includes many more support people. Most experienced bariatric surgeons have learned from their early experiences that each patient who receives a bariatric operation requires hours of support for months from a variety of specialists. If this is not provided, then the surgeon will have a higher complication rate and spend less time operating and more time trying to provide the support these other professionals are better trained to provide.

These operations are behavior-modification procedures that require each patient to make extensive changes in his/her eating and exercise habits to be successful. Long-term success requires the help of exercise specialists, who understand what exercises are practical for the different types of morbidly obese patients who request medical and surgical treatments. Patients need progressive weekly food lists to guide them through their first 3 to 4 months of establishing new eating habits, with a dietician available to support them and answer their questions, and approximately 50% require psychotherapy (see Chapter 6, describing the range of problems most bariatric practices have encountered in the last 10 years). Most of us try to follow our patients regularly for at least 6 months to a year (rather than the two postoperative visits and goodbye associated with other general surgical procedures) and many of our patients need our offices' support for years.

Membership in the ASBS has increased significantly since 1999 and yearly meeting attendance has increased from several hundred to several thousand people, doubling each year for the last three years (2000 to 2002). Senior members of the ASBS are more worried about the general surgeons who are not asking for the organization's help as they start performing bariatric surgery than about the surgeons who attend the yearly meeting or numerous weekend courses, and even mini-fellowships set up by experienced surgeons. In 1999, four hospitals in the state of Louisiana had bariatric surgical programs that were staffed by multidisciplinary teams. At the start of 2003, in the New Orleans metropolitan area alone, bariatric surgery is being performed at nine area hospitals, most without the same level of support the established programs have had for years. Also, only one of the surgeons initiating their hospital's program asked our advice or wanted our help to minimize his learning curve. Alternatively, we have interacted with dozens of hospitals from outside our area.

Additionally, many other Louisiana hospitals are considering starting programs or have surgeons who are seeking to be credentialed to perform bariatric surgery. The Advisory Board Company in Washington, DC, a nationally recognized "think tank" that advises health care entities, prepared a booklet in 2002, *Bariatric Surgery Programs: Clinical Innovation Profile*, which suggests that initiating a bariatric surgical program might be a highly profitable venture for hospital administrative staffs and hospital corporations to consider. This is a very prestigious group outlining what profits are possible in their report, but it does not extensively discuss the risks or the hidden expenses of initiating a modern bariatric surgical treatment program.

Hospital executives who have read this pamphlet and contacted us for advice on how to proceed, have not had a very realistic grasp of the complication profile for this type of surgery or these types of patients. Many smaller hospitals and surgeons want to minimally invest in initiating a program to determine how well it will attract patients and whether the hospital staffs and the surgeons think the financial remuneration is appropriate for the resources all experienced bariatric practices think are necessary to conduct a state-of-the-art bariatric surgical program. We always advise them not to start a half-baked, minimalist program and encourage them to visit successful centers to see the resources these practices have invested in their bariatric programs. Most high-risk surgical procedures have to be performed regularly (high-volume, consistent approach, built-in quality improvement program) and in a consistent manner to obtain the best results.[6] Also, most hospital personnel still do not view surgical treatment of morbid obesity as a necessary procedure like a coronary artery bypass graft to treat coronary artery disease. One early major complication or death can turn the staff against the program quickly unless they have been extensively educated on the morbidity and mortality associated with being morbidly obese. Many medical staffs still see the obese as gluttons and find a death after an elective procedure to treat a "fat person" unacceptable for the hospital's reputation. This is especially true if they think the hospital or surgeon has not approached this endeavor with the proper resources. Additionally, if they are asked to consult on a very ill patient and are told none of the diagnostic equipment in the hospital can accommodate the patient's weight, they are now potentially part of a malpractice case.

HOW TO DETERMINE WHETHER A BARIATRIC PROGRAM WILL WORK

We have discussed the financial obligations that need to be considered before starting a bariatric surgical program. The Advisory Board's publications *Bariatric Surgery Programs: Clinical Innovation Profile* suggests that this type of program can generate a new source of income. Bariatric surgical programs also provide a needed service to an underserved group of patients. If done well, and if there is sufficient patient volume for the local and regional competition, bariatric programs are usually profitable. This is directly dependent on who the major insurers are in the area and what type of contracts the hospital and the surgeons have with these companies. Consultants that may be needed, such as pulmonologists, gastroenterologists, and radiologists, also need to be involved in the planning and need to know how their contracts will affect their reimbursements. Most insurance companies will not reimburse anyone if the primary diagnosis is obesity, although it may for morbid obesity [a different International Classification of Diseases (ICD-9) code] and another significant comorbidity. Consults and diagnostic testing must have the proper diagnoses. If an admitting clerk or a ward clerk enters obesity as the diagnosis because it is what they see and no other diagnoses are provided, neither the hospital nor the physician will receive reimbursement.

It is important to understand that both the field of bariatric surgery and the health care insurance industry's response to this field is in flux. For many insurance companies, both the hospital and surgeon will be able to receive more reimbursement for a patient who has gastric surgery for an ulcer or who has a significant other disease such as renal failure, but the coding system will deny the use of the same modifiers if a bariatric operation is performed. Insurance companies may decrease reimbursement rates for bariatric surgery. There are no hard data within the United States that document the average intensity of service required for bariatric surgery to demand appropriate reimbursement. Many insurance companies are disallowing new bariatric procedures that use FDA-approved devices stating that until 5 years of postmarketing surveillance data is collected, they will consider the procedure experimental.

Several respected surgical organizations, including the American College of Surgeons (ACS), the ASBS, and Society of American Gastrointestinal Endoscopic Surgeons (SAGES), the major laparoscopic surgical society, have published recommended criteria that surgeons should meet to practice bariatric surgery. All recognize the need for a multidisciplinary team approach to the evaluation and follow-up of these patients. The National Institutes of Health (NIH) recently finished accepting applications to identify and fund four to six Centers of Excellence for Bariatric Surgical Research. One goal of this new program is to organize a database to follow bariatric surgical outcomes over decades rather than several years and to organize trials whose outcomes will produce an evidence-based approach to the many unanswered questions in this field.

Generally, senior bariatric surgeons hold the opinion that this field will have to organize so that outcome results are available by hospital program and/or surgeon, similar to transplant centers or cardiac surgery data that in some states is published from administrative databases, and in other states is collected and certified by participating surgeons and hospitals in the Society of Thoracic Surgeons' database. Unfortunately for centers transplanting kidneys or livers, the only criteria that seem to matter to most insurers is that a certain number of cases are performed each year and, more importantly, what the package price is. The 1- and 5-year survival rates for the organs are not usually a consideration. This is partly because most patients stay with the same insurance company for an average of less than 3 years, making 5-year outcome data irrelevant to them for the time being. The insurance industry also is in a constant state of flux so this will also change.

OUR MODEL FOR A BARIATRIC SURGICAL PRACTICE

While there are not many published models of bariatric surgical programs, we published our evaluation and follow-up routines several years ago, and continue to use this multidisciplinary model,[7] which is very similar to that outlined in Chapter 6. We now perform more than 80% of our procedures laparoscopically, often encouraging larger patients to use high-protein, low-calorie diets for up to several months preoperatively to make it possible to use these techniques. Our current breakdown of procedures is 88% gastric bypasses and 12% adjustable gastric bands for new patients. Approximately 5% of our practice is reoperative bariatric procedures for poor results (see Chapter 16).

We consider it optimal to have each surgeon perform at least 20 bariatric procedures per month. Generally, fewer than half of the morbidly obese patients who contact our office have insurance that provides benefits for bariatric surgery. Approximately 25% of the patients who start their evaluation after we have confirmed that they have benefits, drop out before the evaluation is complete, or do not meet all the criteria that their insurance company requires to qualify for a bariatric procedure. More than 67% of the patients who initially request an adjustable gastric band as their treatment have insurance that will not yet cover this procedure, or they become convinced that a gastric bypass may be a better procedure for them once they learn more about the different bariatric procedures.

Our office is an outpatient department of our hospital. We work exclusively in one hospital and our physicians and hospital executives are a team that meet at least weekly to design quarterly and yearly goals. We review our progress weekly and have a continuous quality improvement plan, which has helped us identify problems very quickly. We have approximately 5000 square feet of space. We have four bariatric surgeons supported by two internists, one psychologist, two social workers, two dietitians, one exercise specialist, one nurse practitioner, one rotating surgical resident, four office staffers, a marketing specialist, an administrative assistant for our academic matters, one or two research staffers, and an office manager who is on the executive staff of the hospital. Both the medical school's practice program and the hospital share expenses for the seminars held both at the office and at locations throughout the surrounding 161-km (100-mile) radius each week.

We have four full sets of laparoscopic instruments (50% of which were special orders) and two open sets. Two of the operating rooms are especially designed and equipped for morbidly obese patients, with ceiling mounted equipment and voice-activated computer systems, and are interfaced with our medical school's learning center and all other facilities that can accept and receive data at 10 megabytes per second. We are completing interfacing with the hospital's information network, which will enable the operating surgeons to transmit real-time images to surgeons working in the clinic if consultation to document the appropriateness of a decision is needed. We have an OR light-mounted camera for open cases, as well as our laparoscopic cameras, which are all digital. We also expect to be able to review fluoroscopic procedures on our patients with the radiologist digitally on our 101.6-cm (40-inch) plasma screen in the near future.

We rarely admit patients postoperatively to an intensive care unit (ICU) setting unless intubation with ventilator assistance is required for obesity hypoventilation syndrome or other known serious preoperative problems. Instead, the hospital has built a 10-room bariatric unit with the special features bariatric patients require. All rooms have special spacious bathrooms that are equipped for 294.8+-kg (650+-lb) disabled people, with toilets affixed to the floor, shower seats, handrails, and the other features bariatric patients require, including telemetry of vital signs and pulse oximetry. Only one room is not a private room and this is used as an overflow room for the rest of the hospital or for our nonobese postoperative patients who do not need as much space to move around. All rooms can accommodate a family member overnight. Most importantly, our nurse-patient ratio in this area is 1:3 to 4. The ICU ratio is 1:1 to 2. In the other areas of the hospital, it is 1:8+.

Everyone in the hospital is trained to be responsive to our patients' special needs, fears, and histories that usually include very poor experiences in other hospitals (such as discrimination, verbal abuse, and rudeness). The rooms and the equipment are designed and the staff are trained to meet our patients' needs, so that all furnishings, equipment, and attitudes reflect our belief that on this floor and in our hospital, a 272.2-kg (600-lb) patient is the average patient we are trained to serve, not an oddity or a special needs patient that is a burden to everyone. This is an experience the patients are all too familiar with from prior physicians, hospitals, and other outpatient facilities.

Some of the personnel who work in our office and in our unit were bariatric surgical patients. Positions in our hospital areas are very attractive to those people who like a consistent set of responsibilities and enjoy watching patients improve their quality of life. The staff needs to be tolerant of the psychological issues these patients have and the protective nature of their families, who are sometimes strongly against the patients' decisions to have surgery. Documentation on the hospital record cannot be just vital signs and pregenerated computer phrases. Attitudes such as "buyer's remorse," depression, and paranoia have to be documented, similar to those in a psychiatric ward (see Chapter 8). Sometimes efforts by family members to sabotage the patients' change in behavior must be addressed. Also, our staff has to use part of its time to teach, reinforce, and provide emotional support to the patients.

THE RISKS

We previously reviewed the medical malpractice risk associated with bariatric surgery.[8] Most of the risk occurs during the early stages of a program and during the surgeon's development. This demands that beginner surgeons choose lower-risk patients for at least their first 100 procedures. The accepted mortality rate for bariatric surgery is 0.5 to 1.5% for low-risk patients. It is not as well-documented, but the mortality rate for high-risk patients (i.e., those who weigh more than 181.4 kg [400 lb] or who have a body mass index >55 kg/m^2; those with sleep apnea, cardiac disease, inability to walk one-tenth of a mile, obesity–hypoventilation syndrome, pulmonary hypertension, hypoxia for any reason, long-standing diabetes and/or hypertension; and those with no social support who are relatively impoverished or mentally handicapped) is 5 to 10%. During a malpractice trial, the plaintiff's lawyers have access to the recommendations of the ACS, ASBS, and SAGES, so if a program is deficient, the case becomes harder to win. All jury members know someone who is morbidly obese or have family members who try to convince everyone that their body size is a "life choice" and put up fronts not to attract attention or to be accepted by family and peers. The better notes a practice has on the program planning and the steps it makes to prepare for their program, the more successful the outcome.

HOW TO GET STARTED

Preparing a hospital to become a bariatric surgical center is now a well-established business. Programs provide a range of services from surgery training, proctoring, executive training with onsite support complete with computer software for office records and financial planning, to groups of former patients or bariatric nurse specialists who will recruit patients by advertising, confirm insurance benefits, and complete everything but the surgeon's evaluation under contract to the surgeon or the hospital. Many of these services also provide postoperative patient support in local groups or on the Internet. Most of these vendors are listed on the ASBS Web site, once they have been evaluated by the organization. These groups also advertise themselves on the Web and in locales where they are located. Most senior bariatric surgeons still prefer to control these activities.

The major message of this chapter is that the establishment of a hospital bariatric surgical program is a risky, expensive undertaking that should not be approached casually. The surgeons and hospitals first need to educate their other physicians and staff as to why this is needed and assure them of how professionally it will be developed. The surgeons and hospitals should examine local, regional, and national resources available to help them plan their program, and should try to visit several functioning sites. A shared budget should be developed, as the surgeons will be bringing a new elective service to the hospitals that should provide predictable income and expenses. Insurance contracts should be reviewed and companies contacted to determine their requirements and the number of plans that will cover surgery.

A hospital training schedule needs to be developed to allow all staff members to understand the impact and implications of initiating this type of program. Other major hospital programs have to be assured that they will continue to have the resources they require. Finally, a plan to attract patients must be developed that will demonstrate to potential morbidly obese surgical candidates why your facility should be chosen.

REFERENCES

1. Quesenberry CP Jr, Caan B, Jacobson A. Obesity, health services use, and health-care costs among members of a health maintenance organization. *Arch Intern Med* 1998;158:466–472.
2. Martin LF, White S, Lindstrom W Jr. Cost-benefit analyses for the treatment of obesity. *World J Surg* 1998;22:1008–1017.
3. Martin LF, Smits G, Greenstein R. Laparoscopic adjustable gastric banding to treat morbid obesity: three-year efficacy and six-year safety data from the US Multicenter Trials. *JAMA* (in press).
4. National Institutes of Health. Clinical guidelines on the identification, evaluation, and treatment of overweight and obesity in adults—the evidence report. *Obes Res* 1998;6(Suppl 2):51S–209S.

5. *Obesity: Preventing and Managing the Global Epidemic. Report of a WHO Consultation on Obesity.* Geneva, Switzerland: World Health Organization; 1998.
6. Hannan EI, Kilburn H, Bernard H, et al. Coronary artery bypass surgery: the relationship between in-hospital mortality rate and surgical volume after controlling for clinical risk factors. *Med Care* 1991;29:1094–1107.
7. Hunter SM, Larrieu JA, Ayad FM, et al. Roles of mental health professionals in multidisciplinary medically supervised treatment programs for obesity. *South Med J* 1997;90:578–586.
8. Casey BE, Civello KC, Martin LF, et al. The medical malpractice risk associated with bariatric surgery. *Obes Surg* 1999;9:420–425.

LAPAROSCOPIC AND OPEN BARIATRIC PROCEDURES: WHAT ARE THE DIFFERENCES?

NINH T. NGUYEN /
BRUCE M. WOLFE

HISTORICAL BACKGROUND

In the past decade, the application of laparoscopic techniques to all areas of general surgery has increased greatly, and bariatric surgery is no exception. Roux-en-Y gastric bypass is a commonly performed operation for treatment of morbid obesity in the United States. According to a survey performed by the American Society for Bariatric Surgery (ASBS), 70% of all bariatric operations are Roux-en-Y gastric bypass.[1] Multiple randomized trials have demonstrated the benefits of laparoscopic surgery as compared to open surgery.[2–4] Intuitively, the benefits of laparoscopy also should apply to morbidly obese patients undergoing open gastric bypass and other bariatric procedures if the laparoscopic operation can be performed safely and the fundamentals of the open surgery are adhered to.

In the early years of laparoscopic cholecystectomy, morbid obesity was considered a relative contraindication to laparoscopy. The reluctance of surgeons to perform laparoscopy in morbidly obese patients was based on the increased difficulty in initiating pneumoperitoneum, because the abdominal wall is heavier as a result of the increased fat mass between the skin and muscle, requiring increased pressure to create the gas pocket used to see and remove the instruments, "the working space." It is more difficult to obtain adequate exposure of the operative site because there is an increased intraabdominal fat mass and the small bowel is thicker, taking up more space. Also the disposable and mass-produced laparoscopic instruments are often too short to reach the posterior abdomen in the very obese who have an extra 20 cm (8 inches) of abdominal wall fat. Technical improvement in laparoscopic instrumentation, especially the ability to special order longer instruments and video optics, and advances in operative skill level and technique, however, have overcome the majority of these difficulties. Studies demonstrate the feasibility and safety of laparoscopic cholecystectomy for the morbidly obese.[5,6]

The first description of laparoscopic gastric bypass was reported in 1994 by Wittgrove and colleagues.[7] (see Chapters 10 and 12 for more detailed histories of the evolution of the other bariatric procedures.) In 1996, Wittgrove and colleagues updated their experience of laparoscopic gastric bypass in 75 patients;[8] their technique involved the creation of a transected 15 to 30-mL gastric pouch, a stapled jejunojejunostomy, a retrocolic and retrogastric passage of the Roux limb, and creation of a gastrojejunostomy anastomosis with a circular stapler. In 1996, Lonroth described a technique of laparoscopic loop gastric bypass.[9] During the ensuing 4 years, there was a paucity of reported laparoscopic gastric bypass experience in the literature, but then in 2000, three large outcome studies of laparoscopic gastric bypass were published.[10–12] A year later, the results of two randomized, controlled trials comparing laparoscopic with open gastric bypass were published.[13,14]

This chapter discusses the differences in the instrumentation, patient selection, technique, and outcome between laparoscopic and open gastric bypass. Although there have not been randomized, controlled trials comparing laparoscopic and open techniques for the other major laparoscopic procedures, most of the comparisons would be similar. The technical challenges of mastering laparoscopic versus open bariatric procedures are also very different and it is important when randomized, controlled trials are conducted that the surgeons are equally skilled in both procedures. Although no information exists to document how many open and laparoscopic procedures should be performed on morbidly obese patients before a surgeon develops competence and how often one must perform these procedures to remain competent, most bariatric surgeons feel that one does not become competent and stay competent unless one is performing at least 2 to 4 of each individual type of procedure per month, or 25 to 50 cases per year.

FUNDAMENTAL DIFFERENCES

The fundamental differences between open and laparoscopic gastric bypass procedures are the methods of access and exposure (Table 9–1). These differences account for the different physiologic changes intraoperatively and the different clinical outcomes of the two operations.

Anesthesia and Ventilator Management

Anesthesia for bariatric operations should be performed by an anesthesiologist familiar with the morbidly obese. Endotracheal intubation in obese patients may be difficult, particularly for the superobese, and fiberoptic intubation may

TABLE 9–1. FUNDAMENTAL DIFFERENCES IN THE PROCEDURES OF LAPAROSCOPIC AND OPEN GASTRIC BYPASS (GB)		
CHARACTERISTICS	LAPAROSCOPIC GB	OPEN GB
Anesthesia	Equivalent	Equivalent
Ventilator management	Adjusted to minimize hypercarbia	Standard
Surgical position	Supine and reverse Trendelenburg	Supine and reverse Trendelenburg
Method of access	5 to 6 trocars	Upper midline incision
Method of exposure	CO_2 pneumoperitoneum	Abdominal wall retractor
Visceral manipulation	Minimal	Major
Heat loss	Moderate	Moderate

be necessary because the extra fat mass in the neck makes the airway narrow and decreases flexibility and access. Similar anesthetic agents can be used for patients undergoing laparoscopic gastric bypass (GB) or open bariatric procedures, but ventilator management is different and should be adjusted during laparoscopic GB to accommodate for the increased intraabdominal pressure and systemic absorption of carbon dioxide (CO_2) during the creation and maintenance of the CO_2 pneumoperitoneum.

Carbon dioxide absorption during pneumoperitoneum can result in systemic hypercarbia, hypercapnia, and respiratory acidosis, which can worsen very tenuous situations in patients who already suffer from obesity–hypoventilation syndrome. The increased intraabdominal pressure may lead to cephalad shift of the diaphragm; reduction of lung expansion, which is reduced because of the increased weight of the fat mass of the chest; reduction of diaphragmatic excursion; increase in airway pressure; and reduction in respiratory compliance. Therefore, during laparoscopic bariatric procedures appropriate ventilatory adjustments should be performed to minimize the increase in airway pressure and limit the rise in arterial partial pressure of CO_2.

Method of Access

Access for open bariatric procedures is commonly performed through an upper abdominal midline incision with fixed retractor systems attached to the operating table to help provide exposure (these must be longer and able to hold the larger weights); for laparoscopic gastric bypass, access is performed through five to six abdominal trocars (which may need to be longer) (Figure 9–1).

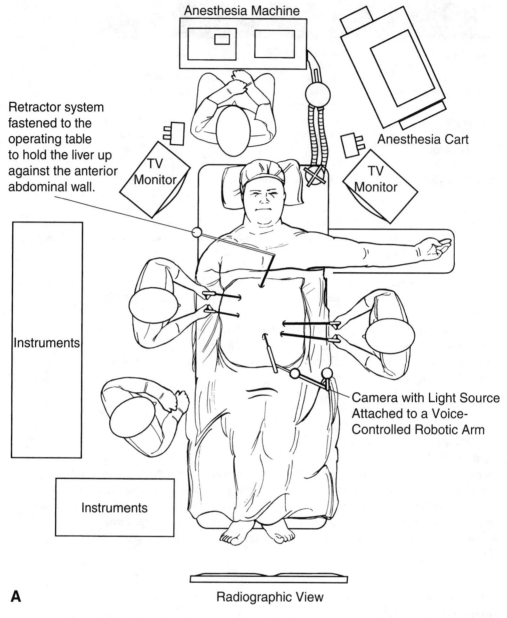

Anesthesia Machine

Retractor system
fastened to the
operating table
to hold the liver up
against the anterior
abdominal wall.

Anesthesia Cart

TV
Monitor

TV
Monitor

Instruments

Camera with Light Source
Attached to a Voice-
Controlled Robotic Arm

Instruments

A

Radiographic View

FIGURE 9–1   Method of access: (**A**) laparoscopic gastric bypass and (**B**)
open gastric bypass.

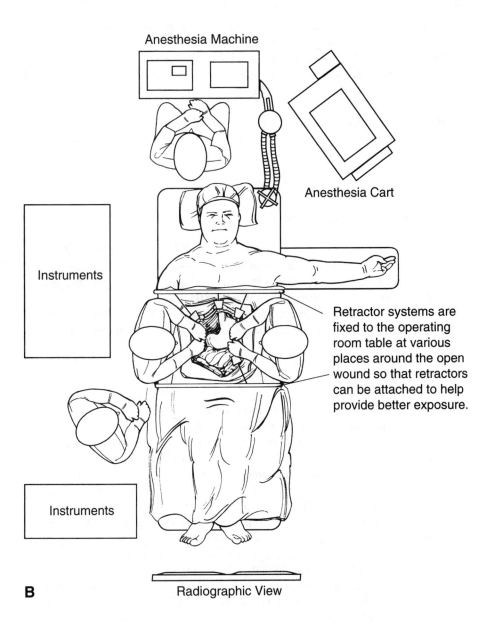

Anesthesia Machine

Anesthesia Cart

Instruments

Retractor systems are
fixed to the operating
room table at various
places around the open
wound so that retractors
can be attached to help
provide better exposure.

Instruments

B

Radiographic View

Method of Exposure

Because the most common method of exposure during open bariatric procedures is through an upper midline incision, there are numerous types of abdominal wall retractor systems that can be used for exposure of the operative
field, which attach to the bed frame of the operating room table. However, the
method of exposure during laparoscopic bariatric surgery is totally dependent

on the use of CO_2 pneumoperitoneum and the method used to retract the liver. The pressure effects of pneumoperitoneum separate the abdominal wall from the abdominal viscera to provide a working space. The left lobe of the liver needs to be elevated and kept as close as possible to the anterior abdominal wall to maximize access to the distal esophagus and stomach. For patients without steatosis of the liver (fatty infiltration), a toothed grasper connected to the diaphragm through a stab wound at the xyphoid maybe adequate. For heavier patients, those with severe steatosis, and especially those with metabolic syndrome X where the liver becomes much thicker and heavier, a specially designed liver retractor attached to the operating room bed frame is used.

Visceral Manipulation

Direct visceral retraction and manipulation of the stomach and other abdominal viscera such as the small and large bowel are required during open bariatric procedures for exposure of the operative field. With laparoscopic bariatric procedures, minimal direct retraction or manipulation of the abdominal viscera is required for exposure, as pneumoperitoneum creates a working space and reverse Trendelenburg position displaces the small bowel caudally by gravity.

Heat Loss

Heat loss occurs during both laparoscopic and open bariatric procedures. However, the mechanisms of heat loss are different between the two procedures. The mechanisms of heat loss during open bariatric procedures include heat loss from the exposed skin surfaces and exposure of the surgical wound and abdominal viscera to ambient room temperature. The mechanisms of heat loss during laparoscopic surgery, however, include heat loss from the exposed skin surfaces and exposure of the abdominal cavity and viscera to large volumes of cool, dry CO_2 insufflation gas. The cool CO_2 gas (typically 21°C [70°F]) delivered intraabdominally is a potential source of significant heat loss during laparoscopic surgery.[15] Gas delivery systems that include heated coils to warm the gas as it is delivered through the plastic tubing from the insufflator to the patient are now available, but it is not clear how effective they are (i.e., there have been no randomized, controlled trials of body temperature maintenance with versus without the coils).

EQUIPMENT

The equipment required to perform laparoscopic bariatric procedures differs from that required to perform open bariatric procedures. Essential laparoscopic equipment includes video optics, a CO_2 insufflator, laparoscopic instruments, endoscopic liver retractor, endoscopic linear staplers, a circular stapler, endoscopic suturing instruments, and the ultrasonic dissector and/or laparoscopic electrocautery devices. Standard laparoscopic instruments have shafts 32 to 35 cm (12 to 14 inches) in length. For morbidly obese patients, it is useful to have instruments with shafts that are 40 cm (15 inches) or longer. In addition to the necessary equipment, the successful performance of laparoscopic gastric bypass requires a well-trained operating team familiar with the equipment, instruments, and techniques of laparoscopic surgery. Also, the hospital facilities must be able to accommodate morbidly obese patients. Basic requirements include operating room tables, hospital beds, commodes, chairs, and wheelchairs capable of handling obese patients. These requirements are more fully described in Chapter 7.

PATIENT SELECTION AND PREPARATION

Preoperative assessment and preparation are critical to the success of any bariatric operation and should be performed similarly for patients undergoing laparoscopic or open bariatric procedures. The indications for laparoscopic procedures are the same as those for open procedures, as established by the 1991 National Institutes of Health Consensus Conference guidelines for treatment of morbid obesity,[16] and are outlined in Chapter 7. Appropriate surgery patients include those who have failed with nonsurgical means of weight loss and who have a body mass index (BMI) greater than 40kg/m^2. In certain instances, patients with a BMI between 35 and 40kg/m^2 can be considered for surgery if they have comorbid conditions such as sleep apnea, pickwickian syndrome, diabetes mellitus, or degenerative joint disease.

Patient preparation for all laparoscopic bariatric procedures consists of a detailed explanation and clear understanding of the risks; benefits; possible need for conversion to open surgery because of an inability to complete a successful procedure secondary to inadequate exposure; complications such as pneumothorax or hemorrhage that can make a laparoscopic approach less safe; inability to technically complete the procedure laparoscopically; other complications; nutritional sequelae; and the need for long-term followup. Preoperative bowel cleansing and antibiotic bowel preparation are instituted 1 day to several days before surgery. Prophylaxis against deep venous thrombosis (DVT) includes the use of perioperative intermittent pneumatic compression devices. The role and dosage of prophylactic subcutaneous heparin or low-molecular-weight heparin and when to initiate and stop such treatment remain controversial. An additional method for DVT prophylaxis is preoperative education about the need for early ambulation after surgery. (A more complete discussion of preoperative preparation is found in Chapter 5.)

Selection of patients to undergo laparoscopic bariatric procedures depends on the experience of the surgeon with the laparoscopic procedure, as not all patients are suitable for the laparoscopic approach. Surgeons with minimal experience in laparoscopic bariatric procedures should select patients with a lower BMI (less than 45), patients with a gynoid body habitus, female patients, and patients without previous upper abdominal surgery. Male patients tend to have more central obesity and intraabdominal adipose deposition, which makes laparoscopic exposure of the operative field more difficult. Certain investigators[12] have made no exclusions to the laparoscopic approach based on BMI, but we routinely do not advocate the laparoscopic approach for patients in the category of superobesity. The surgeons and their operative team usually can increase the body mass index criteria for a laparoscopic procedure with increasing experience. In addition, relative contraindications for laparoscopic procedures include patients with prior gastric, bariatric, or other upper abdominal surgery, and patients with a large ventral hernia defect. Although the laparoscopic approach to revision of previously failed bariatric surgery has been reported, the benefit of laparoscopy for this patient population is uncertain.[17] Absolute contraindications for laparoscopic bariatric procedures include patients with compromised cardiac, respiratory, renal, or hepatic function. The potential adverse consequences of pneumoperitoneum include CO_2 absorption and the effects of increased intraabdominal pressure on various body systems. Depression of cardiac function, alteration of intraoperative respiratory mechanics, and reduction in renal and hepatic portal blood flow have been reported.[18–21] These potential adverse effects of pneumoperitoneum, however, have minimal clinical impact on patients with intact cardiac, respiratory, hepatic, or renal function. The effects of pneumoperitoneum on patients with existing organ dysfunction have not been determined. As discussed in Chapter 5, most patients who can still walk at least half a mile have adequate cardiac and respiratory reserve to undergo bariatric operations. Patients with cirrhosis are rarely candidates for any bariatric procedure. There is no data suggesting that patients with renal failure who can tolerate hemodialysis are not candidates for bariatric procedures, but this is a relatively unexplored area.

SURGICAL TECHNIQUE

The basic Roux-en-Y gastric bypass procedure operation, or other bariatric procedure performed laparoscopically, is similar to that of open procedures except for the method of access and exposure. For gastric bypass, the fundamental procedure for construction of the Roux-en-Y should be adhered to, and the basic operation should not be compromised so that the procedure can be performed laparoscopically. For example, the fundamental procedure of Roux-en-Y gastric bypass was changed when surgeons initially attempting the laparoscopic approach performed the laparoscopic loop gastric bypass because it was technically an easier operation to perform than laparoscopic Roux-en-Y gastric bypass.[9] The loop gastric bypass procedure was first advocated by Griffen et al. in 1977, but was subsequently abandoned because of complications such as alkaline gastritis and esophagitis.[22] Multiple surgical groups[10–14] have shown that with more practice/skill, a Roux-en-Y gastric bypass can be performed with complication rates similar to open procedures. The general consensus among bariatric surgeons is that a surgeon needs to learn how to perform the standard open procedures laparoscopically, rather than performing outdated or discredited procedures because they have not achieved a sufficient skill level to perform the standard procedure laparoscopically.

During open gastric bypass, the gastrojejunostomy is commonly per-

formed by a handsewn technique. Wittgrove et al.[8] described the circular stapler technique to perform the laparoscopic gastrojejunostomy anastomosis.
Subsequently, Champion et al.[23] reported the use of a linear stapler, and Higa
et al.[12] reported the two-layer handsewn technique. Selection of a particular
technique will depend on the surgeon's familiarity, skill, experience with the
technique, and the surgeon's preference. Both circular and linear staplers have
been used to perform the gastrojejunostomy in open gastric bypasses and for
esophagojejunostomies, so these techniques are considered surgeon's preference rather than deviation from standard.

The laparoscopic jejunojejunostomy is usually performed by using the linear stapler, as in most open gastric bypasses, but it can also be handsewn. One
criticism of laparoscopic gastric bypass is the omission of closing mesenteric
defects. Late bowel obstruction was reported, which prompted surgeons to begin closing all mesenteric defects.[10,12,24] The development of numerous intracorporeal knot-tying devices has decreased the difficulty and/or increased the
speed of these maneuvers.

The retrocolic, retrogastric passage of the Roux limb is commonly performed in open GB. In laparoscopic GB, most investigators use the same technique.[8,10] A Penrose drain is sutured to the tip of the jejunal Roux limb. An
opening is created in the transverse colon mesentery, the Penrose drain is
passed through the transverse mesocolon defect into the lesser sac and is re-
trieved above the gastric remnant. As more experience is gained, the three-
dimensional aspects of performing the laparoscopic transfer of the limb behind
the stomach become more obvious and the necessity of using the Penrose drain
is deceased. It is considered prudent to check at least the gastrojejunostomy for
leaks before leaving the operating room. This can be done by placing a colored
dye, such as methylene blue, down a gastric tube or hooking the tube to air or
oxygen to flow by the anastomosis while it is under irrigation fluid, while
watching for bubbles. In both cases, the Roux limb should be occluded with a
noncrushing bowel clamp so that the anastomoses distends.

THE LEARNING CURVE

Certainly, there is a learning curve for all new laparoscopic operations. However, the learning curve for laparoscopic gastric bypass and other bariatric procedures is steeper than for most other advanced laparoscopic operations. Most
laparoscopic surgeons agree that laparoscopic gastric bypass and biliopancreatic bypass are two of the most complex operations performed by the laparoscopic approach. On a relative scale measuring the degree of technical difficulty for laparoscopic operations with 1 considered as the easiest and 10 as the
most difficult laparoscopic procedure, we consider laparoscopic gastric bypass
as being a 9 on this scale. (Laparoscopic biliopancreatic bypass and video coronary artery bypass vein grafting are 10s.) Unlike laparoscopic cholecystectomy,
laparoscopic gastric bypass and biliopancreatic bypass require transection and
reconstruction techniques, a large number of stapling and suturing tasks, and
the creation of two gastrointestinal anastomoses. Therefore, the learning curve

of laparoscopic gastric bypass and biliopancreatic bypass depends on the experience of the surgeon in other advanced laparoscopic operations, experience with open bariatric operations, and experience with laparoscopic suturing and intracorporeal knot-tying techniques. Each surgeon should evaluate his or her own technical ability to perform laparoscopic gastric bypass and acquire the proper training and preceptorship with experienced surgeons before embarking on this complex laparoscopic procedure. Bariatric surgeons familiar with open techniques who want to learn the laparoscopic approach should attend, at the very least, a laparoscopic bariatric surgery course, obtain hands-on experience with the laparoscopic procedures in an animal or cadaver model, and/or obtain a preceptorship with a surgeon experienced in the laparoscopic procedure. Mini-fellowships (1–3 months in length) are now available for experienced surgeons at several university centers. Laparoscopic surgeons with minimal experience with bariatric surgery should not only follow the above guidelines, but should also obtain experience in open bariatric surgery in case there is a need to convert (e.g., pneumothorax, splenic vein injury patient). The operating room must have the retractor system and longer instruments available to perform open bariatric procedures. Equally important, the experienced laparoscopic surgeon who decides to perform bariatric procedures must learn the preoperative and postoperative management of bariatric patients, and use the multidisciplinary approach to obesity, which includes anesthesiologists and nurses who understand the disease, available dietary counseling and exercise programs, psychological assistance, and appropriate support groups. We caution that laparoscopic gastric bypass should not be performed by surgeons who lack proper training in advanced laparoscopic techniques, and who also lack experience in the preoperative and postoperative management of morbidly obese patients. Although a surgeon may have the training and ability to perform laparoscopic gastric bypass procedures, the surgeon should not undertake the operation if there is a lack of multidisciplinary support.

The complexity of laparoscopic gastric bypass has led to the use of hand-assisted laparoscopic gastric bypass.[25,26] Hand-assisted laparoscopic gastric bypass uses the surgeon's hand to provide tactile feedback, improves exposure of the surgical field, aids knot tying and suturing, and may also help to control bleeding. One disadvantage of hand-assisted laparoscopic gastric bypass is that a larger abdominal incision is required than that for a totally laparoscopic GB. However, hand-assisted laparoscopic gastric bypass may have a role for surgeons with limited skills in advanced laparoscopy to possibly decrease the operative time, function as a learning tool before attempting total laparoscopic gastric bypass, salvage difficult laparoscopic gastric bypass cases, or treat patients with high BMI (>60 kg/m^2).

POSTOPERATIVE MANAGEMENT

Postoperative management after laparoscopic gastric bypass should be similar to that of open gastric bypass. Patients are extubated and transferred to the surgical ward postoperatively unless they require ventilatory support or close observation in the intensive care unit. A nasogastric tube is not routinely required in either laparoscopic or open gastric bypass patients by many surgeons. Pain management consists of intravenous morphine administered by patient-controlled analgesia. Patients are encouraged to ambulate on the postoperative night and perform incentive spirometry and deep-breathing exercises. A Gastrografin contrast study is performed on the first or second day postoperatively to make sure that the anastomoses stay intact even after the patient rolls, sits, or stands. (There are significant weight loads on these anastomoses as a result of the increased mesenteric fat mass in the morbidly obese.) A clear liquid diet is started after confirmation of an intact anastomosis without evidence of contrast leak or obstruction. Patients are discharged from the hospital when oral fluid is tolerated. They are scheduled for followup at 1 and 2 weeks postoperatively then at 1, 3, 6, and 12 months, and then yearly thereafter.

CLINICAL OUTCOMES

This section compares the outcomes after laparoscopic and open gastric bypass and relates data collected for our randomized controlled trial of open versus laparoscopic gastric bypass[13] and other supplementary data. Our study was completed in a residency training program where the residents performed the gastric bypasses but a senior surgeon assisted. Residents performed all the laparoscopic gastric bypasses. Our mean operative time of well over 3 hours for the laparoscopic cases reflects the initial learning curve, while the mean time of the open cases (190 minutes) is our standard. Operative time for laparoscopic gastric bypass is generally longer than that for open gastric bypass for the first several hundred procedures. However, the operative time should approach that of open gastric bypass once the surgeon has passed the learning curve of the laparoscopic procedure. Higa et al.[12] reported that their operative time has consistently ranged from 60 to 90 minutes after passing their laparoscopic gastric bypass procedure learning curve, when each of them had performed more than 100 procedures (three surgeons reported performing more than 1000 laparoscopic procedures in 3 years). An operating time for both open and laparoscopic cases of approximately 100 minutes is commonly reported by experienced bariatric surgeons performing more than 100 procedures a year.

Conversion Rate

The conversion rate during laparoscopic gastric bypass is low, ranging from 0 to 1.1%.[10–12] The reasons for conversion to laparotomy include difficulty in initiating pneumoperitoneum, hepatomegaly, difficulty in obtaining exposure, severe abdominal adhesions, pneumothorax, and failure to make progress. Surgeons must have the skill and the equipment to convert to an open procedure when necessary.

Blood Loss

Blood loss during laparoscopic gastric bypass has been reported to be low. It is imperative to maintain meticulous hemostasis during laparoscopic gastric bypass or other bariatric procedures, as intraoperative bleeding can obscure visualization of the operative field. Schauer et al.[10] reported a mean operative blood loss of 115 mL in their series of 275 laparoscopic gastric bypass operations. We reported a higher intraoperative transfusion requirement in open gastric bypass than in laparoscopic gastric bypass patients (3.9% versus 0%), but it was not statistically significant.[13]

Length of Intensive Care Unit Stay

The length of intensive care unit (ICU) stay after laparoscopic gastric bypass has been reported to be low.[27] In our randomized trial, we reported a lower percentage of patients requiring ICU stay after laparoscopic gastric bypass than after open gastric bypass (7.6% versus 21.1%).[13] These percentages, however, were produced in a hospital setting where nurses had extensive experience managing these challenging patients; in newer programs, more patients may need to spend time in settings with lower patient-to-nurse ratios until the hospital establishes its own nursing care plans.

Length of Hospital Stay

The length of hospital stay after laparoscopic gastric bypass is similar to or only slightly shorter than that after open gastric bypass.[28,29] Spanos et al.[28] reported a similar length of stay after laparoscopic and open gastric bypass (4.5 days versus 3.9 days). Conversely, Eagon et al.[29] reported a shorter length of stay after laparoscopic gastric bypass (3 days versus 5 days). Whether the procedure is performed laparoscopically or open, because two enterocuterotomies are performed, it usually takes longer for patients to obtain the return of gastro-intestinal function so that they can be sustained on oral intake alone than it does to wean them from intravenous or intramuscular pain medication.

Mortality

Mortality after laparoscopic gastric bypass has been reported to be low. Higa et al.[12] reported an overall mortality rate of 0.5%. Wittgrove et al.[11] reported no mortality in their series of 500 laparoscopic gastric bypass operations. Both of these programs are established in private California hospitals that do not treat indigent patients. Several studies show that patients of lower socioeconomic status have increased morbidity and mortality rates and higher levels of disease burden on presentation.

Complications

Initial reports suggested a higher leak rate after laparoscopic gastric bypass than after open gastric bypass.[10] The relatively higher leak rate after laparoscopic gastric bypass is likely related to the learning curve of the laparoscopic procedure. Wittgrove et al. reported 9 anastomotic leaks (3.0%) in their first 300 laparoscopic gastric bypass procedures, as compared to only 2 leaks (1.0%) in their last 200 laparoscopic gastric bypass procedures.[11]

The reduced incidence of wound infections after laparoscopic gastric bypass is one of the easily recognized advantages of the laparoscopic approach.[13] Wound infection after open gastric bypass or any other bariatric procedure is a major problem, because it requires a prolonged course of wound care. Conversely, wound infection after laparoscopic gastric bypass can be managed easily with a short course of local wound care.

Another advantage of laparoscopic gastric bypass is the reduced incidence of a late incisional hernia. The incidence of a postoperative incisional hernia after open gastric bypass can be as high as 20%.[30] The majority of these incisional hernias require operative intervention, which is likely to increase the costs associated with open gastric bypass. In our randomized trial, the incidence of ventral hernia after laparoscopic gastric bypass was zero.[13]

Early postoperative bowel obstruction is an infrequent complication after open gastric bypass but has been reported after laparoscopic gastric bypass.[10,12] The reasons for the development of bowel obstruction after laparoscopic gastric bypass include technical narrowing of the jejunojejunostomy anastomosis (the more difficult of the two anastomoses to perform/learn laparosurgically), failure to close all the mesenteric defects, and failure to place the antiobstruction suture at the jejunojejunostomy anastomosis.[24] However, late bowel obstruction from postoperative adhesions should be less frequent after laparoscopic gastric bypass, as one of the benefits of minimally invasive surgery is the reduction of intraabdominal adhesion formations. These comparisons will need to be revisited as laparoscopic techniques reach the same degree of maturity that open techniques have reached (over 30 years of experience).

Stricture of the gastrojejunostomy is a frequent complication after open gastric bypass and laparoscopic gastric bypass.[31] In a comparative study of laparoscopic versus open gastric bypass, Demaria and colleagues[32] reported no significant difference in stomal stenosis rate (24% versus 20%) between the two techniques. Treatment for anastomotic stricture consists of endoscopic balloon dilation under fluoroscopic guidance. The gastrojejunostomy in a gastric bypass is deliberately made to be 10 to 13 mm (0.4 to 0.5 inches) in diameter to help slow gastric emptying. In this range, the tighter the surgeon tries to make the anastomosis, the more often strictures will develop as wound healing is variable. The stricture rate has to be judged against the long-term weight results that the surgeon's patients achieve.

Postoperative gastrointestinal (GI) bleeding after laparoscopic gastric bypass has been reported.[10] The cause for postoperative GI bleeding is presumed to be bleeding from the gastric remnant, gastrojejunostomy, or the jejunojejunostomy staple line. To limit this complication, care must be taken intra-operatively to provide meticulous hemostasis of all staple-line edges, use of a shorter staple height, and oversewing or reinforcement of the staple line if hemostasis is hard to achieve (usually related to the patients prior use of nonsteroidal anti-inflammatory agents or the surgeon's use of deep venous thrombosis prophylaxis).

Postoperative Pain

The degree of postoperative pain after open gastric bypass is multifactorial but to some extent related to the length of the surgical incision, the extent of operative dissection, and trauma of the abdominal wall from surgical retraction. We reported that laparoscopic gastric bypass patients required significantly less self-administered intravenous morphine sulfate than did open gastric bypass patients on the first postoperative day (46 mg versus 76 mg, respectively).[33] Despite the higher amount of self-administered morphine sulfate, open gastric bypass patients had higher visual analog pain scores (reported that they had more pain) than did laparoscopic gastric bypass patients.[33]

Recovery

Recovery is measured subjectively by the patient's response to questions regarding the number of days between the operation and the patient's return to activities of daily living and work. We reported that laparoscopic gastric bypass patients had a significantly more rapid return to these activities than did open gastric bypass patients (Figure 9–2).[13]

Weight Loss

Weight loss after laparoscopic gastric bypass should be equivalent to that achieved after open gastric bypass, as the basic operation is not changed and the only differences between the two techniques are the methods of surgical access and exposure. Spanos et al.[28] reported a similar weight loss after laparoscopic gastric bypass and open gastric bypass (65% versus 60%) at 1 year. Long-term weight loss after laparoscopic gastric bypass has been reported by Wittgrove et al.[11] at more than 80% of excess body weight loss at 5 years, which compares favorably with that of open gastric bypass.

Quality of Life

Quality of life (QOL) is an essential outcome measure to assess the patient's perception of his or her general health. Intuitively, the QOL at long-term followup after laparoscopic gastric bypass should not be different from that after

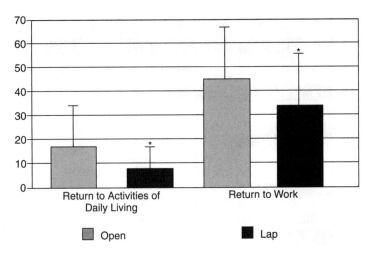

FIGURE 9–2   Time to return to activities of daily living and work after laparoscopic and open gastric bypass (GB). * p <0.05 when compared to open GB.

open gastric bypass. The Moorehead-Ardelt QOL questionnaire assesses self-esteem, physical activity, social life, work conditions, and sexual interest/activity; points are added for positive changes and subtracted for negative changes.[34] We reported that laparoscopic gastric bypass patients had more interest in sexual activity and were able to work more than open gastric bypass patients at 3 months postoperatively.[13] However, these advantages of improved QOL after laparoscopic gastric bypass did not persist when the same questionnaire was administered at 6 months followup (Figure 9–3).

Costs

The major cost difference between the laparoscopic and open gastric bypass operations is the expense of the disposable instruments required by laparoscopic procedure. Liu et al.[35] reported that direct operative cost was 58% greater for laparoscopic gastric bypass versus open gastric bypass. We reported that the operative cost for laparoscopic gastric bypass was 37% higher, but the hospital service cost after laparoscopic gastric bypass was 33% lower than after open gastric bypass (Figure 9–4).[13] The total (direct + indirect) cost, however, was similar for the two operations ($14,087 versus $14,098).[13]

PHYSIOLOGIC OUTCOMES

In addition to the above differences in clinical outcomes, laparoscopic and open gastric bypass are associated with different physiologic response. By limiting

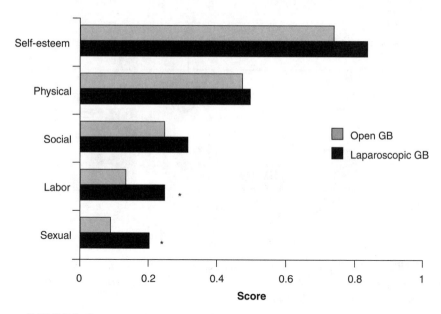

FIGURE 9–3   Moorhead-Ardelt Quality of Life scores after laparoscopic and open gastric bypass (GB) at 3 months postoperatively. * p <0.05 when compared to open GB.

the access incision, one of the physiologic benefits of laparoscopic surgery is the reduction in the extent of operative trauma. Knowing that the systemic stress response after surgical injury correlates with the extent of operative trauma, we previously reported that patients who underwent laparoscopic gastric bypass had an attenuated systemic stress response when compared with open gastric bypass patients.[36] Postoperative concentrations of norepinephrine, adrenal corticol hormone, C-reactive protein, and interleukin-6, were lower after laparoscopic than after open gastric bypass. Our findings suggest a lower degree of operative injury after laparoscopic gastric bypass than after open gastric bypass.

SUMMARY

Laparoscopic gastric bypass is a complex advanced laparoscopic operation that accomplishes the same objectives as open gastric bypass but avoids the large upper midline abdominal incision. We have explained the differences in instrumentation, patient selection, techniques, and outcomes between laparoscopic gastric bypass and open gastric bypass. The main difference between laparoscopic and open gastric bypass are the methods of access and exposure. Laparoscopic gastric bypass is performed through five to six abdominal trocars and uses pneumoperitoneum for exposure of the operative field. These differences account for the adverse consequences of pneumoperitoneum dur-

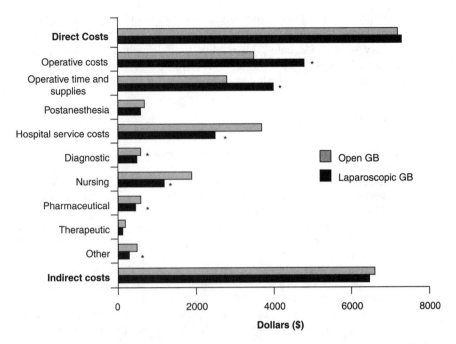

FIGURE 9–4 Cost analysis after laparoscopic and open gastric bypass (GB). *
p <0.05 when compared to open GB.

ing laparoscopic gastric bypass but improved clinical outcomes over the initial postoperative recovery phase. Laparoscopic gastric bypass should not be attempted without the proper equipment, instrumentation, and a dedicated surgical team that understands the technique of laparoscopic gastric bypass. Selection of patients for laparoscopic bariatric procedures is critical, as not all patients are candidates for the laparoscopic approach. The key technical imperative of laparoscopic bariatric surgery is to follow the fundamental principles of the open procedures. If these principles are adhered to, then long-term weight loss and improvement in quality of life after laparoscopic bariatric surgery should be similar to those of the open techniques. The main clinical advantage of laparoscopic GB is not the reduced length of hospital stay, but the reduction in postoperative pain, lower incidence of wound-related complications, and faster recovery to normal life activities.

Given the currently available data, laparoscopic gastric bypass can no longer be considered experimental. However, we advocate that laparoscopic gastric bypass and other bariatric procedures should be a suitable option for treatment of morbid obesity only when performed by surgeons with training in and experience with the laparoscopic techniques who adhere to the principles of open bariatric surgery and perform the operation in centers that have experience in preoperative and postoperative management of the morbidly obese and are committed to the long-term followup of these patients. Both patients and referring physicians should be aware that placing too much importance on the characteristics of the external surgical skin scars and the potential to return to work and/or other daily activities a few weeks to months earlier will not appear very wise if adequate postoperative multidisciplinary assistance is not available as patients try to completely relearn how to eat and maximize their chances of obtaining the healthiest long-term weight.

REFERENCES

1. Schauer PR, Ikramuddin S. Laparoscopic surgery for morbid obesity. *Surg Clin North Am* 2001;81:1145–1179.
2. Laine S, Rantala A, Gullichsen R, Ovaska J. Laparoscopic vs conventional fundoplication: a prospective randomized study. *Surg Endosc* 1997;11:441–444.
3. Milsom JW, Bartholomaus B, Hammerhofer KA, Fazio V, Steiger E, Elson P. A prospective, randomized trial comparing laparoscopic versus conventional techniques in colorectal cancer surgery: a preliminary report. *J Am Coll Surg* 1998;187:46–57.
4. Schwenk W, Bohm B, Witt C, Junghans T, Grundel K, Muller JM. Pulmonary function following laparoscopic or conventional colorectal resection. *Arch Surg* 1999;134:6–12.
5. Ammori BJ, Vezakis A, Davides D, Martin G, Larvin M, McMahon MJ. Laparoscopic cholecystectomy in morbidly obese patients. *Surg Endosc* 2001;15:S91.
6. Miles RH, Carballo RE, Prinz RA, et al. Laparoscopy: the preferred method of cholecystectomy in the morbidly obese. *Surgery* 1992;112:818–823.
7. Wittgrove AC, Clark GW, Tremblay LJ. Laparoscopic gastric bypass, Roux-en-Y: preliminary report of five cases. *Obes Surg* 1994;4:353–357.
8. Wittgrove AC, Clark GW, Schubert KR. Laparoscopic gastric bypass, Roux-en-Y: technique and results in 75 patients with 3–30 months follow-up. *Obes Surg* 1996;6:500–504.
9. Lonroth H, Dalenback J, Haglind E, Lundell L. Laparoscopic gastric bypass: another option in bariatric surgery. *Surg Endosc* 1996;10:636–638.
10. Schauer PR, Ikramuddin S, Gourash W, et al. Outcomes after laparoscopic Roux-en-Y gastric bypass for morbid obesity. *Ann Surg* 2000;232:515–529.
11. Wittgrove AC, Clark GW. Laparoscopic gastric bypass, Roux-en-Y: 500 patients—technique and results, with 3–60 month follow-up. *Obes Surg* 2000;10:233–239.
12. Higa KD, Boone KB, Ho T. Complications of the laparoscopic Roux-en-Y gastric bypass: 1,040 patients—what have we learned? *Obes Surg* 2000;10:509–513.
13. Nguyen NT, Goldman C, Rosenquist CJ, et al. Laparoscopic versus open gastric bypass: a randomized study of outcomes, quality of life, and costs. *Ann Surg* 2001;234:279–289.
14. Westling A, Gustavsson S. Laparoscopic vs open Roux-en-Y gastric bypass: a prospective, randomized trial. *Obes Surg* 2001;11:284–292.
15. Bessell JR, Karatassas A, Patterson JR, Jamieson GG, Maddern GJ. Hypothermia induced by laparoscopic insufflation. A randomized study in a pig model. *Surg Endosc* 1995;9:791–796.
16. Gastrointestinal surgery for severe obesity: Consensus Development Conference Panel. *Ann Intern Med* 1991;115:956–961.
17. Csepel J, Nahouraii R, Gagner M. Laparoscopic gastric bypass as a reoperative bariatric surgery for failed open restrictive procedures. *Surg Endosc* 2001; 15:393–397.

18. Sharma KC, Brandstetter RD, Brensilver JM, Jung LD. Cardiopulmonary physiology and pathophysiology as a consequence of laparoscopic surgery. *Chest* 1996;110:810–815.

19. Beebe DS, McNevin MP, Crain JM, et al. Evidence of venous stasis after abdominal insufflation for laparoscopic cholecystectomy. *Surg Gynecol Obstet* 1993;176:443–447.

20. Morino M, Giraudo G, Festa V. Alterations in hepatic function during laparoscopic surgery: an experimental clinical study. *Surg Endosc* 1998;12:968–972.

21. Chiu AW, Chang LS, Birkett DH, Babayan RK. The impact of pneumoperitoneum, pneumoretroperitoneum, and gasless laparoscopy on the systemic and renal hemodynamics. *J Am Coll Surg* 1995;181:397–406.

22. Griffen WO, Young VL, Stevenson CC. A prospective comparison of gastric and jejunoileal bypass procedures for morbid obesity. *Ann Surg* 1977;186:500–509.

23. Champion JK. Laparoscopic Roux-en-Y gastric bypass with the linear endostapler technique [abstract]. *Obes Surg* 2000;10:131.

24. Nguyen NT, Neuhaus AM, Ho HS, et al. A prospective evaluation of intracorporeal laparoscopic small bowel anastomosis during gastric bypass. *Obes Surg* 2001;11:196–199.

25. Naitoh T, Gagner M, Garcia-Ruiz A, et al. Hand-assisted laparoscopic digestive surgery provides safety and tactile sensation for malignancy or obesity. *Surg Endosc* 1999;13:157–160.

26. Sundbom M, Gustavsson S. Hand-assisted laparoscopic Roux-en-Y gastric bypass: aspects of surgical technique and early results. *Obes Surg* 2000;10:420–427.

27. Nguyen NT, Ho HS, Palmer LS, Wolfe BM. A comparison study of laparoscopic versus open gastric bypass for morbid obesity. *J Am Coll Surg* 2000;191:149–157.

28. Spanos C, Salzmann E, Triglio CM, Shikora SA. A comparative study in percentage of weight loss between laparoscopic and open Roux-en-Y gastric bypass [abstract]. *Obes Surg* 2001;11:384.

29. Eagon CJ, Marin D. Laparoscopic gastric bypass has shorter length of stay and less complications but is more costly compared with open gastric bypass [abstract]. *Surg Endosc* 2001;15:S120.

30. Kellum JM, DeMaria EJ, Sugerman HJ. The surgical treatment of morbid obesity. *Curr Probl Surg* 1998;35:791–858.

31. Sanyal AJ, Sugerman HJ, Kellum JM, Engle KM, Wolfe L. Stomal complications of gastric bypass: incidence and outcome of therapy. *Am J Gastroenterol* 1992;87:1165–1169.

32. DeMaria EJ, Schweitzer MA, Kellum JM, Sugerman HJ. Prospective comparison of open versus laparoscopic Roux-en-Y proximal gastric bypass for morbid obesity [abstract]. *Obes Surg* 2000;10:131.

33. Nguyen NT, Lee SL, Goldman C, et al. Comparison of pulmonary function and postoperative pain after laparoscopic versus open gastric bypass: a randomized trial. *J Am Coll Surg* 2001;192:469–476.

34. Oria HE, Moorehead MK. Bariatric analysis and reporting outcome system (BAROS). *Obes Surg* 1998;8:487–499.

35. Carson Liu. Cost-analysis of laparoscopic versus open Roux-en-Y gastric bypass for morbid obesity [abstract]. *Obes Surg* 2001;11:165.

36. Nguyen NT, Goldman CD, Ho HS, Gosselin RC, Singh A, Wolfe BM. Systemic stress response after laparoscopic and open gastric bypass. *J Am Coll Surg* 2002;194(5):557–566.

GASTRIC RESTRICTIVE PROCEDURES: GASTROPLASTIES AND BANDS

LOUIS F. MARTIN

Gastric restrictive procedures were the last class or group of procedures to develop in the evolution of bariatric surgery in the 20th century, after pure malabsorption procedures and procedures that began to combine less-severe malabsorptive procedures with gastric restrictive procedures, which were classified as combined procedures (see Chapter 2). The incentive to find a purely restrictive procedure that would be an effective bariatric procedure was a reaction to the long-term complications that are always potential problems after the other two types of procedures. Because both of these are designed to bypass part of the normal gastrointestinal (GI) tract as part of their strategy to induce weight loss (creating malabsorption), both types of procedures can lead to vitamin, mineral, and other types of nutritional deficiencies unless supplements are given postoperatively. The problems caused by the current generation of malabsorptive and combined procedures are minimal for intelligent patients who are willing to adjust their dietary intake, take supplemental vitamins and minerals, and/or return to their surgeon or other knowledgeable physician for regular followup and monitoring to make sure nutritional deficiencies do not develop. Not everyone seeking bariatric surgery to help treat their morbid obesity will meet the criteria listed in the prior sentence.

Morbidly obese patients are like any other cross-section of our population sampled by only one of their many characteristics—they have a broad range of intellectual abilities and exhibit degrees of cooperativeness and truthfulness when dealing with authority figures such as physicians. Each also has his or her own system of attitudes and beliefs, especially as it applies to what they will accept as medical and surgical treatments. Obese people who seek medical help to reverse their obesity have personality characteristics that differ from those that do not seek treatment, and those who seek surgical treatments are a separate population from those who will not accept invasive surgical treatments, but who will accept behavior modification, diets, and maybe medications.[1,2]

Relatively severe complications can develop in patients who have had a biliopancreatic bypass or a gastric bypass who do not follow instructions and/or do not take supplements, which include neuropathies and pernicious anemia as a consequence of vitamin B_{12} deficiency; osteoporosis as a consequence of vitamin D and calcium deficiencies; hypoalbuminemia with generalized edema; iron-deficiency anemia; severe diarrhea; gallstones; kidney stones; vitamin K deficiency with abnormal blood clotting; vitamin A deficiencies with abnormal healing; and so on (see Chapters 12, 14, 15, and 16). People of low intelligence who resist medical help or patients who lose their medical insurance can become severely malnourished and can die from the deficiencies they develop. Even patients who are initially cooperative with followup move away from their surgeon (US census data show that 15% or more of Americans move outside of their original communities during each decade). Others will change their habits during times of stress, which can include developing or reestablishing destructive eating behaviors or other signs of psychopathology, including avoiding physicians. Also, these bypass procedures all leave a section of the GI tract unavailable for future radiologic or endoscopic evaluations. Patients need to have physicians who are knowledgeable about how their GI tracts have been rearranged and who know how and when these bypassed segments need to be evaluated as part of the work-up of a patient's symptoms.

Although it can be argued, it is not the surgeon's responsibility to make patients return for followup or to make patients keep their commitments to take supplements; most physicians use the adage "do not harm" whenever possible in providing treatments. Morbidly obese patients may have significantly shorter life spans and poorer quality of life if not treated (see Chapter 1), but their treatments should provide relatively few new medical problems. We maintain contact with more than 95% of our patients for the first postoperative year, but yearly followup drops off to 50% by the fifth postoperative year. We have tried to educate our patients by then to know what tests they should undergo yearly to ensure that their vitamin, mineral, protein, and hemoglobin levels stay within normal limits. We also ask our patients to communicate with their primary care physicians if laboratory abnormalities or other problems develop, encouraging their physicians to contact us so that we can help them know what to do. We do not encourage patients from great distances to seek treatment at our facility unless there is no closer place to receive the treatment they desire. In spite of these values and our attempts to maintain contact, there are people who have misrepresented to us their commitment to followup with the result that we lose contact with them before we are comfortable that they can take adequate care of themselves. These patients often do not respond to our attempts to ensure they have a physician following their progress and helping them remain healthy.

Concerns such as these stimulated the bariatric surgical team at the University of Iowa School of Medicine to begin experimenting with gastric restrictive operations to treat obesity in the late 1960s and early 1970s. Dr. Mason, who described the first gastric bypass procedure in 1966,[3] began performing gastroplasties on patients in 1971[4] (see Chapter 2 and Figure 10–1). A gastroplasty creates a separate small proximal gastric pouch (now less than 20 mL) above the rest of the stomach, with drainage to the rest of the stomach via a narrow outlet that initially was created along the greater curvature of the stomach so the area near the short gastric vessels that connect to the spleen were not disturbed, lessening the risk of splenic injury. A gastroplasty does not bypass any part of the GI tract so that all of it remains available for radiologic or endoscopic evaluation. It is unlikely to be associated with vitamin, mineral, or other nutritional abnormalities if the postoperative patient will eat a balanced diet using a standard food pyramid, but obviously ingesting much smaller quantities of nutritional foods.

The restriction caused by a gastroplasty requires patients to ingest three to six small meals a day of nutritionally balanced foods. Patients who eat high-calorie, low-bulk foods will not feel a restriction. "Sweets eaters"—a phrase coined by Dr. Harvey Sugarman[5] to denote people who drink sugared drinks, carbonated or uncarbonated, consume high-sugar candy snacks, and soft, high-calorie food such as ice cream, cakes, and pies—usually will have difficulty losing weight after a gastroplasty if they cannot eliminate this habit. A gastric bypass or biliopancreatic bypass will usually cause a patient who eats concentrated sweets to develop the "dumping syndrome," which produces severe diarrhea, abdominal cramps, sweating, tachycardia, and other symptoms that discourage this behavior. This is caused when high osmolar solutions have contact

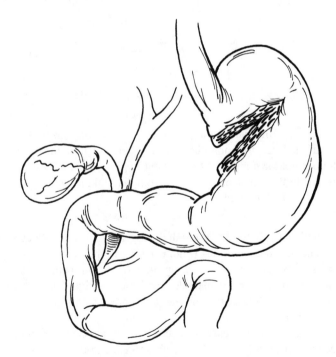

FIGURE 10–1   Original gastroplasty that was described by Printen and Mason in 1973.

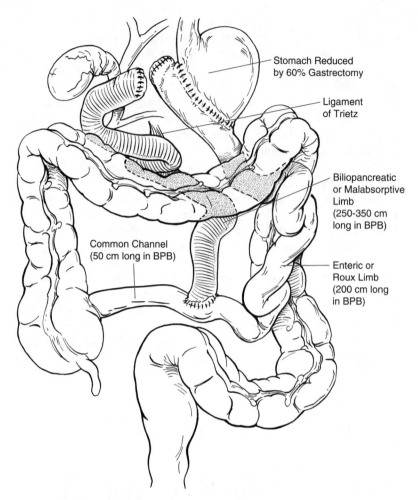

FIGURE 10–2   Biliopancreatic bypass with the enteral limb, the biliopan-creatic limb, and the common channel all labeled. The reduced segment of stomach does not have a pylorus to prevent hyperosmolar solutions from being delivered to the small bowel before complete mixing with gastric secretions leading to the "dumping syndrome."

with the small bowel in the enteral limb of a bypass procedure which is not designed to tolerate such solutions (Figure 10–2). More American patients appear to be sweets eaters than are European patients,[6] probably because more Americans consume more of their daily calories in high-calorie snacks and sugared beverages, while Europeans eat very traditional meals.

As outlined in Chapter 2, the early attempts to use a gastroplasty as a bariatric operation were largely spectacular failures because the initial proximal pouches were too large and were able to expand to accommodate more food, plus the outlets from the upper pouches were either not restrictive enough initially or expanded with use. It took more than a decade of experimentation to learn that the most stable gastric pouches had to be created along the lesser curvature of the stomach as a tube, and that the outlet from the pouch had to be reinforced with a nondistensible material like silicone tubing, polypropylene mesh, or Dacron vascular graft-like materials (Figure 10–3). This type of operation was initially labeled a vertical-banded gastroplasty (VBG) as described by Mason in 1982.[7]

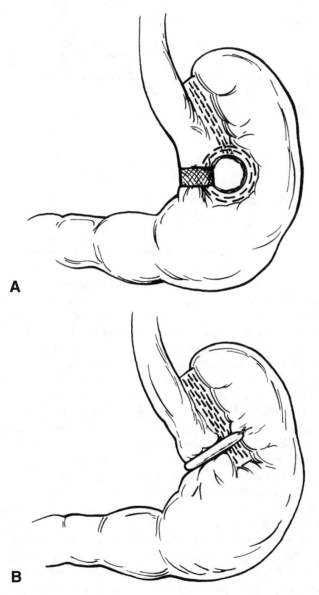

FIGURE 10–3   **A.** Mason vertical-banded gastroplasty (VBG). **B.** Silastic ring vertical gastroplasty (SRVG). **C.** VBG with the pouch separated from the rest of the proximal stomach.

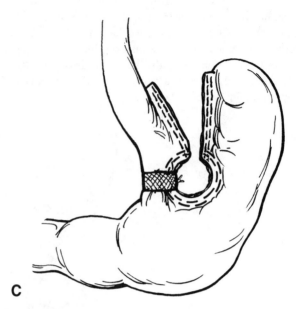

C

FIGURE 10–3   (continued)

The lesser curvature of the stomach is more muscular with several layers of fibers arranged at acute angles to each other, which makes pouches in this area less likely to expand and helps the unidirectional passage of food to lessen the chance of vomiting. Adding a nondistensible material at the distal end of the pouch prevented the restrictive opening to the rest of the stomach from expanding, but increased the incidence of vomiting and staple line disruption if a patient overate. Staple line disruption was decreased if the pouch was divided from the rest of the proximal stomach (see Figure 10–3C), probably because the scar that is created does not depend on the staples remaining in place; that is, once the scar heals, the staples are irrelevant. This was demonstrated in a randomized controlled trial (RCT) initiated by MacLean's group in Montreal, Canada,[8] that showed that an isolated gastric pouch would not fail, while non-divided stable lines would. Although this group only reported the superiority of a divided gastric bypass, Toppino showed that similar results are possible when the VBG staple line is cut, producing a permanent scar.[9]

Gastroplasties have consistently been more acceptable to a group of morbidly obese people than have malabsorptive or combined procedures that rearrange the GI tract. There is a subgroup of the morbidly obese who do *not* want their intestines rearranged, but who can accept the idea of having the capacity of their stomach decreased. This more "physiologic" type of procedure that suggested that a patient would experience less long-term complications was also attractive to a portion of bariatric surgeons, especially since Dr. Mason, considered the "father" of bariatric surgery, decided that he would preferably perform a gastroplasty (the VBG he described in 1982)[7] over a gastric bypass (another operation he initially described and advocated)[3] because he was worried about the complications that noncompliant patients developed after undergoing bariatric operations.

Initially, it was also thought that a gastroplasty, or especially a VBG, would produce less acute complications because not as much of the GI tract was opened. Four prospective RCTs were conducted from the mid-1980s until the early 1990s, comparing the complications and outcomes of VBG against gastric bypass.[5,8,10,11] All of these studies demonstrated that there were no consistent, statistically significant differences in the rates of acute complications (within 30 days of the operation) especially in the life-threatening complications of infection leading to sepsis and pulmonary emboli.

These and other studies[12–14] show that the long-term complications and benefits of these operations are somewhat different. Gastric bypass can cause iron-deficiency and/or vitamin B_{12}-deficiency anemia, causes the dumping syndrome, and eliminates the distal stomach and proximal small bowel from routine evaluation by radiologic or endoscopic studies. It completely cures gastroesophageal reflux disease (GERD), a common comorbid condition associated with morbid obesity, as the small proximal gastric pouch rarely contains any acid-secreting cells (they are located more distal in the stomach) and prevents bile reflux also. The VBG does not as reliably cure GERD, especially if a patient often overeats to the point of vomiting, or if the restriction at the exit of the pouch tightens because of adhesion of the liver or other organs to the foreign materials used to surround the outlet or because of fibrosis. The VBG is not associated with vitamin B_{12} or iron deficiency or the dumping syndrome. The VBG is also quicker and easier to perform. Vomiting and abdominal pain are more common after VBG than after gastric bypass. The outlet to the proximal pouch is more susceptible to obstruction from large boluses of poorly chewed food, multiple pills, or other objects (e.g., popcorn kernels, nuts) because it is not distensible. It also has not been established how long the circumference (usually 40 to 45 mm [1.6 to 1.8 inches]) of the foreign body that is wrapped around the outlet of the proximal pouch to help obstruct the pouch outlet should be, or if there are patient-specific characteristics that should modify this diameter (e.g., a lower esophageal sphincter pressure, history of GERD, motility disorders of the esophagus or stomach).

These four RCTs at these four different sites in the United States and Canada all suggested that the gastric bypass produced a significantly higher degree of weight loss than did a VBG.[5,8,10,11] The studies have 2 to 5 years of followup data, with the majority of patients approximately 3 years after their operations. Weight loss was reported as the percentage of excess body weight (EBW) lost using midpoints in the Metropolitan Life Insurance Tables for ideal body weight (IBW) as a goal so that preoperative body weight (PBW) − IBW = EBW and the percent of EBW lost = PBW − $\dfrac{\text{postoperative body weight}}{\text{EBW}}$ × 100. The weight loss after VBG ranged from a mean of 39% to a mean of 48% of EBW, while the range for gastric bypass was 58 to 67% of EBW. The longest study, which examined patients at 5 years after their procedures, also showed that all gastric bypass patients kept off at least 50% of their EBW while no VBG patient had kept off at least 50% of EBW.[11]

These data have led most surgeons to believe that a gastric bypass will often produce better weight loss for a patient than will a VBG or restrictive procedure. The fact that the gastric bypass makes the stomach smaller, shortens the absorbing length of the bowel, plus is associated with dumping if patients eat concentrated sweets or a high-fat meal while a VBG only makes the stomach smaller, suggests that it is a comparison of a one-dimensional operation versus a three-dimensional operation, which seems unfair. However, many bariatric surgeons feel that the type of operation a patient receives only provides 50% of the mechanism that helps morbidly obese people lose weight. The other 50% is the result of the behavior modifications, dietary, and exercise instruction that the surgeons' office provides, along with the psychological support to help people change their behaviors to allow their operations to maximally help them. The percentage of help provided by the technical aspects of the operation versus the preoperative and postoperative support is a very debatable issue, with no hard data to support either proposition. It is clear, however, that different surgeons have different outcomes when they perform relatively similar bariatric procedures. The volume of cases a month a surgeon performs is related to the complication rate.[15] The expertise in helping people lose weight also increases if an office handles a large volume of patients and is dedicated to providing support services for the patients it serves.

The attitudes and beliefs of the surgeons—that is, whether they believe equal weight loss can be achieved with different procedures—also influences how effectively patients lose weight. Similar to teaching high school students, if the teacher or surgeons believe that their students or patients will achieve a goal, those students or patients are much more likely to achieve that goal. Yale and Weiler[16] reported, in 1991, that their morbidly obese patients lost a mean of 60% of their EBW and kept it off for 5 years, equaling the results of gastric bypass patients in the four RCTs.[5,8,10,11] Buchwald and associates reported on two groups of their patients, the first in 1991[12] and the second in 2000,[13] where they let patients choose between a gastric bypass and silastic ring vertical gastroplasty (SRVG). In both of their series, which included almost 1500 patients having primary bariatric procedures, there was no statistically significant difference in the amount of weight lost, using several different measures, between patients who chose a SRVG versus those who chose a gastric bypass. Their SRVG patients lost more than 55% of their EBW at both 3 and 4 years postoperatively. The only criteria they used to try to guide patients to one procedure or the other was to recommend that all patients with severe GERD have a gastric bypass and all patients with a history of peptic ulcer disease have a SRVG.

Kalfarentizos and colleagues obtained similar weight loss after VBG and gastric bypass in a nonrandomized trial by assigning all sweets eaters to a gastric bypass but allowing other patients their choice.[14] Weight loss after VBG demonstrated a mean of 61% of EBW at 2 years and 50% at 3 years. After a gastric bypass, patients lost a mean of 65% of EBW at 2 years and 63% at 3 years. Both Buchwald and Kalfarentizos had no way of determining whether their weight loss results were a result of differences in technique, a result of the attitudes, beliefs and efforts of the patients who choose the different types of procedures, or a result of differences in the support their offices provide versus the offices of other surgeons who may not be as committed to teaching people how to re-eat and supporting them after VBG. Results from the gastric banding literature presented below also suggest that either the surgeon's office, a country's health care system (socialistic versus fee for service), or the national diet may influence whether or not a purely restrictive operation can be as successful as a combined or malabsorptive procedure.

TECHNIQUES FOR GASTROPLASTIES

The laparoscopic approach differs from what is done at laparotomy although the principles of creating a tube of stomach along the lesser curvature of the stomach remain the same. In both approaches, a bougie, usually 24-French (Fr) or 26-Fr, is inserted orally into the stomach to measure the circumference of the tube that is to be created along the lesser curvature of the stomach. The lower esophagogastric sphincter (LES) needs to be identified. A means to measure a 5- to 7-cm (2- to 2.8-inch) length from the LES along the lesser curvature needs to be established. This is usually a ruler, although a known length of a standard instrument can be used.

At laparotomy, one of the circular stapling devices is usually used to create a circular hole through the anterior and posterior walls of the stomach along the side of the bougie, which also staples this hole shut. Another linear stapling device is then placed through the circular opening, parallel and next to the bougie pointing toward the left crus. Stapling devices that create two separate staple lines, then cut between them, create a permanent scar once the cut ends of the tissue heal, which produces a more long-lasting result in RCTs as compared to not dividing the stomach.[8] A 40- to 70-cm (15.7- to 27.6-inch)–long piece of silicone tubing, or polypropylene mesh, or expanded polytetrafluoroethylene strip is then used to encircle the stomach at the level of the "crow's foot" of the vagus nerve (pes anserinus), attaching itself by suturing the ends together or by passing a suture through the tubing and knotting the suture to secure the circumference.

Alternatively, there is a notched stapling device that is available to be used to create the silicone ring gastroplasty. Figure 10–3 illustrates how the silicone tubing can be placed to complete the procedure without producing a hole in the stomach so that the procedure can be completed as a clean case as opposed to a clean-contaminated case with the hope that infection rates would be lower. This has not necessarily been demonstrated by the studies completed to date.

When a VBG is completed laparoscopically, there is a circular stapler that can be used. The instrumentation to allow the surgeon to push the stem of the circular stapler through the stomach and to position the anvil in place has not been specifically manufactured for laparoscopic surgery. Trying to accomplish this laparoscopically with the available instruments is possible but uncomfortable.

It is easier to create the lesser curvature pouch by resecting a wedge of corpus and fundus using the available linear stapling devices; Figure 10–4 illustrates this. The short gastric vessels are detached from the spleen by using clips. A partial gastrectomy is started by dividing the greater curvature of the

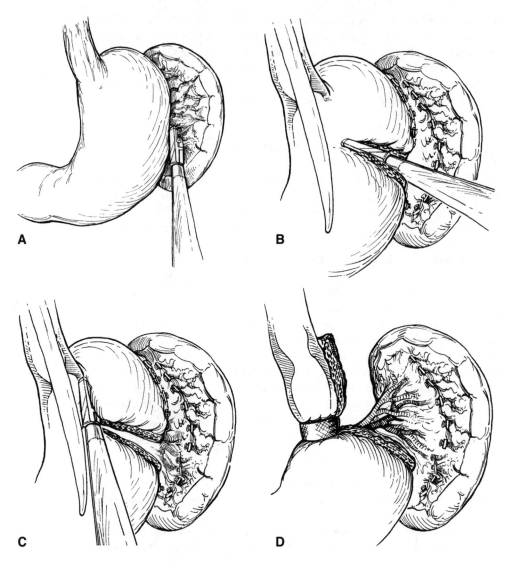

FIGURE 10–4   Technique for laparoscopic vertical-banded gastroplasty.

corpus just below the spleen, angling toward the upper edge of the pes anserinus, using the lateral border of the bougie as the terminal end and inserting
the stapling device from the patient's left side. Then a trocar on the patient's
right side close to the midline is used to complete the gastrectomy by dividing the stomach parallel to the bougie, starting at the point reached by the left-
sided approach to the bougie. Once the ring of nondistensible material is sutured around the lower end of the newly created pouch, the gastric omentum
is used to cover the foreign body in either the laparoscopic approach or at laparotomy.

GASTRIC BANDING AS A FORM OF GASTROPLASTY

Approximately 10 years after the introduction of restrictive operations, the concept of placing a band around the upper stomach of a nonexpandable, but flexible nature was tried in several different ways. One group of surgeons used a band of silicone tubing or polypropylene mesh to reinforce the outlet from a stapled gastric proximal pouch placed horizontally across the upper stomach following the lead of Mason's original idea (see Figure 10–1) but using newly introduced GI tract stapling devices brought to this country initially from the Soviet Union. Another group of surgeons thought it was simpler to use the bands by themselves to make the restriction around the stomach, creating a 50-mL volume (or less) proximal pouch just by the placement location of the band. The early history of this approach is most completely reviewed by Oria[17] who worked with Molena in the group that has performed more simple open-banding procedures than any other practice in the world since the early 1980s (Figure 10–5). Unfortunately, they have never published any peer-reviewed manuscript containing original long-term outcome data from their practice or compared their use of a band to any other bariatric procedure in an RCT, so the reliability of this procedure remains largely unproven.

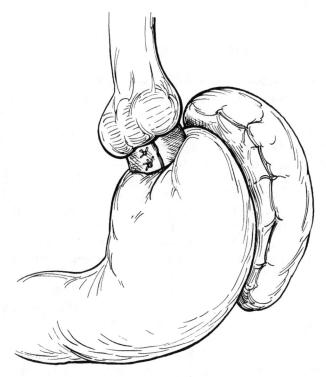

FIGURE 10–5   Molina gastric banding.

TECHNIQUES

Nonadjustable Gastric Banding

The techniques for this approach are taken from the review article written by Oria.[17] He describes using a subxiphoid, midline, mini-laparotomy long enough to emit the surgeon's right hand. The right index finger is used to blindly dissect a retrogastric tunnel from the greater curvature side to and through the peritoneum of the lesser curvature. A 36-Fr bougie calibrates the size of the stomach opening but the pouch is rarely measured because of visibility. They currently use an expanded polytetrafluoroethylene (e-PTFE) strip manufactured by WL Gore & Associates, Phoenix, Arizona, that is available in 2-mm (0.08-inch)–thick sheets with two functionally distinct sides called Gore-Tex Dura Mesh. A rougher side with an open microstructure is placed next to the stomach to encourage adhesions and tissue incorporation, so slippage will not occur. A smoother side is left to face the adjacent tissues to diminish the chance of adhesions. This side has a smaller pore size to reduce cell ingrowth. An 8- to 9-cm (3.1- to 3.5-inch)–long strip of this material is wrapped around the stomach containing the bougie and the band is then sutured to itself using nonabsorbable sutures. The band circumference is then between 6.5 and 8 cm (2.6 and 3.1 inches), depending on the thickness of the stomach wall.

Adjustable Gastric Banding

One problem identified in all restrictive procedures is how to produce a restricted outlet from the proximal gastric pouch that is tight enough to restrict the passage of normally chewed food so that fullness and then pain is produced if consumption is not terminated. The restriction must not dilate and get bigger with use, but also must be big enough so that, even in the immediate postoperative period when posttraumatic edema makes any anastomosis smaller, the anastomosis is wide enough to allow consumption of enough liquids to sustain a patient by the second or third postoperative day in more than 98% of operated patients. In the mid 1980s, Kuzmak,[18] in Livingston, NJ, and Hellers and Forsell,[19] in Sweden, came up with a solution to this problem. They added a balloon to the inside of the band and connected it to tubing that they attached to a reservoir port similar to that used for long-term venous access for chemotherapy that was left in a subcutaneous position attached to the chest or abdominal muscles. This port could then be accessed by using fluoroscopy so that fluids could be added or removed from the outlet to the restrictive gastric pouch, making the outlet adjustable (Figure 10–6).

These new adjustable gastric bands were a curiosity that initially did not have a large impact. In March 1987, however, Philippe Mouret performed the first laparoscopic cholecystectomy in Lyon, France, by using gynecologic instruments, including a scope without video equiptment.[20] Soon, advances in

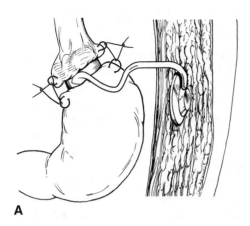 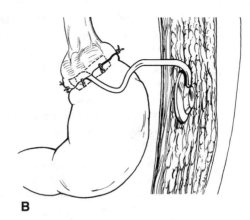

A   **B**

FIGURE 10-6   Adjustable gastric band.

videoendoscopic cameras and instrumentation made it possible to perform many common abdominal operations in addition to cholecystectomy, such as appendectomy, Nissen fundoplication, and highly selective vagotomy, by what was marketed as a laparoscopic.[21] It soon became possible to consider performing bariatric procedures laparoscopically. Suddenly, the adjustable gastric band seemed the ideal medical device to use for a restrictive procedure because it was easier to place this type of device with the first commercially produced instruments designed for laparoscopic surgery than it was to perform a VBG or a gastric bypass. Commercial companies bought the rights to manufacture the Kuzmak and Hellers bands and investment capital was raised to initiate animal and clinical trials and modify the design and manufacturing of these products.[22] Both the excitement of learning to perform new laparoscopic procedures plus the commercial enthusiasm of promoting a new or adjusted product for a new market helped to popularize adjustable gastric banding as a treatment of obesity, first throughout Europe, then Australia, and on to North, South, and Central Americas. It was fortuitous that nonprofit organizations like the Shape Up America! Foundation (created by ex-surgeon C. Everett Koop, MD), and national and international scientific organizations such as the National Institutes of Health and the World Health Organization, developed and promoted practice guidelines for all physicians outlining the need for expanded treatment of obesity.[23–25] The publicity surrounding these documents and the release of more scientific studies on the problems associated with obesity (Chapter 3) helped to advance the use of these devices worldwide for the treatment of morbid obesity.[26]

   The United States has the most organized and rigorous testing of medical devices as part of the mission of the Food and Drug Administration (FDA). US trials were initiated in 1995 by BioEnterics Corporation (Carpenterria, CA) using a modification of the device initially patented by Kuzmak.[18] The device, which is trademarked as the LAP-BAND, was approved by the FDA as an obesity treatment in June 2001, on the basis of a premarket approval application that contained data from a trial of more than 290 morbidly obese Americans plus international data collected in Europe, Australia, and Mexico.

The trial demonstrated that more than 70% (206/292) of the initial group of patients were followed for 3 years, losing and maintaining an average of more than 18% of their initial body weight (approximately 36% EBW). Forty-five patients were lost to follow-up and another 41 had had their band removed by the third year because they felt it was ineffective or had problems with it, usually because of slippage of the band, causing pouch dilation with pain or ineffectiveness.[26] This weight loss represented 40% of their excess body mass index,[27] a representation of how much of their excess weight (above a body mass index of 25) they lost. Better results have been reported in larger, longer-term studies in Australia[28] and Europe.[29]

Remarkably, in this and in another American trial of 193 patients, there were no deaths related to device placement or while the band was in place. This, coupled with the premarket approval application data from Europe,[29] Australia,[28] and Mexico, indicates that the mortality rate for laparoscopic adjustable banding placement maybe one-tenth what the rate was for open VBG or gastric bypass (data on file at the FDA Web site).[26]

The major problems identified with its use are the stability of placement of a medical device and its longevity. Early in the placement experience with the band, almost 20% of the bands moved (or slipped), or the pouch or esophagus dilated in the first year after placement.[26] Technique changes on how to place the band and under what conditions the band should be adjusted have decreased this rate by at least half during the first year. However, these types of problems can occur as long as the band is in place. The overall rate of complications long-term (10-year data) has not been established nor has the longevity of the device (although hundreds of Europeans have now had this model of the LAP-BAND in for 10 years). Leaks where the outside reservoir port connects to the tubing connecting it to the inner band continue to be a problem. The company that owns the patent for Hellers band (J&J Company, New Brunswick, NJ) has patented a design for an adjustable band that would have its own internal reservoir and could adjust the inner balloon diameter by using mechanics initially created by Swiss watchmakers. This is similar to the evolution of the mechanical artificial hearts where an internal design with a moveable reservoir was developed to decrease the risk of infection.

An easy set of rules to produce a successful adjustment schedule of the band has also not been established. DeMaria et al.[30] have shown that if the bariatric treatment team allows the patient to convince them to over-tighten the band rather than teach the patient to not expect the band itself to provide all the restraint necessary to lose weight, then esophageal dilation will be produced. Their report shows the critical need for the surgeon's office to develop a support structure that enhances the patient's chances of benefiting from the procedure rather than have the office develop protocols that add to the patient's chances that the procedure will fail. This site of the US multidisciplinary Trial A was also not as effective at helping their African American patients lose weight as they were helping their white patients, a problem that three other sites with the largest number of African American patients did not experience. DeMaria's site has repeatedly condemned restrictive operations as not being as effective in their hands as gastric bypass.[5] It is not clear to what degree the attitudes and beliefs of the surgeons influence the outcomes of bariatric surgery at their sites. It is also possible that the socioeconomic status and/or education level of their African American patients was significantly different than their other patients, which can influence a patient's ability to learn new habits, affect how much follow-up and support a patient receives, and help to determine the quality of the diet consumed. Additional studies are necessary to define which of these elements has a significant effect on a morbidly obese patient's chances of benefiting from restrictive operations versus a gastric bypass.

The development of a relatively easy laparoscopic bariatric procedure and its marketing by commercial concerns has generated some animosity in this country between older surgeons who have devoted their practices to bariatric treatments and a new generation of surgeons who want to use their training in laparoscopic techniques to help establish a niche in the market. This is more of a controversy in saturated metropolitan areas than it is in rural areas. It is less of an issue in markets where a high degree of managed care penetration prevents new practices from being established. The disagreement has focused on whether the treatment of morbid obesity will suffer another era of unwelcome scrutiny from the insurance industry and the malpractice community of lawyers, if a group of younger surgeons attempt to perform laparoscopic bariatric surgery as a sideline, usually meaning as less than a majority of their practice. Older bariatric surgeons with established practices and a steady stream of patients from "word of mouth" referrals worry that surgeons who devote less than a majority of their time to a bariatric practice will not be able to develop the support apparatus to provide behavioral and dietary instruction that requires a multidisciplinary team and some financial stability for this team. Many investigators have shown that the higher the volume of procedures performed by a surgical team per year the lower the complication rates and the better the outcomes.[15] This correlation has not been established yet for bariatric surgery but there is little doubt among experienced bariatric surgeons that this hypothesis is correct.

These procedures require the patient to modify their behavior to be successful and the majority of people will need a multidisciplinary team to successfully modify their behavior. Also, it is much more difficult to complete abdominal procedures, by laparotomy or laparoscopy, in morbidly obese patients. The surgeons, the anesthesia personnel, and the hospital nursing staff will improve their care of morbidly obese patients only once it becomes routine (there must be a weekly volume of patients to achieve expertise). A part-time practice means that the team is repeatedly trying to remember what it did 2 or 3 weeks ago, rather than continuing to improve its coordination by regular practice. If a group of part-time surgeons create a large group of patients with expensive complications for insurance companies to worry about or an increase in malpractice litigation against a hospital, the whole field of bariatric surgery will come under attack as creating too many expenses and problems. Surgeons older than age 50 years have lived through one such era like this and do not want to see another such era develop. Our system does not have control mechanisms to demand that high-risk procedures be completed in high-volume centers. It is unclear whether common sense among surgeons and their hospitals will win over the desire of inexperienced surgeons to try their luck at the occasional bariatric encounter.

Technique for Placing Adjustable Gastric Bands

The basic technique for successfully placing an adjustable gastric band relies on four principles:

1. Create a position tunnel for the band just below the esophagogastric junction that ensures that the tunnel will remain above the bursa omentalis.
2. Minimize the trauma to the stomach (especially along the greater curvature away from the left *crus*), to the liver, and while tunneling blindly behind the stomach.
3. Minimize the handling of the band and its accessories, avoiding placing stress or any sharp objects near any part of the device.
4. Imbricate the stomach over the band for as much of the arc of the band as possible, but create a tunnel that is tension free without stretching the stomach over any part of the buckle mechanism.

The principles are designed to prevent damage to the band resulting in a leak or a shorter lifetime for the device, to prevent adhesions or tension between the band and the surrounding stomach, which might lead to inflammation and erosion of the band into the lumen of the stomach, and to eliminate any unfettered area of stomach posterior to the band that would be free to slide upward into the space between the band and the circumference of stomach it is surrounding when the patient vomits. If the bursa omentalis is entered, the posterior distal stomach must also be imbricated around the exposed part of the band by entering the lesser sac and closing the area or attaching a foreign body, such as polypropylene mesh, to the distal posterior stomach to prevent it fitting in the potential space between the band and the underlying stomach it circumferences.

Patients also need to be encouraged to take antiemetics whenever they are nauseated to prevent vomiting. A viral illness or sea sickness/inner ear problems can cause vomiting that will break the sutures used to imbricate the stomach over the band, allowing band slippage even years after it is placed. Patients also must avoid using nonsteroidal antiinflammatory agents as these drugs are associated with an increased incidence of erosion of the bands into the lumen of the stomach.

The best way to stay above the bursa omentalis is to create the tunnel using the "pars flaccida" approach. The surgeon identifies where the right crural muscle attaches inferiorly to the vertebra and begins the dissection to create the posterior tunnel just superior to where the muscle attaches inferiorly to the vertebra. The dissection for the posterior tunnel is begun by angling upwards toward the patient's left shoulder, placing the dissecting instrument through a trocar that is lateral and inferior to the esophagogastric junction, lateral to the *midclavicular* line. The bare area of the lesser curvature omentum over the caudate lobe of the liver is opened to expose this space. Before completing the tunnel behind the esophagogastric junction, the attachments of the greater curvature of the stomach to the diaphragm have to be released in the area lateral to the left crural muscle. If the fundus is redundant especially posteriorly, the fundus must be pulled forward and these redundant attachments released to clear an area to emerge from the patient's right side as the posterior tunnel is created behind the esophagogastric junction.

The band should encircle an area of the stomach that is less than 20 mL in volume. The inferior stomach that is used to imbricate tissue over the band must be brought up from enough caudal to the band to create a loose tunnel. At least three individual sutures are used to complete the imbrication. Some surgeons use a running suture instead. We have seen both approaches disrupted by excessive vomiting.

CONCLUSIONS

Not all surgeons and not all patients want their GI tract rearranged or bypassed in their attempts to find a way to lose weight. Gastric restrictive operations were developed as a less invasive and usually reversible way to provide a bariatric surgical approach to help morbidly obese patients lose weight. The adjustable gastric band appears to be the most reversible procedure. Laparoscopic removal of an adjustable band is relatively simple and the stomach usually reverts to its original shape within days.

Restrictive operations do not have as many physiological means to help patients lose weight. Both the patient and the surgeon's office have to work harder to help the patient modify their behaviors. Multiple sites have shown that this approach can be as successful as a gastric bypass, especially if the patient is educated to know how to succeed and how to avoid failure. Centers who do not offer this less-invasive choice must be prepared to lose patients whose beliefs and attitudes may differ from the surgeon's. Although evidence-based medicine is wedded to the RCT as the ideal mechanism to compare therapeutic alternatives to determine which is superior, numerous medical opinion leaders continue to remind the medical field that patient prerogatives remain important to the delivery of medical care in a free society.[31-33] People with strongly held beliefs will often not enter RCTs and this selection bias influences the results of an RCT as much as other important demographic characteristics that influence medical treatment outcomes, such as socioeconomic status or education level. Evidence-based medicine still needs to incorporate a step that demonstrates that the results of an RCT can be duplicated in actual practice environments.

REFERENCES

1. Fitzgibbon ML, Stolley MR, Kirschenbaum DS. Obese people who seek treatment have different characteristics than those who do not seek treatment. *Health Psychol* 1993;12:342–345.
2. Martin LF. The biopsychosocial characteristics of people seeking treatment for obesity. *Obes Surg* 1999:9:235–243.
3. Mason EE, ITO C. Gastric bypass in obesity. *Surg Clin North Am* 1967;47:1845–1852.
4. Printen KJ, Mason EE. Gastric surgery for relief of morbid obesity. *Arch Surg* 1973;106:428–431.
5. Sugerman HJ, Starkey JV, Birkenhauer RA. A randomized prospective trial of gastric bypass versus vertical banded gastroplasty for morbid obesity and their effects on sweets versus no-sweets eaters. *Ann Surg* 1987;205:613–624.
6. Martin LF. Chirurgie de l'obesite: l'experience nord-americaine. In: Dargent J, Pascal JI, eds. *L'obesite morbide: strategie therapeutique.* Paris, France: Springer Verlag, 2002:11–26.
7. Mason EE. Vertical banded gastroplasty. *Arch Surg* 1982;117:701–706.
8. MacLean LD, Rhode BM, Sampalis J, Forse RA. Results of the surgical treatment of obesity. *Am J Surg* 1993;165:155–160.
9. Toppino M, Morino M, Capuzzi P. Outcome of vertical banded gastroplasty. *Obes Surg* 1999;9:51–54.
10. Hall JC, Watts JM, O'Brien PE, et al. Gastric surgery for morbid obesity: the Adelaide study. *Ann Surg* 1990;211:419–427.
11. Howard L, Malone M, Michalek A, et al. Gastric bypass and vertical banded gastroplasty: a prospective randomized comparison and 5-year follow-up. *Obes Surg* 1995;5:55–60.
12. Zimmerman V, Campos CT, Buchwald H. Weight loss comparison of gastric bypass and silastic ring vertical gastroplasty. *Obes Surg* 1992;2:47–49.
13. Buchwald H, Menchaca HJ, Menchaca YM, Michalek VN. Surgically induced weight loss: gastric bypass versus gastroplasty. *Prob Gen Surg* 2000;17:23–28.
14. Kalfarentzos F, Dimakopoulos A, Kehagias I, Loukidi A, Mean N. Vertical banded gastroplasty versus standard or distal Roux-en-Y gastric bypass based on specific criteria in the morbidly obese: preliminary results. *Obes Surg* 1999;9:433–443.
15. Hannan EL, Kilburn H, Bernard H, et al. Coronary artery bypass surgery: the relationship between in hospital mortality rate and surgical volume after controlling for clinical risk factors. *Med Care* 1991;329:1094–1107.
16. Yale CE, Weiler SJ. Weight control after vertical banded gastroplasty. *Am J Surg* 1991;162:13–18.
17. Oria HE. Gastric banding for morbid obesity. *Eur J Gastroenterol Hepatol* 199;11:105–114.
18. Kuzmak LI. Silicone gastric banding: a simple and effective operation for morbid obesity. *Contemp Surg* 1986;28:13–18.
19. Forsell P, Hallberg D, Hellers G. Gastric banding for morbid obesity: initial experience with a new adjustable band. *Obes Surg* 1993;3:369–374.

20. Perissat J. Laparoscopic cholecystectomy: the European experience. *Am J Surg* 1993;165:444–449.
21. Soper N, Brut LM, Kerbl K. Laparoscopic general surgery. *N Engl J Med* 1994;330:409–419.
22. Belachew M, Legrand MJ, Vincent V. History of LAP-BAND: from dream to reality. *Obes Surg* 2001;11:297–302.
23. Shape Up America! Foundation and American Obesity Association. *Guidance for Treatment of Adult Obesity.* Washington, DC: Shape Up America!, 1996.
24. National Heart, Lung, and Blood Institute Obesity Education Initiative Expert Panel. *Clinical Guidelines on the Identification, Evaluation, and Treatment of Overweight and Obesity in Adults. The Evidence Report.* NIH Publ #98–4083, Sept 1998.
25. World Health Organization. *Obesity: Preventing and Managing the Global Epidemic.* Geneva, Switzerland: World Health Organization, 1998.
26. Martin LF, Smits GJ, Greenstein RJ. Laparoscopic adjustable gastric banding to treat morbid obesity: 3-year efficacy and 6-year safety data from the US Multicenter trials. Submitted 2003 *JAMA*.
27. Greenstein RJ, Belachew M. Implantable gastric stimulation as therapy for human obesity: report from the 2001 IFSO symposium in Crete. *Obes Surg* 2002;12(Suppl 1):3S–5S.
28. Dixon JB, Dixon ME, O'Brien PE. Quality of life after lap-band placement: influence of time, weight loss, and comorbidities. *Obes Res* 2001;9:713–721.
29. Belachew M, Legrand M, Vincent V, et al. Laparoscopic adjustable gastric banding. *World J Surg* 1998;22:955–963.
30. DeMaria EJ, Sugerman HJ, Meador JG, et al. High failure rate after laparoscopic adjustable silicone gastric banding for treatment of morbid obesity. *Am Surg* 2001;233:809–818.
31. Kassier JP. Adding insult to injury: usurping patients' prerogatives. *N Engl J Med* 1983;308:898–901.
32. Kassier JP. Incorporating patient's preferences into medical decisions. *N Engl J Med* 1994;330:1895–1896.
33. Solomon MJ, McLeod RS. Should we be performing more randomized controlled trials evaluating surgical operations? *Surgery* 1995;118:459–467.

GASTRIC BYPASS

WALTER J. PORIES /
JOHN SCOTT ROTH

HISTORY

Bariatric surgery is one of the great medical advances. Who would have thought that an operation could achieve durable weight loss along with full and long-term remission of diabetes, hypertension, Pickwickian syndrome, sleep apnea, stress incontinence, and even infertility? This chapter reviews the discovery and evolution of the gastric bypass, the bariatric procedure most often referred to as the "gold standard" for the surgical therapy of severe obesity and its comorbidities.

The discipline of bariatric surgery began quietly in a research laboratory at the Veterans Administration Hospital in Minneapolis when Kremen, Linner, and Nelson observed that shortening of the intestinal tract produced predictable weight loss in dogs. Based on this work, the team performed the first ileojejunal bypass on a 34-year-old woman who weighed 385 lb.[1] At the presentation of the case at the meeting of the American Surgical Association in 1954, Sandblom, in his discussion, stated that Viktor Hendriksson of Sweden performed a similar procedure 2 years earlier, except this procedure involved a resection rather than a bypass: "The procedure produced weight loss," but, he added prophetically, "it also created a difficult situation of nutritional balance."[2]

With that report, Kremen and his associates introduced a startling new concept: severe obesity was such a serious disease that it warranted surgical intervention. The idea spread rapidly, and soon a series of intestinal bypasses (Figure 11–1) with many variations were reported throughout the United States. Unfortunately, these procedures did not live up to their promise. Al-

213

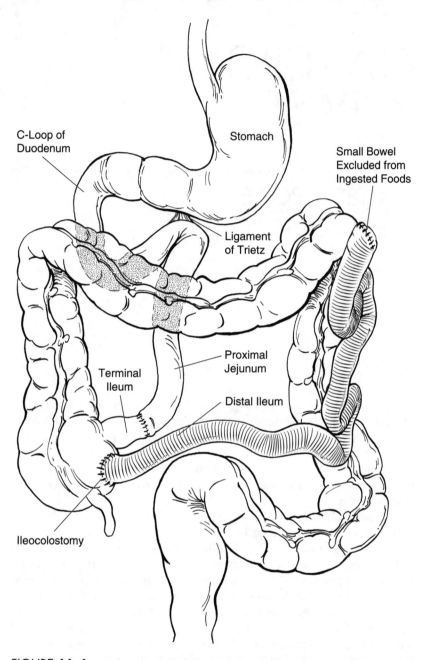

FIGURE 11–1   A late model of the intestinal bypass that excluded all parts of the small bowel except for 35.6 cm (14 inches) of proximal jejunum and 10.2 cm (4 inches) of distal ileum. The excluded bowel was usually drained into the distal colon.

though the intestinal bypasses produced significant weight loss, they were also associated with serious, and sometimes deadly, risks: diarrhea, electrolyte imbalance, enteropathies, intussusception, vitamin deficiencies, trace element deficits, liver failure, hair loss, cholelithiasis, nephrolithiasis, and hypoproteinemia.[3] An operation that produced bald, wrinkled, jaundiced people who smelled bad was not a great advance. Unfortunately, thousands of these procedures were done and almost all had to be reversed.

Mason's Two Solutions

The problem was addressed most successfully by Mason and Ito, in 1969,[4] with the demonstration that a gastric approach could produce weight loss equal to the intestinal bypass but without the many metabolic complications. Mason and his associates developed two operations: (1) the loop gastric bypass (GB) (Figure 11–2) and (2) the vertical-banded gastroplasty (VBG) (Figure 11–3). Both operations limited intake with a reduced gastric pouch and delayed gastric emptying with a gastroenterostomy of limited size. The loop GB, however, increased the efficacy of the approach by interfering with absorption and digestion through the exclusion of part of the foregut, including the antrum, duodenum, and proximal jejunum.

For about two decades, the VBG appears to have been the most commonly performed operation in the United States. Complications associated with the constricting band, leading to intractable vomiting, abdominal pain, and poor food choice because of stricture of the outflow track from the proximal gastric pouch, however, has limited its application, and the procedure has decreased in popularity. The concept of a bariatric operation that restricts intake while maintaining the normal flow of digestion persists with the gradually increasing popularity of the recently introduced adjustable gastric band. This operation is discussed in detail in Chapter 10 and is mentioned here only for historic continuity.

Maturing the Gastric Bypass

Although the loop GB induced weight loss as effectively as the intestinal bypass in some patients, the procedure introduced new problems. Weight loss was variable, and patients complained of biliary emesis and esophagitis because the loop allowed bile to wash back into the stomach.

These issues were addressed at East Carolina University in a series of studies between 1978 and 1980 that developed many of the guidelines still in use today: (1) the gastric pouch must be small, 10 to 30 cc, about the size of a man's thumb; (2) the gastric outlet should be limited to about 1 cm (0.4 inches); (3) drainage from the gastric pouch should be accomplished by a Roux-en-Y arrangement; and (4) the alimentary loop, that is, the jejunum draining the gastric pouch, should be a minimum of 60 cm (23.6 inches) in length (over the last 5 years, the preferred length has risen to 100 to 150 cm [39.4 to 59.1 inches] depending on the weight of the patients). Figure 11–4 diagrams this operation,

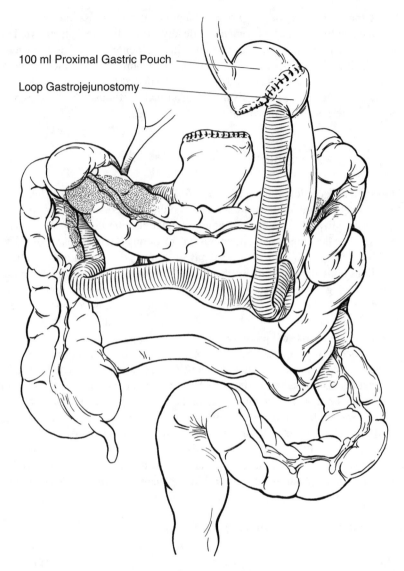

100 ml Proximal Gastric Pouch

Loop Gastrojejunostomy

FIGURE 11–2   Mason's first gastric loop bypass.

which is commonly referred to as the "Greenville gastric bypass." The results for this procedure are given below.

Since then, several other important advances have been introduced, the most important being the application of laparoscopy, a technology that reduces surgical trauma and promotes greater precision in the performance of the surgery. Others have introduced the placement of a silastic ring just distal to the gastroenterostomy to maintain the delay in gastric emptying, and lengthening the alimentary loop to achieve greater weight loss, especially in the super-obese.

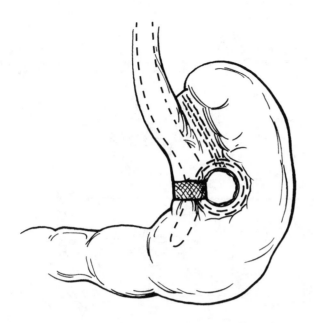

FIGURE 11–3 Mason's vertical-banded gastroplasty. This operation was, for about two decades, the most commonly performed bariatric operation. The adjustable gastric band used today is a modification of that original procedure.

INDICATIONS AND CONTRAINDICATIONS

The basic indications for the gastric bypass were spelled out in the 1993 National Institutes of Health Consensus Conference on the Surgery for Morbid Obesity as follows:

- A body mass index (BMI = kg/m^2) ⩾40
- A BMI ⩾35 if the patient also has comorbidities

In addition, the bariatric surgical community has, through experience, added the following important requirements:

- Patient willing to contract for long-term followup so that long-term nutritional complications can be avoided;
- Patient intelligent enough to understand the procedure and its consequences, that is, well-enough informed to give true informed consent;
- Absence of alcohol and substance abuse or, if previously present, to have these addictions under tight control; and
- Control of other psychiatric disorders, especially depression associated with suicidal ideations or attempts.

The contraindications include the following tenets:

- Uncontrolled medical disease that raises surgical risk to unacceptable levels;

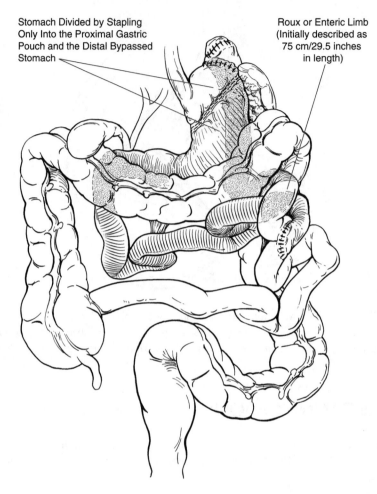

Stomach Divided by Stapling
Only Into the Proximal Gastric
Pouch and the Distal Bypassed
Stomach

Roux or Enteric Limb
(Initially described as
75 cm/29.5 inches
in length)

FIGURE 11–4   The Greenville gastric bypass. The operation is based on Mason's gastric bypass but sharply diminishes the size of the gastric reservoir, decreases the diameter of the gastrojejunostomy, and converts the loop to a Roux-en-Y configuration.

- Uncontrolled emotional disorders including alcoholism and substance abuse;
- Failure to understand the operation and its potential consequences; and
- Lack of family support (a relative contraindication, but an important consideration).

Several potential new guidelines are under intense discussion at this time, including the following:

- Is the gastric bypass an appropriate therapy for severely obese children with major comorbidities, such as type 2 diabetes in a 12-year-old who weighs 300 lb?

- Should the gastric bypass be available for the treatment of severe diabetics with a BMI <35?

Other factors to be considered in the choice of bariatric surgery include the competence and experience of the bariatric surgeon, the capacity of the institution to provide consultants and critical care in the event of a serious complication, the culture of the facility and the team for providing compassionate care to these challenging patients and their families, and the ability to provide long-term follow-up of at least 75% of the individuals for a period of 5 years.

PREOPERATIVE ASSESSMENT AND PREPARATION

If the candidate for the gastric bypass is in apparently good health without any major comorbidities, a workup equivalent to that required for other major operations will generally suffice. This assessment will include a thorough history, physical examination, chest radiograph, electrocardiogram, urinalysis, a complete blood count (CBC), a metabolic panel including a fasting blood glucose, thyroid-stimulating hormone (TSH), and for any woman in her child-bearing years, a pregnancy test, even if the patient denies any sexual activity (see Chapter 5 for a more extensive review of the preoperative evaluation before bariatric surgery). In addition, in the preoperative assessment for gastric bypass, right upper quadrant ultrasonography has become standard practice because of the relatively low sensitivity of gall bladder palpation for the detection of stones. Many of our patients also undergo a barium swallow prior to the laparoscopic gastric bypass to assess any evidence of hiatal hernia that may make the operation more difficult or may sway the surgeon to perform an open approach. At East Carolina University, patients are also screened with a psychiatric instrument. Significant time should be allotted for the discussion of the operation with the patient and family so that true informed consent is obtained.

Patients with comorbidities that cannot be managed by the bariatric surgeon should be seen by the appropriate consultants. Psychiatrists and psychologists trained in the special mental health needs of the morbidly obese can be of great help in the identification of patients who may fare badly, given the great changes that the operations induce in terms of body image and human relationships. Outcomes from bariatric surgery, as with other procedures, are far better if the patients are in optimal condition.

GASTRIC BYPASS: A FAMILY OF OPERATIONS

Even though the gastric bypass is frequently described as the "gold standard" treatment of morbid obesity, the truth is that there are many versions of the gastric bypass. The procedures reported in the literature differ in the following ways:

- Open laparotomy versus laparoscopic approaches;
- Sizes of the gastric pouch;
- Creation of the pouch by division of the stomach into separate structures versus stapling without cutting the tissue to create separate structures;
- Size of the gastrojejunostomy;
- Addition or absence of a silastic ring distal to the gastrojejunostomy in an attempt to further delay gastric emptying;
- Creation of the gastrojejunostomy by stapling or handsewn techniques;
- Length of the intestinal limbs (enteral, biliopancreatic, and common);
- Antecolic versus retrocolic placement of the enteral limb;
- Creation and size of the jejunojejunostomy; and
- Closure versus no closure of sites for potential internal hernias.

If each of these variations is only considered to be a binary choice, then the potential number of gastric bypasses is 2^9 or at least 512 different procedures. The need for standardization of the gastric bypass and other bariatric procedures is evident. Surgeons and the public need to know how to select among these choices to produce the best results.

RESULTS

The most reliable outcomes data for the treatment of morbid obesity with a standardized gastric bypass operation was reported by Pories and his associates.[5] The series included 608 consecutive patients who underwent the operation from 1980 to 1994. Only 17 of the 608 patients (<3%) were lost to follow-up.

The operation, identified as the "Greenville gastric bypass" consisted of a 20- to 30-mL stapled gastric pouch, an 0.8- to 1.0-cm (0.3- to 0.4-inch) gastrojejunostomy handsewn double-layered anastomosis, and a 40- to 60-cm (15.7- to 23.6-inch) alimentary loop attached to the stomach in a Roux-en-Y configuration. (The variations reflect the difficulties of measuring living tissues).

Even though many of the patients were seriously ill, the operation was performed with a perioperative mortality and complication rate of 1.5% and 8.5%, respectively. Of the nine deaths, five patients died of sepsis, three of pulmonary embolism, and one of an unknown cause, possibly dysrhythmia. Perioperative morbidity during the first 30 days after operation included the following complications: minor wound infections, 8.7%; wound seromas, 5.8%; severe wound infections, 3.0%; anastomotic stenoses, 3.0%; splenic tears, 0.5%; and subphrenic abscess 2.5%. Hospital readmission was required of 8.2% of the patients and 2.8% of the patients needed reoperations during the early postoperative period.

The total mortality over the 14 years was 34 of 608, with 9 perioperative and 25 late deaths. The latter were divided into two groups: 13 from emotionally related causes and 12 from "more natural" causes. The emotionally related deaths involved three suicides, three cases of cirrhosis as a consequence of a return to drinking, one case of bulimia, one case of pernicious anemia caused by a refusal to take vitamin B_{12}, one case of alcoholic hepatitis, and four deaths as a result of auto accidents, which we believe also may have been suicides. The other late "natural" deaths included four of cardiac causes, two of cancer, and one each of atherosclerosis, pneumonia, acquired immunodeficiency syndrome, peritonitis, pulmonary embolus, and sepsis from a later operation.

The most frequent late complications were vitamin B_{12} deficiency (40%), anemia (39%), hospital readmission (38%), incisional hernia (23.9%), depression (23.4%), staple-line failure (15.1%), gastritis (13.2%), cholelithiasis (11.4%), and bile reflux (8.7%). In a more recent survey, we also identified 47 patients who developed episodes of symptomatic hypoglycemia with documented levels of plasma glucose of 40 mg/dL or lower and associated acute lethargy. These episodes were unpredictable in onset, occurring as late as 14 years after the gastric bypass. The hypoglycemia was not related to whether or not they had diabetes prior to the surgery. In all of the patients, the symptoms lasted no longer than 2 years and were managed reasonably well by encouraging ingestion of one or more pieces of hard sugar candy (like a Life Saver) until the lethargy resolves. Dumping syndrome (diarrhea, abdominal cramping, tachycardia, etc.) developed in 70.6% of the patients; although this syndrome is sometimes listed as a complication, it is easily controlled by the avoidance of sweets and is actually a desired side effect.

The gastric bypass provides durable weight control. Weights fell from a preoperative mean of 138.1 kg (304.4 lb; range: 89.8 to 279 kg [198 to 615 lb]) to 87.2 kg (192.2 lb; range: 47.2 to 211.4 kg [104 to 466 lb]) by 1 year and were maintained at 93.2 kg (205.4 lb; range: 48.5 to 232.2 kg [107 to 512 lb]) at 5 years, 93.7 kg (206.5 lb; range: 59 to 176 [130 to 388 lb]) at 10 years, and 92.9 kg (204.7 lb; range: 71.7 to 122.5 kg [158 to 270 lb]) at 14 years.

The operation provides long-term control of type 2 diabetes mellitus. In those patients with adequate followup, 121 of 146 patients (82.9%) with diabetes and 150 of 152 patients (98.7%) with glucose impairment returned to and maintained normal levels of plasma glucose, glycosylated hemoglobin, and insulin. In addition to the control of weight and diabetes, the gastric bypass also corrected or alleviated a number of other comorbidities of obesity, including hypertension, sleep apnea, cardiopulmonary failure, arthritis, and infertility. For example, before surgery, 353 of the 608 patients (58.1%) were hypertensive. After surgery, this rate was reduced to 14%.

Livingston et al.[6] evaluated their perioperative results in a series of 1067 consecutive patients over 6.5 years. Unfortunately, the report failed to describe the operations nor was there a differentiation between laparoscopic and open approaches. They reported an operative mortality of 1.3%, with the following complications: anastomotic leak (1.4%), sepsis (0.5%), pulmonary embolus (0.8%), evisceration (0.3%), intestinal bleeding (0.8%), anastomotic stricture (0.1%), respiratory/renal failure (0.8%), and bowel obstruction (0.9%). Univariate analysis revealed that male gender and weight were predictive of severe life-threatening adverse outcomes. Patients older than age 55 years had a threefold higher mortality from surgery than did younger patients.

The Contribution of Laparoscopy

We concur with Buchwald's recent assessment that, "probably the major innovation in bariatric surgery is the laparoscopic revolution."[7] Whittgrove and Clark[8] recently reported 6 years of experience with 500 patients who had undergone their version of the gastric bypass. Their initial excess weight loss (IEWL) at 1 year was 80%, their mean operative time was about 90 minutes, and they had no perioperative deaths (mortality = 0%). Their main complications were bleeding (0.8%) and anastomotic leaks (2.5%).

Schauer and his associates[9] reported their short-term, 2.5 years of experience with 275 laparoscopic gastric bypass procedures. Their IEWL at 2 years was 83% with an operative mortality of 0.4%, a gastrojejunostomy leak rate of 4.4%, and a mean operative time of 260 minutes.

In a comparison of laparoscopic versus open gastric bypass operations, Nguyen and his associates[10] reviewed the outcomes in a group of 155 patients who were randomly assigned to either of the two approaches between May 1999 and March 2001. Despite a longer operative time, patients undergoing laparoscopic gastric bypass benefited from less blood loss, a shorter hospital stay, and faster convalescence. Those patients who underwent the laparoscopic gastric bypass had comparable weight loss at 1 year with those who had the open procedure, but they had a more rapid improvement in the quality of life. The higher initial operative costs for laparoscopic gastric bypass were adequately offset by the lower hospital costs.

A major advantage of the laparoscopic approach is the sharp reduction in the incidence of incisional hernias. With the open approach, several bariatric surgeons, including us, have reported rates of approximately 25%. With the laparoscopic bariatric surgery, the rate for hernias drops to 0 to 2%. (See Chapter 9 for a complete discussion of the benefits of the laparoscopic approach.)

COMPLICATIONS AND THEIR MANAGEMENT

Bariatric surgery is a complex undertaking in a population at high risk. "It takes a village" to care for these individuals, a community of professionals that includes a well-prepared institution, highly trained bariatric surgeons, consultants familiar with the problems of the morbidly obese, a culture that is sympathetic and supportive to these challenging patients, and a staff that does not hesitate to call for help.

The keystone of risk management in bariatric surgery is prevention. Patients must be carefully selected and brought to the most optimal condition. Emotional problems and substance abuse should be brought under full control and remain under control for 6 months to 1 year before offering the surgery to these types of patients. Many patients require diuresis, control of asthma, and treatment of skin lesions or other hygienic problems, as well as adjustment of medications. Families frequently need extra time to adjust; patients seem to do far better when they are surrounded by supportive parents, siblings, and spouses. It is not unusual to require 2 or 3 months to bring these complex patients to the best possible condition for the surgery.

Perioperative Complications

The perioperative complications associated with bariatric surgery reflect those of other abdominal operations, including infection, bleeding, bowel obstruction, cardiorespiratory failure, arrhythmias, pulmonary emboli, dehiscence, atelectasis, and pneumonia. Each of these problems are managed in the same manner as in the nonmorbidly obese, with three major differences: (1) the usual danger signs, such as fever and abdominal pain, are often very subtle in the morbidly obese; (2) these individuals are frequently immunosuppressed (this is actually a comorbid condition in the most morbidly obese or super-obese individuals and should be considered part of their total disease burden) and are unable to mount an appropriate response; and (3) the patients are brittle with little reserve, requiring a more rapid response than do normal individuals.

Preoperative antibiotics, timed to be given within the hour prior to making an incision, are essential. Unless there is a clear indication, antibiotics should be limited to no more than two postoperative doses. One member of our team feels that no postoperative antibiotics are needed.

One complication, the anastomotic leak, deserves special mention. As noted above, even in the best of hands, such as those of Whittgrove and Clark, this potentially catastrophic event occurs in approximately 1 in 45 patients. Because symptoms are often subtle in the postoperative bariatric patient, most surgeons consider a pulse >120 and left shoulder pain pathognomonic of a leak or a developing subdiaphragmatic abscess. Other common signs include unusual anxiety, perspiration, and elevated bands. If any of these signs occur, a gastrographin swallow radiogram should be done. The study is helpful if it confirms a leak; it is not reliable if is negative.

In the past, patients were routinely explored if any of the danger signs were not explained within 4 hours, either through the original mid-line incision for open cases or, for laparoscopic operations, through several of the port sites. Recently, however, some surgeons have reported good outcomes from the routine drainage of the left upper quadrant with suction drains such as Jackson-Pratt or Blake drains combined with intensive antibiotic therapy for a few days. The importance of early intervention cannot be exaggerated.

Late Complications

Three important late complications deserve mention: malnutrition, regain of weight, and depression. One of the few frustrations of bariatric surgery is that the most serious of the complications, malnutrition, is also the easiest to prevent. Even though our group spends considerable time with each patient and the patient's family instructing them that two chewable multivitamin/mineral tablets are absolutely essential for their good health, we have encountered patients with Wernicke-Korsakoff syndrome, kwashiorkor, pellagra, and beriberi severe enough to require hospitalization, even long-term rehabilitation. These nutritional complications, which develop from a lack of compliance with the instructions that are emphasized preoperatively, are the reason that bariatric surgical patients require long-term followup. All too often, classic signs of the above diseases, such as peripheral edema, neuropathies, visual disturbances, and arrhythmias, are missed by primary care physicians who may order many tests but fail to provide the only effective therapy, correction of the nutritional deficits because this is *not* their area of expertise and they do *not* understand how the gastrointestinal tract is rearranged during a gastric bypass so they do *not* know what nutritional deficits to expect.

A few patients will regain their weight. In the past, most of these failures were a result of the breakdown of the staple line used to partition the stomach, but the improvement of stapling devices and surgical technique has reduced this complication to 2%.[11] A more likely cause today is "outeating the pouch," which is a result of continued snacking on "soft calories," such as peanut butter and crackers. Contrast studies of the gastric pouch offer the most rapid and accurate approach to differentiating staple line breakdown from behavioral problems. If the staple line has been disrupted, the patient should be reexplored and repaired. This is not an easy operation and carries a somewhat higher risk than the initial procedure. These operations should only be attempted by experienced bariatric surgeons after a multidisciplinary preoperative evaluation similar to the initial evaluation of bariatric patients.

If the patient is living on soft calories and even if there is some dilatation of the gastric outlet, surgical repair of the anastomosis is likely to prove unsuccessful. The best approach appears to be dietary education, but if this fails lengthening of the enteral or alimentary limb deserves consideration.

Depression and other manifestations of mental illness are common problems in the morbidly obese, seen in approximately 25% of these individuals before and after bariatric surgery. Indications of suicidal ideation, adjustment problems, and abnormal psychosocial behavior deserve early referral to a psychiatrist.

Because each of these complications may appear years after bariatric surgery and because we still do not have enough continuing outcomes data about the various operations, long-term rigorous followup of these patients, by the surgeon, the referring physician, or even through support groups is mandatory.

CONCLUSION

The gastric bypass operation can now be regarded as a well-proven and safe procedure for the treatment of morbid obesity and its comorbidities. The effectiveness of the therapy is startling: durable weight loss of more than 45.5 kg (100 lb) for as long as 14 years postoperatively, full remission of type 2 diabetes, asthma, hypertension, pseudotumor cerebri, infertility, steatosis of the liver, gastroesophageal reflux, and many other conditions that were previously considered untreatable and irreversible.

The operation can be performed with a mortality rate of <1% even though many of the morbidly obese patients who present requesting surgery have multiple, severe comorbid conditions usually associated with a higher perioperative mortality rate. With laparoscopy, lengths of hospital stays have been reduced to 2 to 3 days with few complications. To obtain such results, however, requires a well-prepared institution with a mission to help the morbidly obese, surgeons well trained in bariatric surgery who are performing a high volume of cases monthly (i.e., 5 to 30+ each month), a sophisticated data system, and a determination to provide long-term followup.

REFERENCES

1. Kremen AJ, Linner JH, Nelson CH. An experimental evaluation of the nutritional importance of proximal and distal small intestine. *Ann Surg* 1954;140:439.

2. O'Leary P. Historical perspective on intestinal bypass procedures. In: Griffen WO, Printen KJ, eds. *Surgical Management of Morbid Obesity.*. New York : Marcel Dekker; 1987:294.

3. O'Leary P. Historical perspective on intestinal bypass procedures. In: Griffen WO, Printen KJ, eds. *Surgical Management of Morbid Obesity.*. New York : Marcel Dekker; 1987:294.

4. Mason EE, Ito C. Gastric bypass. *Ann Surg* 1969;170:329.

5. Pories WJ, Swanson MS, MacDonald KG, et al. Who would have thought it? An operation proves to be the most effective therapy for adult-onset diabetes mellitus. *Ann Surg* 1995;222:239.

6. Livinston EH, Huerta S, Arthur D, Lee S, De Shields S, Heber D. Male gender as a predictor of morbidity and age as a predictor of mortality for patients undergoing gastric bypass surgery. *Ann Surg.* 2002;236:576.

7. Buchwald H. Overview of bariatric surgery. *J Am Coll Surg* 2002;194:367.

8. Whittgromve AC, Clark GW. Laparoscopic gastric bypass, Roux-en-Y—500 patients: technique and results, with a 3–60 months followup. *Obes Surg* 2000;10:233.

9. Schauer PR, Ikramuddin S, Gourash W, et al. Outcomes after laparoscopic Roux-en-Ys gastric bypass for morbid obesity. *Ann Surg* 2000;232:515.

10. Nguyen NT, Goldman C, Rosenquist J, et al. Laparoscopic versus open gastric bypass: a randomized study of outcomes, quality of life, and costs. *Ann Surg* 2001;234:279.

11. Pories WJ, MacDonald KG, Chapman W. Staple line breakdown following the open gastric bypass operation. Unpublished data.

CURRENT MALABSORPTION PROCEDURES: BILIOPANCREATIC DIVERSION

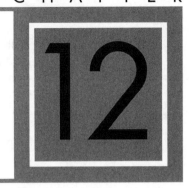

PICARD MARCEAU / SIMON BIRON / FRÉDÉRIC-SIMON HOULD / STÉFANE LEBEL / SIMON MARCEAU

With the increased prevalence of morbid obesity and improved surgical results, the percentage of morbidly obese individuals who are choosing to undergo bariatric surgery is growing rapidly. Collaboration among medical personnel encouraging the morbidly obese to consider surgery as one possible treatment option has slowly replaced resistance to this therapeutic option. Because the success of this surgery greatly depends on adequate postoperative surveillance, it is important that both patients and primary care providers be aware of what this surgical treatment entails. There are two different surgical approaches: one restrains food intake and the other changes intestinal absorption. We believe the latter is more appropriate and more promising. To reduce intestinal absorption surgically, bile and pancreatic juice must be diverted. This chapter discusses the rationale behind this approach, how it is technically performed, and lists the beneficial and detrimental effects of this physiologic change.

In our opinion, three basic facts must be emphasized to fully comprehend the impact of bariatric surgery. First, morbid obesity is a disease; second, it is among the most devastating diseases; and, finally, surgery is its sole efficient treatment.

MORBID OBESITY IS A DISEASE

Even if the exact mechanisms involved in the development of morbid obesity are still unknown, the disease can be defined as the inability of these patients to dispose of daily excess calories in ways other than by fat deposition. Normally, there is a physiologic mechanism by which excess calories taken in daily can be catabolized without needing to be stored as fat, allowing body weight to remain remarkably stable despite considerable variation in food intake. Through a complex mechanism, the system can set itself in a lower or higher gear for calorie consumption to obtain an equivalent energetic result. The organism is able to use more or less calories depending on what is available.[1,2] To prevent accumulation of fat, there is a continuous process by which calories spent will match, with great precision, the amount of calories available, day by day. This is a well-known mechanism that is probably controlled by a set point representing the usual weight. In morbid obesity, this complex mechanism is faulty. Excess calories are preferentially stored as fat instead of being consumed and eliminated. This is not dependent on consciousness, volition, or exercise.[3,4]

The disastrous effect of this faulty mechanism is worsened after weight loss. The weight loss in itself commands the low expenditure gear. The further from usual weight the individual is, the lower the expenditure gear will set itself. So both the low metabolic rate and the absence of the usual mechanism for disposal of excess calories condemn these patients to gain weight rapidly, even with surprisingly low food intakes. This diseased situation is well recognized after bariatric surgery. To maintain weight loss after surgical restriction, calorie intake cannot exceed 1300 kcal/d. This must be permanent, otherwise weight gain will recur.[5] This situation defies any temporary medical or surgical measures aimed at restraining food intake. It needs to be permanent.

Patients have little control over their energy expenditure as 80% is self-regulated.[4] Exercise provides limited help. A brisk, 1-hour walk will consume about 200 calories, representing only a small percentage of the usual daily expenditure (around 2000 to 2500 calories). Eating less, because it reduces the amount of calories needed for the digestion itself, further reduces the threshold above which calories will be considered excessive and stored as fat.

MORBID OBESITY IS A DREADFUL DISEASE

To emphasize the gravity of this disease, it is customary to list the numerous comorbidities that it causes, including diabetes, hypertension, cardiac and pulmonary insufficiency, sleep apnea, angina, osteoarthritis, esophageal reflux and many others.[6] In our experience, despite the frequency and the seriousness of these comorbidities, they do not represent the most dreadful impact of this disease. They are not, in the majority of cases, what drives these subjects to accept the risk of surgery. It is rather a poor quality of life, the feeling of being imprisoned within their body, the living difficulties with personal hygiene, and the profound feeling of suffocation, of being drowned within themselves. This is the motive for seeking help, not the fear of death itself.

Furthermore, their worst suffering comes from the psychological impact resulting from societal prejudices, insinuating lack of discipline, lack of will power, and failure to control their appetite. These notions are widespread, even in the medical profession. The results obtained in many of these patients after successful surgery are eloquent testimony to the contrary.

SURGERY IS THE ONLY EFFICIENT TREATMENT

Until an efficient life-long medication is available, treatment of morbid obesity will remain surgical. To cure these patients, the amount of weight that needs to be lost is such that drastic measures are required. For that, there are only two approaches: forceful restriction of food for life or changing intestinal absorption. Restriction must be permanent and so severe that it is hardly compatible with normal life and it often fails in more obese patients. Changing intestinal absorption has become more appealing because long-term risks are better known and found to be reasonable, preventable, and curable.

Today, there is only one reversible way available for changing intestinal absorption. It is by diverting bile and pancreatic juice to decrease their role in the digestive process. This is called a biliopancreatic diversion (BPD).

WHAT IS A BILIOPANCREATIC DIVERSION?

BPD (Figure 12–1) changes the patient's anatomy to reduce absorption of fat, a particularly important source of calories and known to be taken in excess in our society. Bile is necessary for fat absorption. Limiting its contact with food decreases fat absorption. By a simple reversible technique, the contact between bile and food can be delayed. Normally, the entrance of bile is at the beginning of the intestine where food arrives. In BPD, it is moved down closer to the end of the intestine. A segment of intestine is used for conveying bile from one site to the other and no food is allowed in this segment. The longer this segment, the shorter the segment that is left for the passage of food. The shorter the segment left for the passage of food, the greater the decrease in absorption. The further down bile is allowed to be in contact with food, the greater the specific decrease in fat absorption. In this process, pancreatic juice is also involved because pancreatic juice and bile share the same point of entry into the intestine. The concomitant diversion of pancreatic juice further reduces food absorption.

The transfer of bile from one site to the other is in itself a simple, reversible procedure, but, unfortunately, removing bile from its normal entry at the outlet of the stomach prevents its role as buffer of gastric acid and predisposes the patient to peptic ulcer. Consequently, it is necessary to decrease the amount of acid from the stomach. This can be accomplished in different ways. Part of the stomach can be removed or bypassed. This is discussed in the sec-

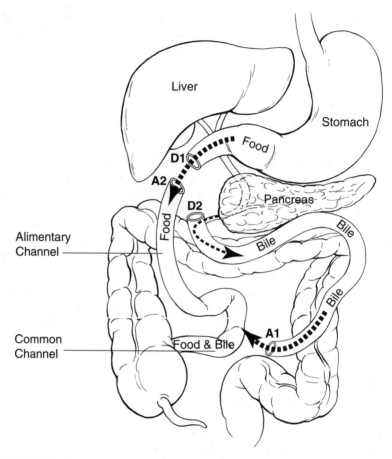

FIGURE 12–1 A biliopancreatic diversion is created by sectioning the small bowel and using the distal segment for food (alimentary channel or limb) and the proximal segment as a conduit for bile and pancreatic juice (biliopancreatic limb) to be connected further down for food and bile to mix. The level at which the section is made determines the length of intestine for food absorption (common channel) and the site at which the distal end will be connected determines the role given to bile in the digestive process.

tion on the gastric remnant. This part of the operation will also greatly contribute to the results of the operation.

A biliopancreatic diversion is composed of three modules, each influencing results in term of weight loss, side effects, and complications. All three determine its efficiency in reducing intestinal absorption. First, the segment of intestine left for food contact, called the "alimentary channel," determines the capacity of absorption as a whole. Second, the site of bile reentry, more or less distant from the end of the alimentary tract, leaves a segment called the "common channel" where bile and food are mixed. It determines the capacity of fat absorption. Finally, the size and the quality of the gastric remnant determines satiety and the volume of food ingestion at a meal.

EVOLUTION OF
BILIOPANCREATIC DIVERSION

The concept of BPD and the demonstration of its safety and efficiency must be credited to an Italian team led by Scopinaro.[7,8] After more than 20 years of performing this procedure, despite great resistance, these investigators have established a place for this approach in bariatric surgery. Previous attempts with jejunoileal bypass, another malabsorptive procedure, turned out to be fiascos after initial encouraging results. This earlier experience had left skepticism and fear of any new attempt at changing intestinal absorption and no change was to be considered unless proved to be safe after a very long period of observation.

For 20 years there was a place only for "restrictive procedures." The malabsorptive approach was retained by only a few centers that continued to believe in its merits and believed that the reduction of intestinal absorption was more desirable for better quality of life than imposing abnormal food restriction. Twenty years have passed since BPD was first proposed and time has proved this approach to be reliable, safe, and profitable, and Scopinaro's results have been confirmed.[9–11] BPD is a procedure very different from the previously unsuccessful jejunoileal bypass. Indeed, the basic mechanism is different, the malabsorption is directed primarily toward fat; the surface of absorption is four times larger; bile turnover remains undisturbed; and, finally, BPD does not leave a blind loop, an element later recognized as the most detrimental feature of jejunoileal bypass. Over the years, the basic principle of BPD has been used in various ways by different authors and BPD has become increasingly popular.

HOW BPD WORKS

BPD is composed of three functional parts: the alimentary channel, the common channel, and the gastric remnant (Figure 12–1). Each has positive and negative effects and influences the results, which depend essentially on harmonizing the three components. It is not yet established what is the best construction. Whether the arrangement needs to be individualized depending on patient characteristics such as age, size, and sex, is not presently known. Variations in all three parts have been tried by various authors in small numbers of patients with limited follow-up. While these different trials are of great interest, they have not yet given sufficiently strong data to impose a definite rule for the construction of a BPD.

Alimentary Channel

Initially, based on the fact that only half the intestine is necessary for normal life, Scopinaro used half the intestine for the "alimentary channel." Subsequently, to simplify the technique, he adopted a fixed 250-cm (98.4-inch) alimentary channel, which, in most cases is close to half the intestinal length. Oth-

TABLE 12–1. CHARACTERISTICS OF PATIENTS TREATED BY BILIOPANCREATIC DIVERSION: 1982–2002	
Sex (f/m)	4/1
Age (years)	38 ± 10
Initial weight (kg)	131 ± 30
Body mass index	48 ± 1
Initial excess weight (kg)	107 ± 42

Note: The table reflects some of the basic characteristic of our 1289 patients who had a biliopancreatic diversion during the last 20 years. Up to 1990, 250 of them had a Biliopancreatic diversion, Scopinaro type. We then moved to biliopancreatic diversion with duodenal switch. This became our sole procedure for nearly all patients.

ers have used different lengths but no comparative studies have been performed. We believe that the length of the alimentary tract does not need to be that precise, it must only be sufficiently short to temporarily create a "short-bowel syndrome" but long enough to allow patient recuperation by meeting individual needs. Although the intestine is initially too short after the procedure, this produces substantial weight loss. Absorption will improve through cellular multiplication until individual need is met, resulting in weight stabilization. Presently, there are no predictors of physiologic recuperation on which to decide the ideal length of the alimentary channel. However, we believe that older people may not have the same capacity to recuperate as do younger people, and therefore may require a longer length of the alimentary channel.

The Common Channel

This is the segment where food and bile are mixed and which is responsible for most fat absorption. Undigested fat will cause fatty diarrhea (steatorrhea). The goal is to obtain the maximum decrease in fat absorption without diarrhea. Scopinaro, after animal and human experimentation, chose to return bile 50 cm (19.7 inches) before the iliocecal valve (ICV) at the end of the intestine, because at this site fat absorption decreased nearly 70% without major diarrhea. We and many others have found that, at that level, with an American-style diet, the prevalence of diarrhea and hypoalbuminemia is too high, and have chosen to insert bile at 100 cm (39.4 inches) from the ICV. This significantly decreases side effects without compromising weight loss.

The Gastric Remnant

Removing bile from the outlet of the stomach predisposes the duodenum to development of peptic ulcer. Gastric acid needs to be decreased for the BPD to be relatively complication free. How this is done will determine patient well being and how well they will eat. Distal gastrectomy was proposed initially because this was known to be an efficient way to treat ulcer disease and prevent new ulcer formation. This would allow normal eating habits after surgery. Because distal gastrectomy has been performed regularly for over a century, the short- and long-term side effects are well defined. For years, this has been the classic treatment for peptic ulcer, a disease much less debilitating than morbid obesity. Despite the irreversibility of the gastrectomy, the well-known long-term risk appeared to be minimal considering the seriousness of the disease. Over the years, many variations have been attempted by different surgeons. To avoid gastrectomy the stomach was left in place and only bypassed (Figure 12–2). This added another factor of potential morbidity because of the inaccessibility of this vulnerable organ left in place below the staple line. Other surgeons have added restriction to malabsorption by converting the part of the stomach still in contact with food into a small pouch that can contain as little as 15 mL with an obstructing outlet, in an attempt to produce early satiety. This addition undermines the major advantage of BPD, which is the allowing of normal eating habits. Furthermore, it adds the inconveniences of both malabsorptive and restrictive approaches.

More than 10 years ago, an easier and a more physiologic gastrectomy was proposed by our group and by others. A sleeve of stomach was removed along its greater curvature, protecting nerves and the whole mechanism of food delivery. The harmonious function between the antrum, the pylorus, and the duodenum was preserved. Distal gastrectomy was replaced by this new sleeve gastrectomy. It created a smaller, normally functioning stomach that was more suitable for inducing early satiety. This procedure, called "duodenal switch," is gaining popularity.

RESULTS OBTAINED WITH BPD

Results of a BPD depend on the harmonization of its three components: the alimentary channel, the common channel, and the gastric remnant. Each influences weight loss and side effects, as well as complications. Each type of construction gives its own results. For the past 12 years, BPD with duodenal switch, a 250-cm (98.4-inch) alimentary channel and a 100-cm (39.4-inch) common channel has been our construction of choice and used in almost all our patients. Most results reported here concern this type of procedure. Patient characteristics are given in Table 12–1.

Operative Risk

The risk of major complication is the same with BPD as with any other bariatric operation that opens the gut. Operative death is approximately 1%. Patients stay in the hospital about a week. The incidence of complications that prolong hospital stay is approximately 15%. Only "simple banding" is a less-dangerous procedure.

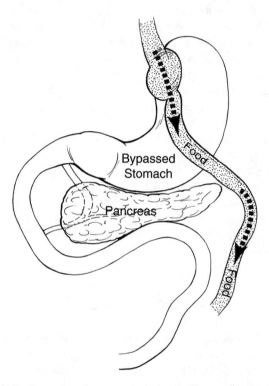

A

FIGURE 12–2   With BPD, food passes from the stomach to a segment of intestine that is deprived of the normal buffer role of bile. To prevent intestinal
mucosal damage, gastric acid must be reduced. It can be obtained by gastric
bypass (A) or by distal (Scopinaro) (B) or sleeve (duodenal switch) (C) resection.

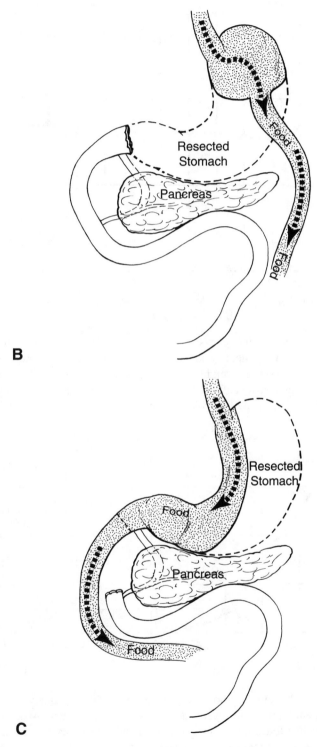

B

C

FIGURE 12–2   (continued)

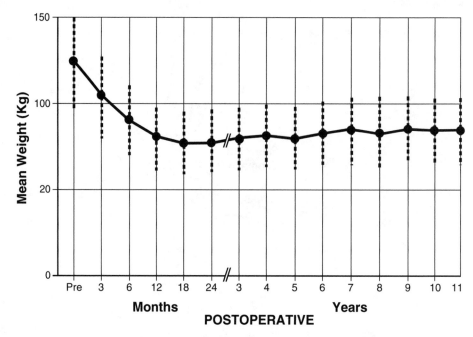

FIGURE 12–3   The graphic shows weight loss after duodenal switch. It is based on 450 consecutive patients who have been operated on and followed for more than 5 years. Maximum weight loss occurs around 18 months. It is followed by a slight regain so that after 10 years, there is still a mean lost of about 45.4 kg (100 lb). Recurrence of morbid weight is rare.

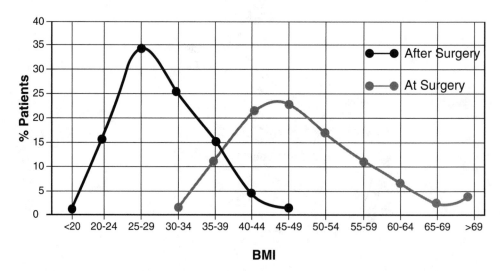

FIGURE 12–4   This graphic shows the changes in body mass index of 569 consecutive patients, a mean of 8 years after biliopancreatic diversion–duodenal switch. Note that fewer than 5% of patients remained surgically obese according to National Institutes of Health criteria.

Weight Loss

Most weight loss (Figure 12–3) occurs within 6 months. Weight continues to decrease, but progressively less, for another 12 months. It reaches a plateau after 18 months. Weight loss is expected to reach approximately 40 to 45% of the initial weight or 70 to 75% of the initial excess weight. Average BMI decreases from approximately 50 to 30. After 2 years, more than 85% of patients are no longer morbidly obese and have a BMI below 35. Ten percent will continue to have a BMI between 35 and 40 and less than 5% above 40 (Figure 12–4). There will be a mean weight gain of 1.4 kg (3.1 lb) per year during the following years. More than 85% of patients declared themselves satisfied with their weight loss.

Quality of Life

In our view, better quality of life is the greatest asset of BPD. Almost all patients find increased self-confidence, with better social, marital, and sexual relations. Undoubtedly, the major weight loss is responsible for the improvement in quality of life, but we believe that "free diet" is also a major factor. Patients appreciate being able to eat normally. Their attitude toward food changes. They see the good results from this physiologic operation as living proof that their disease was physiologic and not psychological. This further increases their satisfaction.

Side Effects

The most annoying side effect of BPD is malodorous stool and gas. It is a major problem in 33% of patients and forces them to decrease fat intake and to avoid certain foods. This problem is relieved by the intermittent use of antibiotics, particularly metronidazole. It subsides over the years but can remain intermittently annoying in a few patients. The number of stools after surgery is about three a day. Some patients retain a susceptibility to diarrhea. Our database shows diarrhea requiring intermittent use of metronidazole to be present in about 10% of patients. There are other, less important, side effects after BPD. They usually are temporary and easily treatable. Fatigue is common and often is caused by iron deficiency. Persistent stomach burning/gastritis is rarely a problem, but patients use H_2 blockers occasionally. The prevalence of kidney stones is not increased after BPD. Because gallstones frequently develop postoperatively, we have elected to remove the gallbladder routinely at surgery.

LONG-TERM COMPLICATIONS

The efficiency of BPD to produce better weight loss and a better quality of life than other bariatric operations has never been challenged in a randomized controlled trial format. The long-term metabolic complications of BPD have concerned many physicians and patients considering their treatment options. It is evident that normal physiology cannot be changed without paying a price, and BPD is no exception. Many surgeons and patients believe that the price is reasonable for the great improvement in quality of life. This is an exchange of an intolerable and untreatable disease for a tolerable and treatable one. This fundamental notion must be kept in mind by both patients and care providers so that long-term surveillance remains an essential part of postoperative surgical care. After BPD, patients are exposed to complications that are predictable, preventable, and curable. The success of this surgery greatly depends on the quality of the followup care.

BPD can be a source of complications in several different ways: by insufficient absorption of vitamins and minerals; by decreased absorption of proteins; and by the change in intestinal bacterial flora. It also renders the diagnosis of intestinal obstruction more difficult.

These complications must be understood and their presence continuously suspected in the care of these patients. Furthermore, because of the tendency for these patients to underestimate the importance of these complications they must be emphasized and the patients must be willing to comply with life-long followup at least yearly. The natural desire of these patients is to consider themselves normal or cured. Their physicians must maintain empathy for the patient but demand compliance so that total protein levels and vitamin levels remain within normal limits.

Decreased Absorption of Vitamins and Minerals

By decreasing fat absorption, BPD also decreases absorption of fat-soluble vitamins (vitamins A, D, E, and K), and patients must take supplements. They are asked to take one multivitamin, one vitamin A (25,000 IU), and one vitamin D (50,000 IU) tablet. *Vitamin A* is measured yearly. It is present in the serum in the form of carotene or retinol. While serum carotene levels fall below normal, the serum retinol levels remain normal. Deficiency in vitamin A, in the form of retinol, is rare and responds to increased supplement. *Vitamin D* supplementation is imperative for the protection of bone and is discussed with calcium. No additional *vitamin E* is given outside of the 50 IU contained in most multivitamins. We are not aware of any clinical manifestation as a result of its deficiency. Supplementation of *vitamin K* is not necessary. There is a slight raise in the international normalized ratio (INR) in some patients, but the overall mean INR value does not change after BPD. Rarely, administration of vitamin K is indicated if INR levels rise above 1.4.

Iron and calcium absorption is compromised. These metals are normally absorbed by the first part of the intestine (the second and third portions of the duodenum), which is bypassed in a BPD. In the majority of patients, improved absorption by the rest of the intestine is insufficient to compensate. Daily supplement of both iron and calcium is advised for life.

Iron supplementation is particularly important for menstruating women who are more susceptible to anemia. Iron deficiency causes fatigue. It is responsible for anemia in 6% of patients. Taking iron every day is not easy. It causes constipation, increases flatulence, and causes nausea in some people. Eight percent of patients choose intermittent intramuscular injections to avoid having to take iron by mouth.

Calcium deficiency can also cause fatigue. In 33% of patients, it will cause a rise in parathyroid hormone (PTH). More calcium and vitamin D by mouth will lower the PTH level. The simultaneous decreased absorption of both calcium and vitamin D after BPD increases concern about bone physiology. However, previous experience with jejuneoileal bypass demonstrates that bone is relatively tolerant to this metabolic change. No increased bone fractures have been noted after jejuneoileal bypass. Our own study with BPD confirms this resistance. With appropriate followup and adjusted supplement, bone density was found to be remarkably stable 10 years after surgery. The density has even improved in almost 33% of these patients.[17]

Decreased Protein Absorption

After BPD, protein absorption is compromised.[18,19] Twenty percent of patients show a deficit in S-albumin during the first year, with levels between 32 and 36 (normal: 36 to 50) g/L. With improved intestinal absorption as the intestine adapts, S-albumin normalizes. On the other hand, this operation increases endogenous protein loss. Normally, daily intestinal nitrogen loss is the equivalent of about 6 g of our own protein. After BPD this can be increased by four or five times for reasons that are still unclear. Therefore, even with improved protein absorption and normalization of serum protein levels, these patients remain susceptible to protein deficit when facing any additional cause of protein loss.

After BPD, only a percentage of what is eaten is absorbed and additionally there is a greater loss of already absorbed protein so that the minimum daily protein requirement must be increased. It increases from 40 to 90 g or more daily. A normal diet of 2000 to 2500 kcal can contain as much as 100 to 120 g of protein. The minimum requirement can usually be met if patients are taught how to monitor their protein intake. However, in the face of dietary stress, deficits can result. Patients inherit a permanent susceptibility for protein deficit. Serum albumin levels should be frequently monitored, even in the absence of any related symptoms. A low albumin level (below 36 g/L), present in approximately 5% of our patients, was found to be an indicator of liver fibrosis and bone damage. If it resists medical treatment, revision should be considered. In our series, this occurred in fewer than 1% of our patients and many of them had to be convinced that a reversal of their BPD was absolutely necessary to treat their medical conditions. It was very important to them not to regain their weight and any condition that is not life-threatening may not be severe enough for them to consider reversal.

Change in Intestinal Flora

Another source of complications after BPD is the change in intestinal bacterial flora.[18,19] The level of bacteria in the intestine is astronomic (levels of 10^9 bacteria per mL in the colon) but remains in a balanced state. This is a result of a complex mechanism by which both the quality and quantity of this flora is maintained stable. The absence of bile in a segment of intestine, the presence of undigested food in the colon, and the fact that the gut is shorter after BPD are all factors that may compromise both the quality and the quantity of the bacterial population. Change in bacterial flora can cause many clinical manifestations such as flatulence, diarrhea, and bad breath, and more seriously, fever, chills, and arthalgia. Mild symptomatology will respond to dietary adjustment and fasting. Often, it will require the use of an antibiotic to control the quality of bacteria or to return the distribution and amounts to the normal flora. Metronidazole by mouth is prescribed to these patients; it will relieve most symptoms efficiently in the majority of cases. Approximately 10% of patients use this antibiotic occasionally, for a day or two at a time. They learn when and how to use it. We encourage the use of yogurt and even pharmaceutical preparations of lactobacillus (probiotic agent).[20,21]

In our opinion, bacterial overgrowth after BPD occurs more often than initially thought. Serious manifestations such as chills, fever, and arthalgia sometimes require aggressive antibiotic therapy. It can be a life-threatening situation if unrecognized. Fortunately, this is rare. Greater experience with this operation is needed to better define the impact of this complication. When major manifestations of bacterial overgrowth is recognized, it should be treated aggressively. If it is recurrent, a total reversal of the diversion is indicated. Reversal was necessary in 1% (12/1400) of patients in our series.

Difficulty in Diagnosing Intestinal Obstruction

Intestinal obstruction is not more frequent after BPD than after any bariatric operation. However, its clinical manifestation can be different and its diagnosis more difficult. Care providers must be aware of these problems. Obstruction of the bypassed segment is sometimes unrecognized on simple abdominal radiographs because of the absence of swallowed air in this segment. It is only evident on a computed axial tomography scan. An obstruction of this biliary segment may perturb liver and pancreatic enzymes because of the back pressure it causes. This makes differential diagnosis of abdominal pain more difficult. Patients and physicians must keep this in mind.

CONCLUSION

Morbid obesity is a dreadful disease treatable only by surgery. To be effective, treatment needs to be for life, otherwise morbid weight will recur. The disease defies any temporary measures and recurrence is a discouraging experience. The choice is between restriction of food for life or changing intestinal absorption.

For a better quality of life, allowing normal eating habits, and better maintenance of weight loss, we favor malabsorptive procedures. However, these patients pay a price by being made vulnerable to certain situations and good medical surveillance is imperative. Both physically and psychologically, these patients find themselves much more normal after surgery despite these side effects. The patients who choose this believe the benefits far exceed the inconvenience of taking vitamins, the need for medical surveillance, and the presence of certain calculated risks. Increased experience with this operation is needed to minimize its impact. Presently, BPD duodenal switch type is our procedure of choice in the treatment of morbid obesity.

REFERENCES

1. Lowell BB, Spiegelman BM. Towards a molecular understanding of adaptive thermogenesis. *Nature* 2000;404:652–660.
2. Liebel RL, Rosenbaum M, Hirsch J. Change in energy expenditure resulting from altered body weight. *N Engl J Med* 1995;332:621–628.
3. Levine JA, Eberhardt NL, Jensen MD. Role of nonexercise activity thermogenesis in resistance to fat gain in humans. *Science* 1999;283:212–214.
4. Kopelman PG. Obesity as a medical problem. *Nature* 2000;404:635–643.
5. Brolin RE, Robertson LB, Kenler HA, Cody RP. Weight loss and dietary intake after vertical banded gastroplasty and Roux-en-Y gastric bypass. *Ann Surg* 1994;220:782–790.
6. Kellum JM, DeMaria EJ, Sugerman HJ. The surgical treatment of morbid obesity. *Probl Surg* 1998;35:791–858.
7. Scopinaro N, Gianetta E, Cevalleri D, Banalumi V, Bachi V. Biliopancreatic bypass for obesity: II. Initial experience in man. *Br J Surg* 1979;66:618–620.
8. Scopinaro N, Adami GF, Marinari GM. Biliopancreatic diversion. *World J Surg* 1998;22:936–946.
9. Holian DK, Clare MW. Biliopancreatic bypass for morbid obesity: late results and complications. *Clin Nutr* 1986;5(Suppl):133–136.
10. Clare W. Equal bibliopancreatic and alimentary limbs: an analysis of 106 cases over 5 years. *Obes Surg* 1993;3:289–295.
11. Lemmens L. Biliopancreatic diversion: 170 patients in a 7 years follow-up. *Obes Surg* 1993;3:179–180.
12. Marceau S, Biron S, Lagacé M, et al. Biliopancreatic diversion with distal gastrectomy 250-cm and 50-cm limbs. Long-term results. *Obes Surg* 1995;5:302–307.
13. Hess DS, Hess DW. Biliopancreatic diversion with a duodenal switch. *Obes Surg* 1998;8:267–282.
14. Marceau P, Hould FS, Simard S, et al. Biliopancreatic diversion with duodenal switch. *World J Surg* 1998;22:947–954.
15. Anthone GJ, Harrison M. The duodenal switch as primary surgical treatment for morbid obesity [abstract]. *Obes Surg* 1999;9:142–143.
16. Rabkin LA. Distal gastric bypass/duodenal switch procedure Roux-en-Y gastric bypass and biliopancreatic diversion in a community practice. *Obes Surg* 1998;8:853–859.

17. Marceau P, Biron S, Lebel S, et al. Bone change after biliopancreatic diversion? *J Gastrointest Surg* 2002;6:690–698.

18. Marceau P, Biron S, Hould FS, Lebel S, Marceau S. Changing intestinal absorption for treating obesity. In: Surgerman HJ, Cie Dekker M, eds. *Management of Morbid Obesity*. In preparation.

19. Marceau P, Hould FS, Lebel S, Marceau S, Biron S. Complications specific to biliopancreatic diversion. *Curr Surg*. In preparation.

20. Fuller R. Probiotics in human medicine. *Gut* 1991;32:439–442.

21. Vanderhoof JA, Young RJ, Murray N, Kaufman SS. Treatment strategies for small bowel bacterial overgrowth on short bowel syndrome. *J Pediatr Gastroenterol Nutr* 1998;27(2):155–160.

C H A P T E R

13

GASTRIC PACING

SCOTT A. SHIKORA / JIANDE CHEN / VALERIO CIGAINA

Over the last 50 years, surgery has evolved into a safe and effective treatment for intractable morbid obesity. A number of procedures have evolved over years of development from the trial-and-error approach described in Chapter 2, and at least four procedures are frequently performed in the United States as "accepted" surgical treatments. Furthermore, the introduction of minimally invasive techniques, such as the use of laparoscopy, has also increased the safety and popularity of these surgeries. However, despite all the advances in surgical technique and instrumentation, all of the currently popular procedures still create major alterations of the gastrointestinal tract, which can lead to both early operative complications, as well as long-term nutritional and gastrointestinal consequences. These untoward events have dampened the enthusiasm for surgery for the extremely obese, among those who qualify for this surgery, and some of their physicians and family members. Thus, a significant number of morbidly obese patients have not come forth for surgical therapy, which is considered the only reliable treatment currently available. Fewer than 1% of those who meet standard criteria for eligibility for surgical therapy have bariatric surgery in any given calendar year. This may be partially a result of a lack of medical insurance coverage, or a lack of knowledge about the efficiency of these treatments, but it is also because of fear of the consequences of invasive treatments.

Implantable gastric stimulation (IGS), electrically stimulating the stomach, offers a fresh and unique approach to treating obesity. It is a new concept that is currently undergoing international investigation. Preliminary results in both animals and humans are encouraging. Unlike other forms of bariatric surgery, it involves minimal manipulation of normal gastrointestinal anatomy. Additionally, it can almost always be performed laparoscopically. Both of these beneficial characteristics should minimize the potential for both early operative complications and long-term development of nutritional/gastrointestinal consequences, thereby being more palatable to many obese patients who currently would not consider the more invasive procedures.

Exactly how electrical stimulation of the stomach results in weight loss is unknown. However, the limited experience with the device demonstrates that it can be safely placed and is efficacious for many patients. This chapter reviews the consequences of traditional bariatric surgeries, the physiology of gastric electrical stimulation, the history and development of the modality, and its current status worldwide.

COMPLICATIONS ASSOCIATED WITH TRADITIONAL BARIATRIC SURGERY

Currently, all traditionally accepted surgical procedures to treat morbid obesity alter the gastrointestinal tract to cause nutrient restriction, nutrient malabsorption, or a combination of both. These conditions are accomplished by partitioning or dividing the stomach and/or by bypassing a segment of the small intestine. Consequently, complications can occur from many sources. First, all abdominal surgical procedures expose patients to complications such as hemorrhage, organ injury, and peritonitis. The more complex the procedure, the greater the likelihood of technical complications. Second, most surgeons would agree that obese patients are more prone to operative problems because of hepatomegaly and increased intraabdominal adiposity. Additionally, the large abdominal cavities of the most obese patients increase the technical difficulties of abdominal surgery because the instruments may not reach adequately. Finally, the unique characteristics of each category of surgical procedure has its own unique complications (see Chapters 14 and 16).

In contrast to the procedures described in other chapters, IGS only involves the placement of electrical leads into the stomach wall to deliver the electrical stimulation from an energy generator very similar to a cardiac pacemaker (see Figure 13–1). The generator is placed in the subcutaneous adipose tissue just above the abdominal muscular wall. While the other procedures induce weight loss by physically restricting meal size and/or limiting nutrient absorption, this modality is thought to induce weight loss by causing early satiety (feeling full). The absence of staple lines, anastomoses, and the need to manipulate the intestine, along with the ability to perform this procedure quickly and via a laparoscope have enabled it to be extremely safe and with few long-term consequences. As detailed later in this chapter, the worldwide experience with IGS in more than 200 patients, plus the experience with tens of thousands of patients who have received cardiac pacemakers and other implantable generator systems, confirms the safety of this type of treatment. However, we must still determine how such stimulation affects eating behavior and how to maximize this effect before we can expect to master the most efficacious way to use this as an obesity treatment.

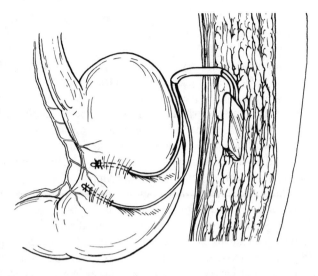

FIGURE 13–1   Gastric electrical stimulator with two bipolar leads inserted in the muscular layer along the lesser curvature. The leads are placed close to the pes anserinus.

PHYSIOLOGIC BASIS FOR IMPLANTABLE GASTRIC STIMULATION

Gastric Motility and Gastric Emptying

Motility is one of the most critical physiologic functions of the human gut. Without coordinated motility, digestion and absorption of dietary nutrients could not occur. To accomplish its functions effectively, the gut needs to generate not just simple contractions but contractions that are coordinated to produce the transit of luminal contents (peristalsis) of nutrients to a position where they are maximally absorbed without inadvertently bypassing the point of absorption by hypermotility. Thus, coordinated gastric contractions are necessary for the emptying of the stomach. These contractions are generated by the native gastric electrical activity.

The patterns of gastric motility are different in the fed and the fasting states.[1] In the fed state, the stomach contracts at its maximum frequency, 3 cycles/min (cpm) in humans and 5 cpm in dogs. The contraction originates in the proximal stomach and propagates distally toward the pylorus. In healthy humans, 50% or more of the ingested food is usually emptied from the stomach by 2 hours after the meal and 95% or more has been emptied by 4 hours after the meal.[2] When the stomach is emptied, the pattern of gastric motility changes. The gastric motility pattern in the fasting state (nonfed) undergoes a cycle of periodic fluctuation divided into three phases: phase I (no contractions, 40–60 minutes), phase II (intermittent contractions, 20–40 minutes), and phase III (regular rhythmic contractions, 2–10 minutes).

Gastric Myoelectrical Activity

Gastric motility (contractile activity) is, in turn, regulated by the myoelectrical activity of the stomach. Normal gastric myoelectrical activity consists of two components: slow waves and spike potentials.[3] The slow wave is omnipresent and occurs at regular intervals, whether or not the stomach contracts. It originates in the proximal stomach and propagates distally toward the pylorus (Figure 13–2). The gastric slow wave determines the maximum frequency, propagation velocity, and propagation direction of gastric contractions. When a spike potential (similar to an action potential) is superimposed on the gastric slow wave, a strong lumen-occluding contraction occurs. The normal frequency of the gastric slow wave is about 3 cpm in humans and 5 cpm in dogs.

Gastric dysrhythmias represent aberrations from the normal gastric myoelectrical activity. Similar to cardiac dysrhythmias, they include abnormally rapid contraction (tachygastria) and abnormally slow contraction (bradygastria). For example, there can be an ectopic pacemaker in the distal stomach in addition to the normal pacemaker in the proximal stomach (Figure 13–3). The ectopic pacemaker generates slow waves with a higher frequency than normal (tachygastria), and with a retrograde propagation toward the proximal stomach. These abnormal waves may interfere with the normal slow wave propagation and possibly disrupt normal gastric contractions.

Recently, the prevalence and origin of various gastric dysrhythmias were investigated by one of the authors (JC, unpublished communication). It was found that the majority of bradygastria (80.5 ± 9.4%) originated in the proximal stomach (p <0.04 versus other locations) and propagated all the way to the distal antrum. That is, bradygastria is attributed to a decrease in the frequency of the normal pacemaker. In contrast, tachygastria mainly originated in the dis-

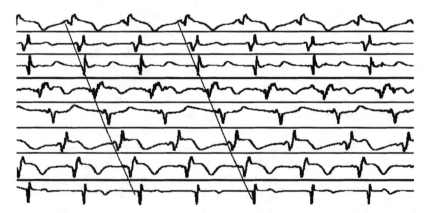

FIGURE 13–2   Gastric slow waves recorded from electrodes implanted on the serosa of the stomach along the greater curvature in a healthy dog (1.5-minute recording). The top tracing was obtained from a pair of electrodes 16 cm (6.3 inches) above the pylorus and the bottom tracing was obtained from the electrodes 2 cm (0.8 inches) above the pylorus.

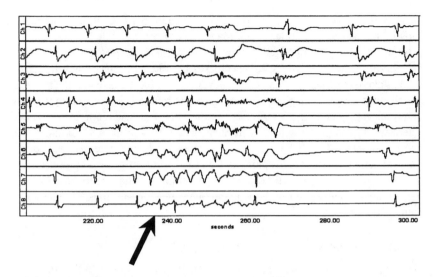

FIGURE 13–3   Tachygastria. Gastric slow waves recorded from electrodes implanted on the serosa of the stomach along the greater curvature showing the ectopic tachygastrial activity in the distal stomach (*arrow*). The top tracing was obtained from a pair of electrodes 16 cm (6.3 inches) above the pylorus and the bottom tracing was obtained from the electrodes 2 cm (0.8 inches) above the pylorus.

tal antrum (80.6 ± 8.8%) (p <0.04 versus other locations) and propagated partially or all the way to the proximal stomach. Meanwhile, the normal pacemaker in the proximal stomach may still be present. That is, it is not uncommon that the proximal stomach is dominated with normal slow waves, whereas the distal stomach is dominated with tachygastria. The prevalence of dysrhythmia was highest in the distal antrum and lowest in the proximal part of the stomach.

Gastric Emptying and Obesity

Gastric emptying plays an important role in regulating food intake. Several studies show that gastric distension acts as a satiety signal to inhibit food intake[4] and that rapid gastric emptying is closely related to overeating and obesity, especially in animals with lesions in the hypothalamic region of the brain.[5] In a study of 77 humans comprised of 46 obese and 31 age-, sex-, and race-matched nonobese individuals, obese subjects were found to have a more rapid emptying rate than nonobese subjects.[6] Obese men were found to empty much more rapidly than their nonobese counterparts. It was concluded that the rate of solid gastric emptying in the obese subjects is abnormally rapid. Although the significance and cause of this change in gastric emptying remains to be definitively established, Carlson proposed that a relationship existed between the gastrointestinal tract and the hypothalamus that regulated dietary intake based on work he performed at the University of Chicago in 1913.[7] It has also been shown that several peptides, including cholecystokinin (CCK) and corticotropin-releasing factor (CRF), suppress feeding and decrease gastric transit. Peripherally administered CCK-8 decreases the rate of gastric emptying and food intake in various species.[8] CRF also decreases food intake and the rate of gastric emptying by peripheral injection.[9] More recently, it was shown that in ob/ob mice (a genetic model of obesity), the rate of gastric emptying was accelerated, as compared with that in lean mice.[10] Urocortin, a 40-amino-acid peptide member of the CRF family, dose-dependently and potently decreased food intake and body weight gain, as well as the rate of gastric emptying, in ob/ob mice. This suggests that rapid gastric emptying may contribute to hyperphagia and obesity in ob/ob mice and opens new possibilities for the treatment of obesity.

GASTRIC ELECTRICAL STIMULATION (PACING)

Gastric pacing involves the application of an electrical current to the stomach to influence or change gastric emptying. This may involve stimulating the stomach from proximal to distal (antegrade pacing) or from distal to proximal (retrograde pacing). The goal of antegrade stimulation is to improve normal gastric emptying whereas the goal of retrograde stimulation is to retard or adversely impact normal gastric emptying. Antegrade pacing may be potentially beneficial for patients with persistent gastric dysrhythmias and retrograde pacing may be of benefit for patients with abnormally rapid gastric emptying, such as those patients with dumping syndrome and the morbidly obese.[11] The utility of gastric pacing would only be realized if artificially generated electrical current could entrain normal gastric pacesetter potentials. This has been demonstrated in canines[12] and in humans.[13]

ANTEGRADE GASTRIC ELECTRICAL STIMULATION

A number of papers have been published on gastrointestinal electrical stimulation for the treatment of gastrointestinal motility disorders in both dogs and humans. These disorders are characterized by poor contractility and delayed emptying (in contrast with obesity) and the aim of electrical stimulation in this setting is to normalize the underlying electrical rhythm and improve these parameters. In general, this is done by antegrade or forward gastric (or intestinal) stimulation.

Previous work on antegrade gastrointestinal stimulation has been focused on its effects on gastric myoelectrical activity, gastric motility, gastric emptying, and gastrointestinal symptoms.[14–21] These studies show that entrainment of gastric slow waves is possible by using an artificial pacemaker. Recent studies in our laboratory indicate that such entrainment is dependent on certain critical parameters, including the width and frequency of the stimulation pulse.[14] We have also shown that antegrade intestinal electrical stimulation can entrain intestinal slow waves by using either serosal electrodes or intraluminal ring electrodes.[17,20] In a study of nine patients suffering from gastroparesis, McCallum and coworkers demonstrated that antegrade gastric pacing could entrain gastric slow waves in all the patients. They paced the greater curvature of the stomach at frequencies approximately 10% higher than the slow wave frequencies measured. In two patients, it converted tachygastria to normal slow waves. Most importantly, it significantly improved gastric emptying and symptoms.[18] In a case report, Familoni et al. found that they were able to improve gastric emptying and symptoms in a patient with severe diabetic gastroparesis by pacing the stomach at a high frequency (12 cpm).[22] However, Hocking et al. were unable to treat postgastrectomy gastric dysrhythmias with pacing in a patient who underwent vagotomy and gastrojejunostomy for an obstructing duodenal ulcer.[23]

RETROGRADE GASTRIC ELECTRICAL STIMULATION

The principle of retrograde gastric electrical stimulation is the opposite of what has been described for patients with impaired gastric emptying. Retrograde gastric electrical stimulation employs retrograde pacing with the aim of retarding the propulsive activity of the stomach and slowing down gastric emptying (Figure 13–4). This may be useful in the treatment of obesity where it is postulated that a delay in gastric emptying will lead to early satiety and decreased food intake. Retrograde gastric electrical stimulation is equivalent to placing an artificial ectopic pacemaker in the antrum. This artificial ectopic pacemaker results in electrical waves propagating retrogradely from the antrum to the proximal stomach, fighting against the normal and physiologic electrical waves that propagate from the proximal to the distal stomach. Consequently, gastric dysrhythmia is induced and the regular propagation of gastric electrical waves is impaired. The severity of impairment is determined by the strength of electrical stimulation.

Recently, there has been considerable interest in retrograde gastric electrical stimulation for the treatment of obesity. In the late 1980s, an Italian surgeon, Valerio Cigaina, conceptualized the use of electrical gastric stimulation as a potential treatment modality for morbid obesity. This concept was based on an observation made in a 6-month-old infant.[24] The child had recurrent vomiting and associated failure to thrive. The cause of the condition was determined to be an abnormal ectopic gastric pacemaker located in the antrum of the stomach. This pacemaker was thought to cause abnormal gastric emptying leading to vomiting. At that time, the authors hypothesized that exogenous electrical impulses could be used to dysregulate normal gastric electromotor activity in obese patients, mimicking this clinical syndrome, resulting in weight loss. Furthermore, the intention was to induce weight loss with minimal derangement of physiology and as few of the side effects as possible that are associated with conventional bariatric procedures.[25]

CLINICAL STUDIES WITH GASTRIC PACING FOR WEIGHT LOSS

Studies investigating the potential for gastric electrical stimulation to induce weight loss began in 1992 in a porcine model. The results showed that retrograde gastric electrical stimulation was both safe and effective in moderating

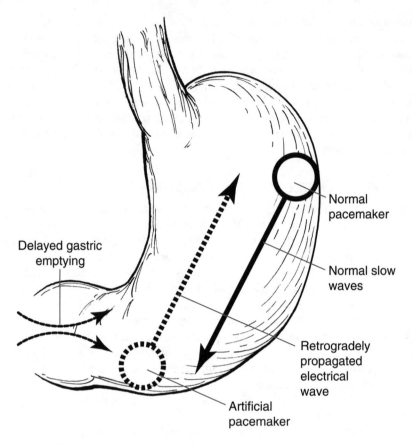

FIGURE 13–4   Retrograde gastric electrical stimulation. Electrical stimulation from an ectopic gastric pacemaker located in the distal stomach might delay gastric emptying.

weight gain in growing swine.[26] Animals were divided into three groups, two of which had electrodes implanted into the muscle layer of the distal antrum. Control animals received sham surgery. Implanted swine experienced either 3 or 8 months of electrical antral stimulation at 5 or 100 hertz (Hz) respectively. All animals were fed ad libitum. As expected, immature swine in the control group progressively increased feeding and gained weight. Over the first 12 weeks of the study, there were no differences in animal feed intake or weight between the groups (both control and stimulated groups increased intake and weight). After 13 weeks, animals subjected to high-frequency stimulation decreased their feed intake relative to the control group and then their weight. After 8 months, the swine stimulated at 100 Hz weighed 10.5% less than the control animals. The overall feed intake in the group stimulated at 100 Hz was 12.8% lower than in the control group. However, animals in the group stimulated at the lower frequency (5 Hz) for only 3 months demonstrated dramatically less change than the control group.[26] Gastric peristalsis has also been studied in the swine model. Peristalsis was noted to be altered with electrical stimulation. Swine stimulated at 40 Hz were noted to have decreased peristalsis.[27] However, the exact mechanism of action was not elucidated and gastric emptying not evaluated.

As a consequence of the animal study results, the initial human studies began in 1995.[28] Four women with a BMI 40 kg/m^2 or greater were implanted and followed for up to 40 months. Via laparoscopy, patients had platinum electrodes implanted intramuscularly on the anterior gastric wall, adjacent to the lesser curve and proximal to the pes anserinus. The system was "bipolar" in design so that two electrodes, one an anode and one a cathode, were inserted into the gastric muscle layer. A prototype electrical stimulator was implanted in a subcutaneous pocket of the anterior abdominal wall. All four patients were permitted food and drink ad libitum. At 40 months after implantation, one patient had lost 32 kg (70.5 lb), and a second had lost 62 kg (136.7 lb). In the other two patients, malfunctions occurred in their stimulator systems. One patient had a fracture of the lead, which compromised its effectiveness. At 40 months after implantation, the patient had lost only 2 BMI units. Similarly, in a second patient there was also an apparent fracture of the lead, and that patient did not lose weight. In both of these patients, lead fracture led to unipolar pacing (only one electrode was presumed to be functional) versus the intended bipolar stimulation. The two subjects who had no lead problems and received bipolar pacing had much better results. Therefore, it was concluded that bipolar electrical stimulation was necessary. In addition, chronic gastric electrical stimulation was considered safe as no side effects were reported.

In 1998, a second study was performed in human subjects to investigate the safety and efficacy of a first-generation, dedicated, gastric stimulator, the Prelude implantable gastric system.[29] All patients had a BMI greater than 40 kg/m^2, a history of unsuccessful weight loss, absence of serious cardiac, and respiratory or psychiatric problems; patients with cardiac pacemakers were excluded. Ten patients underwent a minimally invasive surgical procedure to implant the system. Stimulation was initiated 30 days after implantation. After implant, all subjects were permitted food and drink ad libitum during three regular meals, but told not to eat between meals. Only sweets and alcoholic beverages were discouraged. Patients were followed at approximately monthly intervals. The stimulator was interrogated using transcutaneous radiofrequency telemetry that linked the implanted device to a computerized programmer. Data collected included stimulation parameters, lead impedance, and residual battery charge. Patients were followed for a mean of 340 days postimplant.

This study demonstrated both safety and efficacy. There were no deaths or other significant medical problems during the study, no complications related to the procedure, and no long-term complications. Specifically, there were no lead fractures or failures of the electrical components of the system. To date, three patients have had their generators replaced following battery depletion. After receiving 15 months of stimulation, the mean weight loss was 14.9 kg (32.8 lb) and the mean body mass loss was 5.0 BMI units. At 36 months, mean weight loss increased to 19.1 kg (42.1 lb) (Table 13–1).

In 2000, an additional study was performed in 10 patients using the

TABLE 13–1. RESULTS OF 1998 STUDY BY DR. V CIGAINA						
WEIGHT AND BODY MASS LOSS*						
	MONTH 1	MONTH 6	MONTH 12	MONTH 18	MONTH 24	MONTH 30
No. of subjects	10 (100%)	10 (100%)	10 (100%)	10 (100%)	10 (100%)	10 (100%)
Weight loss (kg)	−5.1 ± 2.9	−12.3 ± 6.3	−15.7 ± 6.3	−14.4 ± 9.2	−14.9 ± 10.7	−19.5 ± 13.7
%EBL	−7.3 ± 5.2	−18.8 ± 11.8	−24.1 ± 10.7	−21.6 ± 13.2	−22.3 ± 16.4	−28.5 ± 20.3
% Weight loss	−3.5 ± 1.9	−8.7 ± 4.4	−11.2 ± 4.3	−10.1 ± 5.8	−10.4 ± 7.2	−13.5 ± 9.2

* Data presented as mean ± standard deviation.
Abbreviation: %EBL = % excess body mass lost, where preoperative BMI − 25 = 100%. Excess body mass = amount of BMI (kg/m^2) greater than 25.

TABLE 13–2. PRELIMINARY RESULTS OF 2000 STUDY BY DR. V. CIGAINA					
WEIGHT AND BODY MASS LOSS*					
	MONTH 1	MONTH 3	MONTH 6	MONTH 9	MONTH 12
No. of subjects	10 (100%)	10 (100%)	10 (100%)	10 (100%)	7 (70%)
Weight loss (kg)	−3.6 ± 2.6	−9.2 ± 3.9	−15.1 ± 8.3	−20.6 ± 13.3	−24.7 ± 19.4
%EBL	−5.4 ± 3.6	−14.6 ± 6.7	−23.5 ± 11.7	−29.8 ± 17.4	−33.5 ± 23.3
% Weight loss	−2.7 ± 1.7	−7.1 ± 3.1	−11.6 ± 5.8	−15.3 ± 9.3	−17.8 ± 13.4

* Data presented as mean ± standard deviation.
Abbreviation: %EBL = % excess body mass lost, where preoperative BMI − 25 = 100%. Excess body mass = amount of BMI (kg/m^2) greater than 25.

second-generation gastric stimulator, Transcend.[29] Entry criteria were identical to the earlier investigation. Again, patients demonstrated consistent weight loss. To further prove that the weight loss achieved was secondary to gastric electrical stimulation and not placebo, patients demonstrated weight gain with battery exhaustion or lead dislodgment and renewal of weight loss with lead reinsertion or battery replacement (Table 13–2).

Current International Trials with Gastric Electrical Stimulation for Weight Loss

Prompted by the results achieved by Dr. Cigaina in Italy, several studies were initiated in both Europe and in the United States. In Europe, the investigations were predominantly open label and nonrandomized. In the United States, a multicenter, randomized, controlled, double-blinded trial was developed to evaluate both the safety and efficacy of the IGS system. Since the investigation began in February 2000, 100 patients have been enrolled. The entry criteria were similar to that employed by Dr. Cigaina. The IGS lead was laparoscopically placed in all patients. One month after insertion, patients were random-

TABLE 13–3. COMPLICATIONS ENCOUNTERED DURING THE US TRIAL	
Gastric perforation at implant	15
Complete lead dislodgment	10
Abdominal pain/discomfort	9
Upper respiratory infection	8
Sinus infection	7
Headache	6
Nausea/vomiting	6
Connection problem	5
Depression	5
High impedance	5
Indigestion	5
Bloating	4
Diarrhea	4
Discomfort during impedance test	4
Partial lead dislodgment	4

ized to device activation or to having the device remain in the "off" mode. After 7 months, the nonfunctioning devices were also activated. Patients were seen in clinic monthly for 24 months and carefully monitored for complications and for weight loss.

Although the investigation confirmed the safety of the procedure, the results were inconsistent. For the 100 patients, there were no deaths or complications from implantation (Table 13–3). One patient was unable to have the device lead inserted laparoscopically because of adhesions, and was withdrawn from the study. The duration of the procedure was approximately 1 hour (range: 22 minutes to 2.5 hours). Midway through the investigation, it was discovered that the lead design was inadequate to maintain its proper position in the gastric muscular wall. Several patients were found to have had lead dislodgment. There were two types of lead dislodgment. First there was total lead dislodgment where the two electrodes were no longer inside the stomach muscle layer. The second type of dislodgment was a partial dislodgment in which the lead doesn't completely pull off the gastric wall, but one of the electrodes is pulled outside of the gastric muscular tunnel. With partial dislodgment, some food-related satiety might remain, yet it is unknown whether this condition is less effective than when both electrodes are in good position. Total lead dislodgment is always associated with weight regain. Total dislodgment is easier to diagnose as patients may experience symptoms such as abdominal discomfort (because of peritoneal stimulation) and/or mild burning or muscular fasciculation in the generator pocket. Partial dislodgment is generally asymptomatic but may be discovered by endoscopic ultrasonography.[30] In the first 41 patients, 10 complete dislodgments (25%) were discovered, which led to a change in the operative technique. Surgical clips were subsequently placed on the lead and no complete dislodgments were discovered in the remaining 59 patients. It is not known how many partial dislodgments were present.

At this time, it is premature to analyze the success of this device for achieving and maintaining weight loss. The preliminary results showed no difference in weight loss between placebo-treated patients (those with a system in place but not turned on for the first 7 months) and those with treatment. Some patients did quite well (n = 23), with a mean weight loss at 13 months of 13.6 kg (30 lb) (10.3%), while others failed to lose weight. Although the reason for this finding and the better results seen in the open-label European studies are still not known, many possible explanations can be made. Obviously, lead dislodgment contributed. In Europe, lead suture sleeves were used to increase lead security. This device was only recently approved for use in the United States, unfortunately too late to be used in the trial. In addition, the study design may have contributed to the inconsistent results. Blinded randomization with half of the participants having their device remain inactive for 7 months led many patients to experiment and overeat to see if they could elicit symptoms to suggest whether their device was activated. The design of the study also prevented the investigators from offering diet and behavioral support, which is vital for any weight-loss therapy. Furthermore, patients were not screened preoperatively for abnormal eating behavior, such as binge eating, which might adversely affect the results. Finally, all patients received the same stimulation parameters and only minor changes were made after 10 months of stimulation. The initial wave amplitude was 6 milliamperes (MA) while 10 MA was shown to be more effective in Europe. It may also turn out that parameters should be individualized for each patient. The mean weight of US patients was significantly higher than that of patients entered in European studies. This technology may not be appropriate for the superobese (BMI >50 kg/m^2) or much higher parameters of stimulation may be required to have an effect. It would be helpful to have an objective test that could demonstrate that a patient ate less of a standardized meal once a certain level of stimulation was achieved.

Lessons Learned from the First US Trial

Despite the inconsistent results from the first US trial, there was enough success to maintain interest in future investigations. Some patients did very well, with one man losing almost 45.4 kg (100 lb). Others reported less appetite and snacking, even without significant weight reduction. Many of the patients who had not lost meaningful weight at least did not gain weight during the trial, despite the natural tendency for the obese to chronically gain weight. Any future endeavors will need to address these issues. Identifying the most effective means for lead security, the most effective lead insertion location, and the optimal stimulation parameters may be best investigated in an animal model prior to human investigation. In addition, better patient selection to exclude those predicted to do poorly with this technology, such as binge eaters, should be considered. The addition of dietary and behavioral counseling may also improve results. Lastly, it is critical that the actual mechanism of action be identified so that we can establish how to apply the technology; that is, where should the stimulus be placed, how much stimulus should be placed, and what parameters can be measured to determine that the stimulus is producing the desired effect.

The Future

Presently, there is active animal investigation to answer many of the above questions. Concurrently, new human trials are beginning in Europe, Australia, and the United States. In all centers, the study will include higher output settings, improved lead fixation, improved patient selection, and behavioral and dietary modules. In the United States and Australia, a novel four-electrode device will be used, which has two bipolar leads connected to the same stimulator where each lead can be stimulated independently or from one lead to the other increasing the potential permutations of the stimulation options. In addition to the above study improvements, patients will also benefit from more rapid changes in the protocol when stimulation parameters can be changed monthly or bimonthly based on the weight loss results achieved under the protocol variations. Two investigational centers in the United States will enroll 30 patients into this nonrandomized, open-label investigation. The results should be available within a few years. Other designs for stimulator leads and pacing protocols and tests that predict weight loss outcomes will undoubtedly be tested by other investigators interested in this type of manipulation.

CONCLUSION

Gastric electrical stimulation for weight loss offers an exciting new surgical approach to intractable obesity. Animal and human study over almost a decade has confirmed its safety in contrast with most traditional bariatric surgical options. Weight-loss results have thus far been encouraging but inconsistent. This is a result of many factors, which can be attributed to the "newness" of this technology. This field is at a similar level of expertise as that of cardiac pacemaker technology in the 1960s. The theoretical possibilities are impressive, but the clinical experience and technological expertise is minimal. There remains a significant amount of knowledge about this modality that needs to be gained, and many questions that must be answered. Gastric electrical stimulation as a concept is still in its infancy. Only time will tell whether it leads bariatric surgery into a new era of treatment.

REFERENCES

1. Hasler WL. The physiology of gastric motility and gastric emptying. In. Yamada T, Alpers DH, Owyang C, Powell DW, Silverstein FE, eds. *Textbook of Gastroenterology*. 2nd ed. Philadelphia: Lippincott Williams & Wilkins; 1995:181–206.
2. Tougas G, Eaker EY, Abell TL, et al. Assessment of gastric emptying using a low fat meal: establishment of international control values. *Am J Gastroenterol* 2000;95:1456–1462.
3. Chen JDZ, McCallum RW, eds. *Electrogastrography: Principles and Applications*. New York: Raven; 1995.

4. Phillips RJ, Powley TL. Gastric volume rather than nutrient content inhibits food intake. *Am J Physiol* 1996;271:R766–R779.

5. Duggan JP, Booth DA. Obesity, overeating, and rapid gastric emptying in rats with ventromedial hypothalamic lesions. *Science* 1986;231:609–611.

6. Wright RA, Krinsky S, Fleeman C, et al. Gastric emptying and obesity. *Gastroenterology* 1983;84:747–751.

7. Carlson AJ. *The Control of Hunger in Health and Disease*. Chicago: University of Chicago Press; 1916.

8. Moran TH, McHugh PR. Cholecystokinin suppresses food intake by inhibiting gastric emptying. *Am J Physiol* 1982;242:R491–R497.

9. Sheldon RJ, Qi JA, Porreca F, et al. Gastrointestinal motor effects of corticotropic-releasing factor in mice. *Regul Pept* 1990;28:137–151.

10. Asakawa A, Inui A, Ueno N, et al. Urocortin reduces food intake and gastric emptying in lean and ob/ob obese mice. *Gastroenterology* 1999;116:1287–1292.

11. Eagon JC, Soper NJ. Gastrointestinal pacing. *Surg Clin North Am* 1993; 73:1161–1172.

12. Kelly KA. Differential responses of the canine gastric corpus and antrum to electrical stimulation. *Am J Physiol* 1974;226:230–234.

13. Miedema BW, Sarr MG, Kelly KA. Pacing the human stomach. *Surgery* 1992;111:143–150.

14. Lin ZY, McCallum RW, Schirmer BD, et al. Effects of pacing parameters in the entrainment of gastric slow waves in patients with gastroparesis. *Am J Physiol* 1998;274:G186–G191.

15. Eagon JC, Kelly KA. Effects of gastric pacing on canine gastric motility and emptying. *Am J Physiol* 1993;265:G767–G774.

16. Hocking MP, Vogel SB, Sninsky CA. Human gastric myoelectrical activity and gastric emptying following gastric surgery and with pacing. *Gastroenterology* 1992;103:1811–1816.

17. Lin XM, Peters LJ, Hayes J, et al. Entrainment of segmental small intestinal slow waves with electrical stimulation in dogs. *Dig Dis Sci* 2000;45:652–656.

18. McCallum RW, Chen JDZ, Lin ZY, et al. Gastric pacing improves emptying and symptoms in patients with gastroparesis. *Gastroenterology* 1998;114:456–461.

19. Qian LW, Lin XM, Chen JDZ. Normalization of atropine-induced postprandial dysrhythmias with gastric pacing. *Am J Physiol* 1999;276:G387–G392.

20. Abo M, Liang J, Qian LW, et al. Normalization of distention-induced intestinal dysrhythmia with intestinal pacing in dogs. *Dig Dis Sci* 2000;45:129–135.

21. Bellahsene BE, Lind CD, Schlimer BD, et al. Acceleration of gastric emptying with electrical stimulation in canine model of gastroparesis. *Am J Physiol* 1992;262:G826–G834.

22. Familoni BO, Abell TL, Voeller G, et al. Electrical stimulation at a frequency higher than usual rate in human stomach. *Dig Dis Sci* 1997;42:885–891.

23. Hocking MP. Postoperative gastroparesis and tachygastria-response to electrical stimulation and erythromycin. *Surgery* 1993;114:538–542.

24. Telander RL, Kelly KA. Human antral tachygastria with gastric retention: a new syndrome. *Gastroenterology* 1997;13–23:A117–A140.

25. Pories WJ. The surgical approach to morbid obesity. In: Sabiston DC, ed. *Textbook of Surgery*. 15th ed. Philadelphia: WB Saunders; 1997:933–946.

26. Cigaina V, Saggioro A, Rigo V, et al. Long-term effects of gastric pacing to reduce feed intake in swine. *Obes Surg* 1996;6:250–253.

27. Cigaina V. Gastric peristalsis control by mono situ electrical stimulation: a preliminary study. *Obes Surg* 1996;6:247–249.

28. Cigaina V, Rigo V, Greenstein RJ. Gastric myo-electrical pacing as therapy for morbid obesity: preliminary results. *Obes Surg* 1999;9:333.

29. Cigaina V. Gastric pacing as therapy for morbid obesity: preliminary results. *Obes Surg* 2002;12:12S–16S.

30. Shikora SA, Knox TA, Bailen L, et al. Successful use of endoscopic ultrasound (EU) to verify lead placement for the implantable gastric stimulator (IGS). *Obes Surg* 2001;11:403.

MANAGING POSTOPERATIVE COMPLICATIONS AFTER BARIATRIC SURGERY

LOUIS F. MARTIN

The recognition of obesity as a national epidemic[1-3] and the efficacy of gastric bypass in producing reliable and reproducible weight loss[4-6] have brought bariatric surgery to the forefront of medical care. The increase in the number of morbidly obese patients treated with surgery since the introduction of laparoscopic Roux-en-Y gastric bypass[7-10] and laparoscopic adjustable gastric banding, has mandated that physicians of varying specialties remain abreast of the management of these challenging patients. This chapter addresses the complications that develop short-term (within the first month) and long-term (after 1 month) postoperatively in caring for patients who have undergone gastric bypass surgery and the other procedures mentioned in the preceding chapters. Additionally, Chapter 16 presents issues that pertain to unsatisfactory outcomes after bariatric procedures including when patients should be considered for revisional surgical procedures.

IMMEDIATE SHORT-TERM POSTOPERATIVE MANAGEMENT

Regardless of the approach (open or laparoscopic), the postoperative management of bariatric patients centers around aggressive return to activity and pulmonary toilet, as well as vigilant surveillance for the signs and symptoms of surgical complications. Patients are required to sit in a chair as early as the night of surgery and ambulate by the morning of the first postoperative day. Incentive spirometry is strongly promoted and the hospital bed is placed at 30 degrees of reverse Trendelenburg position to enhance pulmonary function. Adequate pain control is essential to maximize respiratory mechanics and compliance with activity; our patients are routinely managed with intravenous narcotic analgesics administered via a patient-controlled analgesia (PCA) system.

Postoperative Diet

Patients who undergo bariatric operations are routinely examined by a double contrast (water-soluble contrast followed by barium sulfate) upper gastrointestinal (UGI) series in the immediate postoperative period. If the study does not reveal any evidence of a gastrojejunal leak, or of a Roux or enteral limb obstruction after a gastric bypass or any kind of malabsorptive procedure (Figure 14–1), a clear liquid diet not to exceed 60 mL per hour is initiated. Leaks also must be looked for after restrictive procedures plus it is important to make sure the new gastric stoma is not obstructed from edema. When a gastric band has been placed, it is also important to know how it looks (i.e., the angle of the band compared to the spinal processes in the anterior–posterior and lateral directions) so there is a reference point if the patient returns with new digestive complaints. The size of the new proximal stomach is also noted. The size can be expected to almost double in most patients with use. Once clear liquids are tolerated for 24 hours, the diet is advanced to pureed food without added sugar and supplemented by high-protein, low-calorie protein drinks. The patient is instructed to continue the pureed diet and/or the protein drinks for 1 month after surgery, at which time regular food may be gradually reintroduced. Patients are required to abstain from foods or liquids high in sugar content.

Anastomotic Complications

The gastric suture lines and the anastomoses (gastrojejunostomy, jejunojejunostomy, or duodenojejunostomy) performed during Roux-en-Y gastric bypass and the other malabsorptive procedures may be the source of early complications and present a diagnostic challenge to clinicians caring for these patients.[8,10,11]

We routinely test each anastomosis intraoperatively by endoscopic insufflation of the anastomosis under external submersion in saline or with methylene blue dye under pressure infusion. Unfortunately, postoperative leaks may still present in a minority of the patients with negative intraoperative leak tests, probably as a consequence of the force vectors pulling on the anastomoses, once the patient is mobile (i.e., rolling over, changing positions, walking) or once the patient begins their diet. The closed-suction drain, routinely placed posterior to the gastrojejunostomy or other anastomoses, is removed after the postoperative UGI series does not demonstrate a leak *and* the patient tolerates a liquid diet for at least 24 hours. We have been successful in managing carefully selected patients with contained or a controlled anastomotic leak or gastric suture line leak without signs of sepsis with drainage, antibiotics, and parenteral nutrition without the need for subsequent surgery.

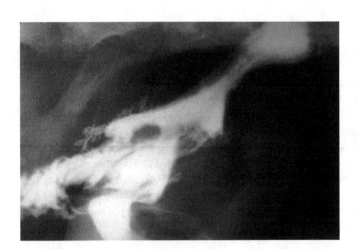

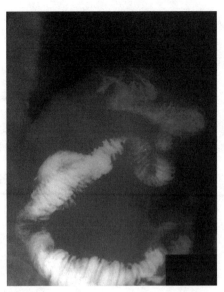

FIGURE 14–1   Radiograph of a normal barium contrast study of a patient who had a gastric bypass one day prior to this film.

Leakage may also occur at the jejunojejunostomy. These leaks often present a significant diagnostic challenge because of the extreme difficulty in imaging this anastomosis. Alternatively, a narrowed jejunojejunostomy may result in bowel obstruction.

While patients with intestinal leak may present with peritonitis and the hemodynamic derangements of sepsis, they frequently demonstrate more subtle signs and symptoms of intraabdominal sepsis. These patients may present with fever, tachycardia, hiccoughs, leukocytosis, oxygen desaturation, left-shoulder pain, decreased mentation, or impending sense of doom. Clinical suspicion must be maintained in patients who demonstrate any of these signs, as early reexploration averts the potential devastation of continuing intraabdominal sepsis.

Patients with bowel obstruction from a narrowed jejunojejunostomy or postoperative adhesions anywhere along the small bowel may present with abdominal pain, nausea, or vomiting. These symptoms may be difficult to distinguish from expected postoperative complaints, but persistence or extended duration of these symptoms should prompt a diagnostic workup. Plain abdominal radiography or contrast UGI series may aid in diagnosing this complication by demonstrating jejunal distension or slowed transit of contrast material. While obstruction because of anastomotic edema should resolve early in the postoperative period, long-standing obstruction must be surgically decompressed to prevent gastric dilatation of the excluded stomach/biliopancreatic limb leading to a leak or compromise of one of the anastomoses or the proximal staple line of the biliopancreatic limb or excluded stomach. The radiologist must be reminded that the biliopancreatic limb usually will not fill with contrast and when obstructed, may be fluid filled rather than be filled with ingested air depending on where the obstruction is relative to the jejunoje-junostomy.

Thromboembolism

Obese patients are at increased risk for lower extremity deep venous throm-bosis in the perioperative period. Our routine practice of administering low-molecular-weight heparin (enoxaparin 40 mg subcutaneously) preoperatively and daily during the hospital stay seems to reduce the occurrence of deep ve-nous thrombosis and pulmonary embolism. Sequential compression stockings are used during the surgery and the hospital stay. Patients at highest risk for venous thromboembolism (e.g., previous history of thromboembolism) and those at highest risk for a poor outcome following a pulmonary embolism (e.g., patients with pulmonary hypertension) are considered for placement of a vena caval filter prior to surgery.

LATE POSTOPERATIVE MANAGEMENT

Patients who have undergone bariatric surgery require lifelong follow up. The significant lifestyle changes that occur following bariatric surgery demand long-term medical guidance to identify potential complications, prevent nutri-tional disturbances, and provide a psychosocial support structure.

Gastrojejunostomy or Duodenojejunostomy Complications

Anastomotic stenosis may occur at the gastrojejunostomy or duodenojejunos-tomy (after biliopancreatic diversion with duodenal switch) and may present with dysphagia, nausea, or vomiting. Frequently, these patients may experi-ence these signs immediately after eating. Workup may include UGI series, but upper esophagogastroscopy is usually diagnostic and confers the therapeutic advantage of allowing the performance of concomitant balloon dilation, which usually corrects the problem. Stenoses respond well to endoscopic dilatation as long as the patient is alerted to return for help as soon as these symptoms occur, and this complication rarely requires surgical intervention. Although ap-proximately one-third of these patients will require more than one dilation and 1–5% will require multiple dilations in the months after a stricture develops, this complication is almost always able to be treated without surgery to revise the anastomosis.

Marginal ulcers frequently present with epigastric abdominal pain. While these patients may present with signs and symptoms similar to those of stomal stenosis, the presence of abdominal pain steers the diagnosis toward this complication. Less commonly, signs of GI hemorrhage will occur with the vomiting of blood or loose, dark brown or black, tarry stools. The ulcer is frequently located on the jejunal side of the anastomosis. Upper endoscopy is the diagnostic modality of choice. Once the diagnosis is confirmed, the presence of a gastrogastric fistula must be entertained, even if the stomach has been completely divided to create the gastric pouch. Although this fistula may occasionally be identified on endoscopy, a UGI series is often required to definitively exclude this complication. Patients without counterindications may receive H_2 antagonists for 1 month after surgery, beginning immediately postoperatively, as prophylaxis against this complication, although a fistula can occur even years after bariatric surgery, especially in gastric bypass patients where the proximal pouch is only separated from the distal stomach by staples and not by completely dividing the stomach sections where a more permanent scar forms. Marginal ulcers respond well to therapy with proton pump inhibitors when a gastrogastric fistula is not present. Infrequently, marginal ulcers refractory to medical therapy may require revision of the gastrojejunostomy.

Internal Hernia

The potential spaces created during gastric bypass and other malabsorptive surgery provide the opportunity for development of intestinal obstruction from internal herniation of the small bowel.[9–12] We routinely close the three spaces: the defect in the small-bowel mesentery at the jejunojejunostomy, the mesocolic defect through which the Roux/enteral limb passes, and the "Petersen" defect between the mesentery of the Roux/enteral limb and posterior portion of the transverse mesocolon.

Patients present with intermittent, cramping abdominal pain with or without nausea, vomiting, or other signs of obstruction. A UGI series with small bowel follow-through may be diagnostic if performed during the episode of abdominal pain. More often, the diagnosis is based on the history of the complaint.

Management of this complication depends on the clinical scenario. Patients who are determined to have incarceration of the bowel in the hernia require urgent admission and operation to reduce the hernia and prevent strangulation and perforation. On the other hand, patients who present with complaints of intermittent abdominal pain without evidence of obstruction can be electively reexplored. If the original operation was performed laparoscopically, laparoscopic reexploration is usually possible.

Cholelithiasis

Regardless of the approach to gastric bypass, patients have a significant risk (32%) of developing gallstones during the rapid-weight-loss phase.[13] This risk is significantly reduced (2%), however, when patients are treated postoperatively with a 6-month course of ursodiol.[13] All patients with gallbladders should be evaluated preoperatively or intraoperatively for cholelithiasis and should usually undergo concomitant cholecystectomy at the time of bariatric surgery if gallstones are present especially if the patient is symptomatic.

Wound Complications

Wound complications are a significant source of morbidity for obese patients regardless of the operative procedure. When wound infections occur in patients who have undergone open bariatric surgery (7% have some wound complication), the resulting disability may be significant, and management of the open incision often presents a wound-care challenge. The laparoscopic approach seems to have significantly diminished the rate of development of this complication. Several series report that the overall wound infection rate for laparoscopic Roux-en-Y gastric bypass is 1 to 5%, while the incidence of major wound infections is closer to the lower end of that range.[14]

While the reasons for this difference have not been completely elucidated, several technical factors may contribute to this phenomenon. The incisions used for laparoscopic gastric bypass cover a much smaller area of the abdominal wall than the upper midline laparotomy incision used for the open approach. Furthermore, all instrumentation and tissues are withdrawn via laparoscopic trocars, limiting direct exposure of the wound to contamination.

Obese patients are also at increased risk of developing incisional hernias. The incidence of this complication also seems to have been significantly reduced by the advent of laparoscopic gastric bypass. Series of Roux-en-Y gastric bypass performed via the laparoscopic approach report this complication to occur at a rate of 1% or less.[7–11,14] In our experience, we have identified incisional hernias at 12-mm (0.5-inch) trocar sites in two patients who presented with postoperative bowel obstruction. No hernias have been identified in 5-mm (0.2-inch) trocar sites. It is our routine practice to close the fascia of all 12-mm (0.5-inch) trocar sites, although other surgeons restrict this practice to trocar sites ≥ 18 mm (0.7 inches).

Dumping Syndrome

Many patients who undergo Roux-en-Y gastric bypass or biliopancreatic bypass develop dumping syndrome. This condition is characterized by diaphoresis, tremulousness, nausea, and a sensation of intense generalized malaise following ingestion of sugar. Although unpleasant, this consequence of gastric bypass surgery aids the patient in adhering to the prescribed dietary restrictions by providing a negative feedback to intake of sugar.

Nutritional Considerations

The success of bariatric surgery depends on dietary retraining for a lifelong commitment to healthy dietary intake and on dedication to a regular exercise program. Patients are asked to refrain from sugar intake and are encouraged to obtain a significant portion of their calories from protein (50 to 60 g/d). As protein deficiency may be insidious, the role of patient education in preventing this complication cannot be overemphasized. Patients often rely on fish, dairy products, and protein supplements to meet daily protein requirements.

Daily nutritional supplementation also includes 500 μg of vitamin B_{12}, 1200 mg of calcium, and a multivitamin tablet. Menstruating females are also asked to take 650 mg of ferrous sulfate each day. The serum levels of these supplements are checked during clinic appointments (see Chapter 15 also).

Lifelong Followup

Most experienced bariatric surgeons concur that patients who have undergone Roux-en-Y gastric bypass and other malabsorptive procedures require lifelong followup in the bariatric surgery clinic. While a significant number of medical issues, including weaning from medications, may be handled in the primary care setting, patients will continue to require surveillance for nutritional abnormalities and identification of complications.

MANAGING POSTOPERATIVE COMPLICATIONS SPECIFIC TO ADJUSTABLE GASTRIC BANDING

Since the release of the adjustable gastric band (LAP-BAND System, Inamed Corporation, Santa Barbara, CA) in June 2001, after the FDA approved its pre-market approval application, this device has penetrated all areas of the United States and more than 90,000 have been implanted worldwide (data on manufacturer's web site, www.inamed.com). There are a number of complications associated with this type of adjustable band that are unique to these types of devices (there are at least three other models of an adjustable band available in other parts of the world which have not yet undergone FDA evaluation) and a few others that can occur anytime a band of polypropylene or Dacron mesh, silicone or silastic tubing, or other medical-grade material is wrapped circumferentially around part of the GI tract (Figure 14–2).

The most common complaint in the first year after placement of an adjustable gastric band is nausea and vomiting (23 to 38%), followed by a gastroesophageal reflux disease (GERD) in 15% of patients in the US multicenter trials.[15] These data documented how often patients complain about symptoms that are often the result of overeating but that can also be the result of primary stomal obstruction from postoperative edema, overfilling of the band, or improper placement of the band. Secondary stomal obstruction can occur after band slippage when the band moves relative to its initial placement around the stomach or the inferior stomach is pushed upward into the band usually as the result of vomiting. Obstruction often leads to pouch dilation or esophageal dilation if the lower esophageal sphincter becomes incompetent.

As noted in Chapter 10, the adjustable gastric band is a new therapy that has not been used as long as the other established bariatric procedures. It requires more interaction between patients and the multidisciplinary team in the surgeon's office for the patient to be successful because there are not as many mechanisms helping the patient to control their diet and lose weight as there are in the mixed restrictive–malabsorptive procedures. These interactions should include normal postoperative followup by the surgeon plus behavior modification, using a support group, where postoperative patients gather weekly to talk about the problems together and in consultation with a dietician; an exercise plan; and adjustments to the balloon in the band system to tighten or relax the opening from the upper gastric pouch into the rest of the stomach.

Most Americans receive an average of three to four adjustments to their band in the first postoperative year and then may average one to two adjustments every 2 years because, over time, the system usually loses some fluid. Plus, the muscles in the GI tract above the band usually become hypertrophic to overcome some of the resistance (this happens more during than after the first year). In countries with a socialized system of medical care (i.e., without fee-for-service arrangements), adjustments tend to be made more frequently. There is currently no current procedural terminology (CPT) code that allows a physician to charge specifically for a band adjustment and no International Classification of Diseases (ICD)-9 codes for a diagnosis that will or could be matched to a CPT code to assure payment in our insurance system.[16] An adjustment can cost as much as $800 if it is associated with a radiologic fluoroscopic exam using barium. In the United States, this tends to prohibit all but the most essential adjustments. It is still not clear what the ideal schedule or protocol is to maximize the cost-effectiveness of the adjustments.

Currently, when a patient complains of reflux, it is important to obtain a careful history of food intake and try to determine if the patient is overeating. It is important to have people with an adjustable gastric band not vomit regularly from overeating, motion sickness, or any other condition that can be prevented by education or medication. Vomiting will often cause GERD with burning pain. It also can force an additional portion of the stomach up inside the ring and it's enclosed stomach from the part of the stomach that is caudal to the band. This extra tissue often will fill enough of the space within the ring to obstruct the original opening that is now trapped beside it in the band (Figure 14–3). The patient will then become obstructed and have nausea and vomiting. If the band has more than 0.5 mL of saline in the balloon, removing the saline will usually allow the prolapsed stomach to fall out of the ring and relieve the obstruction. This will also sometimes change the position of the band on X-ray evaluation (Figure 14–4).

Initially, during the period 1993 to 1996, when the proximal gastric pouches created by the band were bigger and the posterior tract for the band might transverse the bursa omentalis, slippage rates as high as 25 to 30% were recorded at

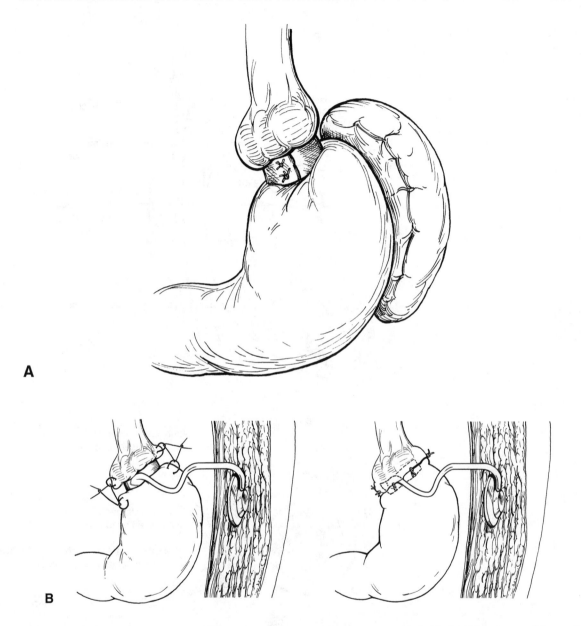

FIGURE 14–2   Gastric bands. **A.** Molina nonadjustable gastric band. **B.** LAP-BAND system of Inamed Corporation.

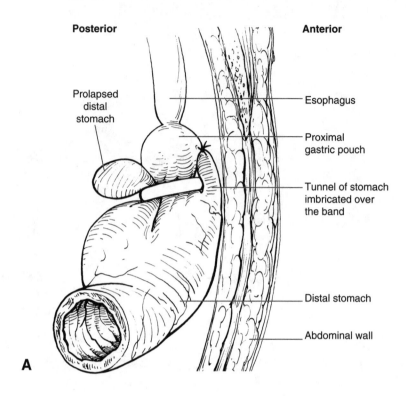

Posterior

Anterior

Prolapsed
distal
stomach

Esophagus

Proximal
gastric pouch

Tunnel of stomach
imbricated over
the band

Distal stomach

Abdominal wall

A

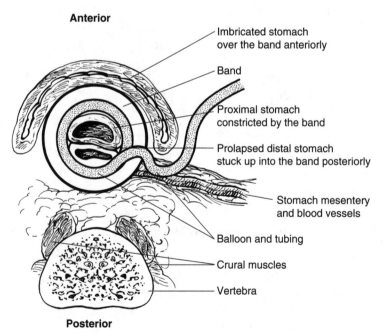

Anterior

Imbricated stomach
over the band anteriorly

Band

Proximal stomach
constricted by the band

Prolapsed distal stomach
stuck up into the band posteriorly

Stomach mesentery
and blood vessels

Balloon and tubing

Crural muscles

Vertebra

B

Posterior

FIGURE 14–3   Slippage or prolapse of the stomach through the band. **A.**
Lateral view with the distal stomach prolapsed back up into the ring after an
episode of vomiting. **B.** Cross-sectional view.

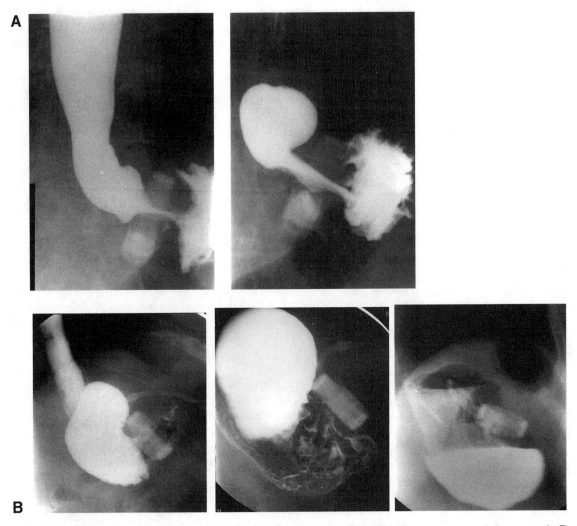

FIGURE 14–4   **A.** Radiographs of a band in a normal position for band placement around the stomach. **B.** Several patients with a slipped-prolapsed lower stomach causing a larger proximal pouch and the band to be "flipped" over.

some of the American study sites in the US multicenter trials and in other international sites.[15,17] Newer placement techniques have decreased this to 5% in the US trials.[15] Experience also decreases the risk of this complication. O'Brien reported a reoperation rate for slippage of 24% in the first 350 patients he treated with an adjustable gastric band (many with the old technique), but only 0.6% in his last 350 patients through May 2000.[17] Prolapse can happen at any time during the life of the patient as the stitches used to imbricate the band over the stomach can break with extensive vomiting from a viral illness (personal case history of one author's [Martin] patient). This is less likely to occur after the first several years and the incidence O'Brien reports is a significant difference in the rate of slippage per patient month of having a band even though his first 350 patients

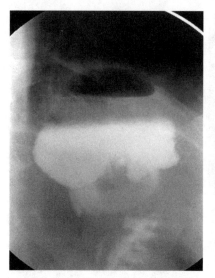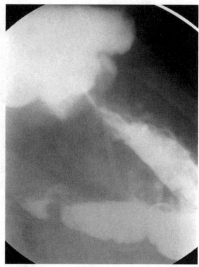

FIGURE 14–5   Radiograph of two patients who have forced the band down onto the more distal stomach from overeating and who have partial obstruction with a layer of barium nearest the outlet, then a mixed layer, and then saliva on top.

have been followed for an average of more than 3 years, while his second set of 350 patients had been followed for only 2 years.

Patients can also force the band further down onto their stomach where the band is forced to encircle a larger section of the stomach and can become obstructed (Figure 14–5). This will also lead to reflux, nausea, and vomiting. Often, these patients have to sleep sitting up because when they lay down the fluid trapped above the band no longer has gravity helping it stay in place and the patient begins to vomit. If the balloon can be emptied and the patient can change his or her habits, this can resolve. Often, however, the band has become fixed and reoperation is necessary. We do not think it is wise to replace a band at a higher location for someone who overeats and forces their band down further on their stomach as their behavior has defeated the idea of the band once. For patients who have been compliant but had their band slip because of vomiting, O'Brien's group has had good results replacing the band relocating it to a more cephalad position closer to the esophagogastric junction (the results were similar to those obtained by his patients who did not have revisional surgery).

Even when the band does not leave its initial position, it can contribute to the development of obstructive symptoms if it is overtightened, creating too narrow of a lumen through the band. This can lead to loss of lower esophageal sphincter pressure, reflux, and ultimately to dilation of the esophagus (Figure 14–6). Patient's pressure whoever is making an adjustment to "make it tight" not always understanding that the band can be made "too tight." If this error is made and the patient does not return to have it loosened because they are content to not be able to eat any solid food, over time, the esophagus dilates and

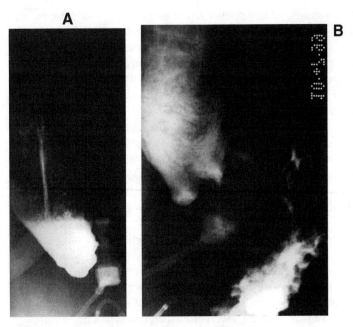

FIGURE 14–6   Radiographs of two patients with a dilated esophagous above the band with no lower esophageal sphincter tone. **A.** Enlarged esophagous with swallowed barium streaming through space. **B.** Dilated esophagous being used to store food.

loses its ability to contract. Often, the patient can gradually eat more solid food because the dilated esophagus begins to work as a storage organ and it retains partially digested food (Figure 14–6B). This increases the changes of an aspiration and usually results in the patient not being able to lay down without vomiting. If not caught before this stage in which the esophagus "gives out," it may become impossible to correct just by removing the fluid from the band and the band itself may have to be removed. When corrected early enough, esophageal function will return when the band is loosened, although the patient may begin to regain lost weight. When a degree of tightness cannot be found where the patient can feel full on small amounts of solid food without enlarging the esophagus, yet gains weight whenever enough fluid is removed from the band so that the esophagus regains its original size, then the patient should be considered for conversion to another type of weight-loss operation that does not depend on restriction alone to help the patient lose weight.

Another complication that can develop, that may be partially related to having the band too tightly wrapped around the stomach, is erosion of the band through the wall of the stomach into the lumen of the stomach. All the foreign bodies that have been used to wrap around the stomach to restrict intake as a mechanism for weight loss are associated with erosion and perforation. Nonadjustable bands have been eroding into the stomach since they began being used in the early 1980s. This does not usually result in peritonitis because the stomach, omentum, liver, or other tissue often adheres to these foreign bodies, covering them so that when an erosion into the stomach occurs, the adhered tissue prevents gastric acid from escaping the stomach lumen. With the adjustable gastric bands, the tubing, which connects the adjustable band to the subcutaneously placed access port (see Figure 14–1), provides a pathway for gastric acid to track along this pathway and may change how this complication presents in patients with this operation. Whenever erosion occurs, the restriction around the outside of the stomach no longer exists, so patients usually begin gaining weight. With an adjustable gastric band, the patient may present with an open, draining fistula near the access port caused by gastric acid eroding through the tissue by tracking along the path of the connecting tubing. Because the fistula is not usually infected, a culture of this draining wound may be negative for bacterial growth or colonized by skin flora.

It is not clear why erosions occur in patients who do not have an overtightened band. It occurs more frequently in patients who have had perforations at initial placement of a band presumably as a result of adhesions occurring between the foreign body and the stomach.[15] It is assumed that if the band is attached firmly to the stomach as a consequence of inflammation, that contractions of the stomach associated with normal digestion produce a "sanding" motion between the band and the stomach wall. Alternatively, if a patient uses nonsteroidal antiinflammatory agents, these medications may irritate the mucosa, especially as they have to transverse the restriction caused by the band, leading to an erosion occurring from the inside out.

The most common cause for removal of an adjustable gastric band is dissatisfaction from patients who cannot adjust to changing their behavior in response to the restriction provided by the band or because of inadequate weight loss associated with maladaptive behavior. Patients who eat soft, high-calorie foods or beverages will not lose weight. Others may complain that they cannot eat regular food, usually because they eat too fast or do not chew their food adequately, and will ask to have the band removed or demand conversion to another weight-loss procedure. This is a situation that physicians hope will improve with better patient education materials or selection tools to prevent patients who will refuse to adjust their behavior from having this treatment. Surgeons who offer this treatment also must be prepared to provide their patients with the support of psychotherapists, dietitians, and exercise specialists who can assist these patients in their efforts to change their behavior and successfully use these devices to lose weight. Referring physicians will, it is hoped, become sophisticated enough to only refer their patients to practices that demonstrate patient outcomes that prove that the practice has the support services necessary to help patients use these devices successfully.

SUMMARY

Roux-en-Y gastric bypass offers an effective, lasting treatment for morbid obesity and its associated comorbidities. Other bariatric procedures are still being measured against the long-term efficacy of gastric bypass usually accompanied by modest postoperative problems (see Chapters 10 to 12). All patients require significant education regarding the specifics of the bariatric procedure they receive and its expected outcomes, the potential complications, and the significant lifestyle modifications that follow surgery.

The laparoscopic approach affords patients an early recovery and a decrease in wound complications. The efficacy of the laparoscopic operations seems to be similar to that of their open counterpart. Careful management of these patients in the immediate and distant postoperative period helps to assure the best possible outcomes.

REFERENCES

1. NIH conference. Gastrointestinal surgery for severe obesity. Consensus Development Conference Panel. *Ann Intern Med* 1991;115:956–961.
2. Kuczmarski RJ. Prevalence of overweight and weight gain in the United States. Am J Clin Nutr 1992;55:495S–502S.
3. Colditz GA. Economic costs of obesity. *Am J Clin Nutr* 1992;55:503–507.
4. Sugerman HJ, Kellum JM, Engle KM, et al. Gastric bypass for treating severe obesity. *Am J Clin Nutr* 1992;55:560S–566S.
5. Sugerman HJ, Starkey JV, Birkenhauer R. A randomized prospective trial of gastric bypass versus vertical banded gastroplasty for morbid obesity and their effects on sweets versus non-sweets eaters. *Ann Surg* 1987;205:613–623.
6. Brolin RE. Critical analysis or results: weight loss and quality of data. *Am J Clin Nutr* 1992;55:577S–581S.
7. Wittgrove AC, Clark GW. Laparoscopic gastric bypass, Roux-en-Y—500 patients: technique and results, with 3–60 month follow-up. *Obes Surg* 2000;10:233–239.
8. Schauer PR, Ikramuddin S, Gourash W, et al. Outcomes after laparoscopic Roux-en-Y gastric bypass for morbid obesity. *Ann Surg* 2000;232(4):515–529.
9. Higa KD, Boone KB, Ho T. Laparoscopic Roux-en-Y gastric bypass for morbid obesity: technique and preliminary results of our first 400 patients. *Arch Surg* 2000;135:1029–1033.
10. DeMaria EJ, Sugerman HJ, Kellum JM, et al. Results of 281 consecutive total laparoscopic Roux-en-Y gastric bypasses to treat morbid obesity. *Ann Surg* 2002;235:640–647.
11. Schauer PR, Ikramuddin S. Laparoscopic surgery for morbid obesity. *Surg Clin North Am* 2001;81:1145–1179.
12. Serra C, Baltasar A, Bou R, et al. Internal hernias and gastric perforation after a laparoscopic gastric bypass. *Obes Surg* 1999;9:546–549.
13. Sugerman HJ, Brewer WH, Shiffman ML, et al. A multicenter, placebo-controlled, randomized, double-blind, prospective trial of prophylactic ursodiol for the prevention of gallstone formation following gastric-bypass-induced rapid weight loss. *Am J Surg* 1995;169:91–96.
14. Nguyen NT, Goldman C, Rosenquist CJ, et al. Laparoscopic versus open gastric bypass: a randomized study of outcomes, quality of life, and costs. *Ann Surg* 2001;234:279–291.
15. Martin LF, Smits GJ, Greenstein RJ. Laparoscopic adjustable gastric banding to treat morbid obesity: 3-year efficacy and 6-year safety data from the US multicenter trials. Submitted.

16. Martin LF, Robinson A, Moore A. The socioeconomic issues affecting treatment of obesity in the new millennium. *Pharmacoeconomics* 2000;18:335–353.

17. O'Brien PE, Dixon JB, Brown W, et al. The laparoscopic adjustable gastric band (LAP-BAND): a prospective study of medium-term effects on weight, health, and quality of life. *Obes Surg* 2002;12:652–660.

CHAPTER 15

METABOLIC DEFICIENCIES AND SUPPLEMENTS FOLLOWING BARIATRIC OPERATIONS

ROBERT E. BROLIN

Operations currently performed for treatment of morbid obesity can be divided into three categories. First, there are pure gastric-restrictive operations that compartmentalize the stomach into a small upper pouch with a calibrated conduit or stoma leading to the remaining stomach and digestive tract. The currently performed gastric-restrictive procedures—gastroplasty and gastric banding—reinforce the stoma with a prosthetic band to prevent dilatation (see Figure 15–1A and B and Chapter 10). Second, Roux-en-Y gastric bypass (RYGB), which can best be considered a combined restrictive–malabsorptive operation in that weight loss occurs primarily via restricted calorie intake but produces certain metabolic deficiencies that result from exclusion of nearly all of the stomach and the entire duodenum from gastrointestinal (GI) continuity (Figure 15–1C and Chapter 11). At present there is no operation performed for treatment of severe obesity that relies entirely upon malabsorption of ingested food to produce weight loss. However, there are several procedures that employ biliopancreatic diversion to produce malabsorption of fat and starches. These procedures include the biliopancreatic bypass (BPB) designed by Scopinaro (Figure 15–1D and Chapter 12) and the pylorus-preserving modification of biliopancreatic diversion dubbed the duodenal switch, plus there are modifications of the gastric bypass, including both the distal (or very, very long Roux limb) gastric bypass, with a common channel of 150 cm (59.1 inches) or less (Figure 15–1F), and the more standard long-limb gastric bypass that extends the Roux limb to over 100 cm (39.4 inches) but does not typically create a common channel that is less than 250 cm (98.4 inches) (see Chapter 2).

275

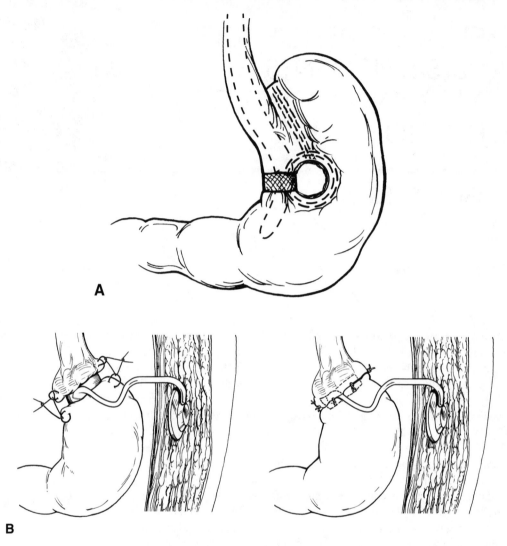

FIGURE 15–1   The standard bariatric procedures performed as of 2003. **A.** Vertical banded gastroplasty; (**B**) adjustable gastric band; (**C**) Roux-en-Y gastric bypass with a retrocolic, retrogastric Roux limb via a laparoscopic approach; (**D**) Scopinaro biliopancreatic bypass (BPB) with the limbs identified; (**E**) BPB with duodenal switch; and (**F**) distal gastric bypass.

PURE RESTRICTIVE OPERATIONS: GASTROPLASTY/GASTRIC BANDING

Although there is no rearrangement of GI tract anatomy in purely restrictive operations, vitamin and mineral deficiencies have been reported following these procedures.

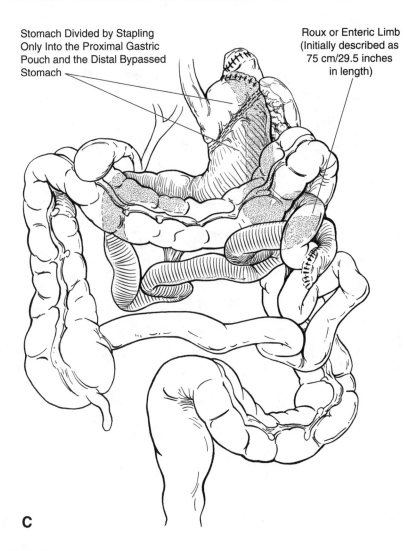

Stomach Divided by Stapling
Only Into the Proximal Gastric
Pouch and the Distal Bypassed
Stomach

Roux or Enteric Limb
(Initially described as
75 cm/29.5 inches
in length)

C

FIGURE 15–1

Incidence of Metabolic Deficiencies

There are virtually no published reports that focus on the incidence of metabolic deficiencies following pure restrictive operations. However, several independent reports show inadequate intake of potassium, calcium, magnesium, phosphorus, iron, zinc, copper, iodine, and vitamins A, C, D, E, K, B_1, B_2, and B_6, as shown in Figure 15–2.[1-3] Many of these deficiencies were noted in patients who were regularly taking multivitamin supplements. MacLean et al. measured various vitamins in 17 patients who were admitted for either malnutrition or excessively rapid weight loss after horizontal gastroplasty, and found significantly reduced serum levels of thiamin, serum folate, and red

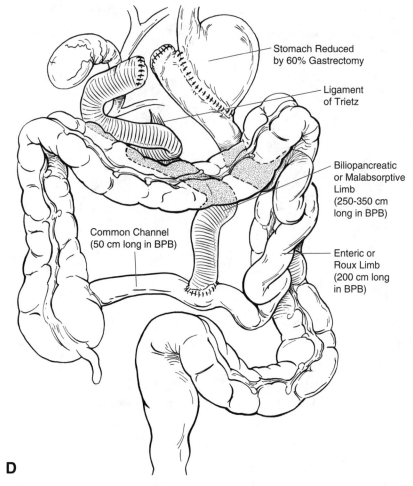

Stomach Reduced
by 60% Gastrectomy

Ligament
of Trietz

Biliopancreatic
or Malabsorptive
Limb
(250-350 cm
long in BPB)

Common Channel
(50 cm long in BPB)

Enteric or
Roux Limb
(200 cm long
in BPB)

D

FIGURE 15–1   (Continued)

blood cell folate in comparison with preoperative levels. Thiamin levels were low in 50% of these "selected" patients, whereas folate levels were decreased in 65% of these patients.[4]

Although severe nutritional deficiencies appear to be rare and isolated after pure restrictive procedures, cases of protein-calorie malnutrition have been reported.[4,5] MacLean et al. measured body composition in 167 patients who had horizontal gastroplasty in the early 1980s.[4] These investigators reported a nearly 30% incidence of malnutrition defined by a >10% decrease in body cell mass. Nearly 40% of the malnourished group in MacLean's report required reoperation to enlarge the outlet stoma whereas the remainder responded to other measures of supplemental nutrition support including gastrostomy tube feedings. Similarly, Raymond et al. measured body composition after stapled gastroplasty and reported losses of significant amounts of lean body tissue during the first 3 months.[6] However, these reductions were corrected at 1 year postoperation.

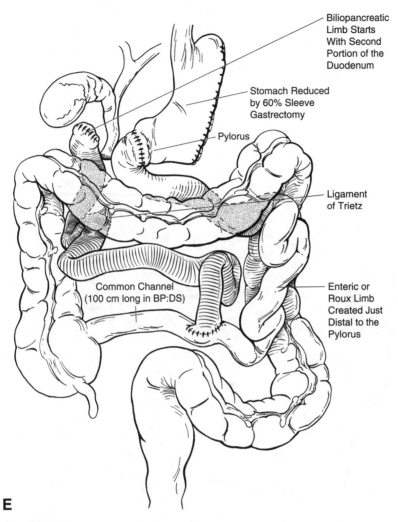

E

FIGURE 15–1

Causes of Deficiencies

There are two basic causes for development of metabolic deficiencies after restrictive operations: (1) excessive, protracted vomiting and (2) the so-called soft-calorie syndrome that results from intolerance and avoidance of nutritious foods such as meat, vegetables, and fresh fruit. The "soft-calorie" syndrome is likely a consequence of postprandial vomiting (see chapter 14). Sugerman and colleagues were the first group to suggest that gastroplasty may influence postoperative eating behavior. They reported that sweet eaters showed significantly less weight loss than did nonsweet eaters following vertical-banded gastroplasty (VBG).[7] Our group also showed significant changes in pre- versus postoperative food choices and eating behavior following VBG. In our study, 30

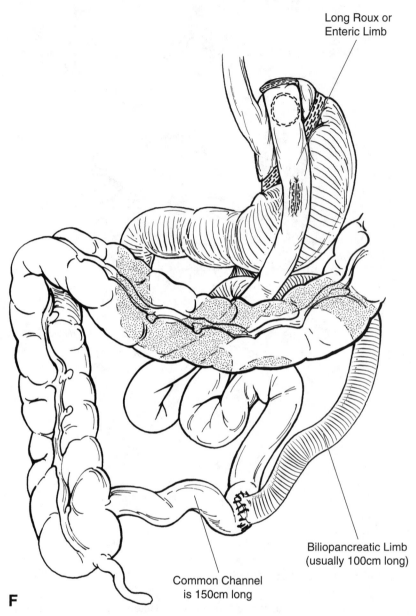

Long Roux or
Enteric Limb

Biliopancreatic Limb
(usually 100cm long)

Common Channel
is 150cm long

F

FIGURE 15–1   (Continued)

patients were selected to have VBG rather than gastric bypass on the basis of
their preoperative eating patterns.[8] Patients who ate large quantities of food at
mealtime (big meal eaters) with an average of no more than one snack per day
were assigned to the VBG group. The remainder had RYGB. We found that patients who had VBG frequently became sweet and junk food eaters because
they could not consume more nutritious foods without developing pain or vom-

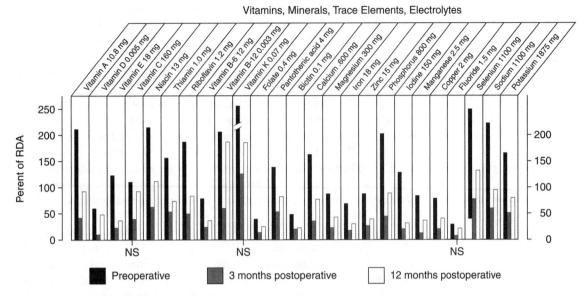

FIGURE 15–2 Median daily intake of vitamins, minerals, trace elements, and electrolytes before and after gastroplasty, expressed as percentage of the lower level (at top) of recommended dietary intake (RDA). The difference in pre- versus postoperative intake was significant ($p < 0.05$) except for vitamin C, vitamin K, and fluoride, indicated by NS. Reproduced with permission from Miskowiak et al.[1]

iting, even if they had previously been big meal eaters. The majority of our VBG patients could not eat meat. Our study describes the evolution of the "soft-calorie" syndrome after a pure gastric-restrictive operation.

There are conflicting results among reports that have correlated stoma diameter and weight loss after pure gastric-restrictive procedures. Generally, investigators who measured emptying of the gastric pouch failed to show a correlation between emptying rate and weight loss, whereas studies that employed endoscopy to measure the outlet showed a positive relationship between weight loss and stoma diameter.[4,5] MacLean et al. found that patients with a stoma diameter ≤10 mm (0.4 inches) frequently required readmission for troublesome vomiting, whereas patients with stomata measuring ≥10 mm (0.4 inches) had fewer problems tolerating solid food. It seems likely that substantial reductions in the recommended dietary allowance (RDA) of most vitamins, minerals, and trace elements parallel the decrease in consumption of solid foods after pure gastric-restrictive operations.

Clinical Consequences/Symptoms

Although a wide variety of nutritional deficiencies have been reported after pure restriction operations, the prevalence of symptoms or illness related to these deficiencies is poorly documented in the literature. The one exception, however, is thiamin (vitamin B_1) deficiency. In the early 1980s, there were several reports of acute thiamin deficiency causing Wernicke's encephalopathy following stapled gastroplasty.[5,9] By 1990, there were 21 reported cases of acute thiamin deficiency following gastric-restrictive operations.[5] All of these cases were a result of protracted vomiting.

The early symptoms of thiamin deficiency include generalized weakness, ataxia, and numbness in the extremities. Clinical signs include nystagmus, ophthalmoplegia, and the loss of position sense. If untreated the condition can progress to Wernicke-Korsakoff's encephalopathy, which is characterized by mental confusion, memory loss, progressive paralysis, and coma. Because symptoms are produced by demyelinization of nerves, neurologic changes are often permanent unless the syndrome is recognized and treated early in its course.

Because advanced Wernicke-Korsakoff encephalopathy is frequently fatal, the urgency of treatment cannot be overemphasized. Unfortunately, the laboratory diagnosis is based on a test that is not performed at most medical centers (serum erythrocyte transketolase), so treatment should be initiated on the basis of the clinical presentation. Thiamin should be given intravenously in doses of 50 to 100 mg diluted in 500 to 1000 cc of normal saline. Intramuscular injections are also effective but less reliably absorbed. Oral thiamin is not recommended for treatment in the acute stages of the syndrome.

Treatment/Prevention

Patients who develop vomiting to the point of intolerance of liquids should immediately be hospitalized. I found that rehydration and cessation of oral intake for as little as 24 hours is frequently all that is needed to reverse edema of the outlet stoma, which is invariably associated with protracted emesis in patients with a VBG or nonadjustable gastric band. However, when resumption of oral liquids is met with further nausea or vomiting, upper endoscopy should be performed. Protracted vomiting and food intolerance occasionally resolve after endoscopic dilatation of the outlet stoma and/or band deflation in patients with adjustable bands. Total parenteral nutrition (TPN) can be used as an adjunct during hospitalization or, in some cases, at home. Intractable cases that do not respond to several attempts at endoscopic dilatation or deflation of adjustable bands should be taken down (reversed) or converted to Roux-en-Y gastric bypass.

Multivitamin supplements should be given to all gastroplasty and banding patients because the RDA of many vitamins and minerals is rarely attained postoperatively in the reduced intake of a restricted diet. Because vitamin and mineral deficiencies are uncommon after gastric-restrictive procedures, laboratory tests are not routinely performed postoperatively. However, patients who are experiencing chronic problems with postprandial emesis should have a complete blood cell count and chemistry profile that includes electrolytes, protein, and albumin levels.

COMBINED RESTRICTIVE–MALABSORPTIVE OPERATIONS

Nearly all of the stomach and the entire duodenum are excluded from the functional digestive tract, causing patients who have RYGB to be prone to deficiencies in iron, vitamin B_{12}, and folate.[1-5]

Incidence of Metabolic Deficiencies after RYBG

Table 15–1 summarizes data in several published articles that focus on vitamin and mineral deficiencies after RYGB. Our 1998 report extensively reviewed several hematologic parameters in 348 patients who had RYGB during a 10 year period, including 321 patients who had primary RYGB and 27 (7.7%) who had revision procedures[10]. Our technique of RYGB incorporated a $\leq$ 30cc capacity upper pouch with Roux limbs ranging from 50–150 cm in length. Follow-up in that series ranged from 6 months to 10 years with a mean follow-up of 42.3 months. Deficiencies were recognized in 268 of the 348 patients (82%) postoperatively including 155 patients with iron deficiency (47%), 122 (37%) with vitamin B-12 deficiency, 115 (35%) with folate deficiency and 177 (54%) patients with anemia. All of our patients are told to take multivitamin supplements daily for the rest of their lives.

In our 1998 report,[10] the incidence of anemia and deficiencies in iron and folate were substantially higher than in previously published series,[11,12] including our earlier 1991 report.[13] Longer postoperative followup in our most recent series likely explains the greater incidence of these deficiencies, as the incidence of low iron, folate, and hemoglobin levels nearly doubled with a proportional increase in followup time.[10] The incidence of anemia also is a re-

TABLE 15–1. PUBLISHED REPORTS OF METABOLIC DEFICIENCIES AFTER GASTRIC BYPASS					
REPORT/YEAR/#PATIENT	MEAN FOLLOWUP	IRON	B_{12}	FULATE	ANEMIA
Halverson[11] (N=69)	20 mo	20%/17 mo	26%/20 mo	9%/13.0 mo	18%/—
Amaral[12] (N=150)	33.2 mo	49%/15.6 mo	70%/13.0 mo	18%/—	35%/20 mo
Brolin[13] (N=124)	24.2 mo	33%/13.4 mo	37%/12.8 mo	16%/10.7 mo	22%/12 mo
Brolin[10] (N=348)	42.3 mo	47%/11.0 mo	37%/12.8 mo	35%/11.5 mo	54%/10.8 mo

Mean incidence and time of deficiency recognition are listed under each micronutrient with mean follow up shown in right column.

flection of the proportion of menstruating women in each series, as it is much more difficult for these women, who have to both replace the blood they lose monthly as well as consume enough iron and related nutrients to compensate for the 90-day life cycle of all red blood cells in patients with an intact spleen. Conversely, the incidence of B_{12} deficiency remained constant over time. There was little difference in the mean time of recognition of iron, B_{12}, and folate deficiency among these reports.[10–13]

Table 15–2 shows the time-related changes of iron, B_{12}, and folate levels in our 1998 report.[10] The onset of deficiencies was rapid in many patients, as the median time interval for recognition of low iron, B_{12}, folate, and hemoglobin (HGB) levels was the 6-month visit. Serum iron levels remained relatively stable through the first 3 years postoperatively. Although mean iron levels at ≤36 months were significantly lower than at previous intervals, they remained well within the normal range. Changes in the total iron-binding capacity were generally consistent with serum iron levels throughout the study. Although microcytic, hypochromic indices were found in the majority of anemic patients, only 63% of low iron levels were associated with microcytic indices. Moreover, 50% of low HGB levels were not associated with iron deficiency.

As mentioned, iron deficiency and anemia are far more common in women than men after RYGB. In our 1998 report,[10] the mean time of recognition of anemia in men was at 29 months postoperatively, nearly 2 years later than in women. This finding explains why anemia was not recognized in men in two earlier reports.[12,13] Iron saturation levels were significantly lower in women than in men throughout the study. The incidence of folate deficiency was higher in women (35%) than in men (22%), at a level that approached significance ($P = 0.058$).[10] There was no significant difference in the incidence of B_{12} deficiency or anemia between men and women in our 1998 report.[10] Megaloblastic anemia was not recognized in any of our patients as compared with a respective incidence of 5% and 7% in two earlier reports.[2,5] Only three patients in our study (0.8%) had macrocytic indices.[10]

TABLE 15–2. CHANGES IN HEMATOLOGIC PARAMETERS OVER TIME						
TIME	HGB (G)	HCT (%)	IRON (μG/DL)	TIBC (μG/DL)	VITAMIN B_{12} (PG/DL)	FOLATE
Preoperative (N=348)	13.8 ± 1	41.4 ± 4	79 ± 35	343 ± 61	450 ± 341	5.5 ± 3.4
12 mo (N=304)	13.2 ± 2*+	39.5 ± 4*+	74 ± 31	328 ± 62*	350 ± 205*	8.1 ± 5.2*
24 mo (N=213)	12.8 ± 2*+	38.4 ± 5*+	77 ± 37	352 ± 73	337 ± 192*	9.0 ± 5.2*
≥36 mo (N=195)	12.4 ± 2*+	37.7 ± 5*+	65 ± 36*+	378 ± 217*	357 ± 217*	9.2 ± 5.2*

Abbreviations: HCT = hematocrit; HGB = hemoglobin; TIBC = total iron-binding capacity.
Data expressed as mean ± SD. * indicates significant difference versus preoperative measurement (p <0.05 by analysis of variance with Student-Newman-Keuls test). + indicates significant difference versus the preceding time interval(s) (p <0.05 by analysis of variance with Student-Newman-Keuls tests).

Causes of Post-RYGB Deficiencies

Postgastric bypass vitamin B_{12} deficiency occurs primarily as a consequence of maldigestion of dietary B_{12}. The minimum daily requirement for vitamin B_{12} is 5 ìg with body stores estimated at 5000 ìg. The main dietary source is red meat, particularly liver. Other important sources include eggs, milk, fish, oysters, and clams. Dietary B_{12}, which is protein bound, must be enzymatically cleaved from the protein before absorption can occur.[14] Both pepsin and hydrochloric acid (HCl) are required to separate food-bound B_{12} from the protein moiety in the stomach. Enzymatic cleavage of the food-bound B_{12} moiety is limited after gastric bypass as a consequence of absence of HCl in the upper gastric pouch and exclusion of the distal stomach and duodenum where pepsin and pancreatic secretory enzymes facilitate binding of the freed B_{12} to intrinsic factor. Several investigators have demonstrated that food-bound vitamin B_{12} is less-well absorbed than orally administered crystalline B_{12} after both parietal gastrectomy and RYGB.[15–17] Other investigators report normal Schilling tests in RYGB patients, suggesting that secretion of intrinsic factor occurs in the bypassed stomach.[18,19] Consequently, oral supplements of crystalline B_{12} should provide effective treatment for vitamin B_{12} deficiency after RYGB. The megaloblastic anemia associated with both B_{12} and folate deficiency is manifested in erythroid precursor cells which express nuclear maturation and nuclear-cytoplasmic dissociation as a consequence of impaired DNA synthesis. These marrow granulocyte precursors show large, horseshoe-shaped nuclei, the so-called megaloblasts.

Iron deficiency after RYGB results from both malabsorption and maldigestion of dietary iron. Only 5 to 10% of ingested iron is absorbed. The primary source of dietary iron is red meat, which is the most difficult type of food to consume after RYGB. Other iron-rich foods include shellfish, lima/brown beans, and prune juice. The RDA for iron in adults is 15 to 18 mg with requirements decreasing to approximately 10 mg in postmenopausal women and men older than age 50 years. Although a balanced diet should provide these requirements, it is estimated that 25 to 30% of Americans consume an iron-deficient diet. Iron is stored in the marrow, liver, and spleen. Stores in adult males are typically 1000 mg, whereas 10 to 20% of menstruating women have virtually no iron reserves. Dietary iron is absorbed primarily in the duodenum and upper jejunum, which are excluded from the functional digestive tract in RYGB. In the normal stomach, absorption of dietary iron is facilitated by hydrochloric acid. Several investigators have shown that there is markedly reduced acid production in the upper pouch of gastric bypass patients, which typically does not include very many parietal cells, those cells that secrete acid.[17,19] Additionally, the corpus, where most of the parietal cells reside, does not secrete as much acid because this part of the stomach no longer receives stimulation from the distension caused by food. Hence, it seems likely that decreased acid secretion in the small gastric pouch and in the distal bypassed stomach contributes to development of iron deficiency after RYGB.

There are remarkably few studies of iron metabolism after RYGB. Rhode et al. performed iron-absorption tests in 55 patients at a mean of approximately

3 years after RYGB and found that patients with normal absorption of iron had a significantly higher incidence of anemia and lower serum ferritin levels than did those with below-normal absorption.[20] These investigators also found that adding 500 mg of vitamin C to a daily regimen of oral iron that contained 50 mg in the elemental form, significantly increased serum ferritin levels postoperatively.

Menstrual blood loss clearly contributes to development of iron deficiency and anemia after RYGB. In our 1998 report,[10] iron deficiency was significantly less prevalent in women who had a total abdominal hysterectomy prior to RYGB than in those women who did not. This finding supports the notion that menstrual blood loss is an important contributing factor to development of post-RYGB iron deficiency. However, low HGB levels did not correlate with having a total abdominal hysterectomy, suggesting that post-RYGB anemia in some women has causes other than menstrual blood loss. Low iron stores in menstruating women are probably the primary cause of iron deficiency and anemia in this group.

Our group performed a prospective randomized study of oral iron versus placebo in 56 menstruating women who were followed a mean 34 months after RYGB.[21] Prophylactic oral iron supplements consistently prevented development of iron deficiency postoperatively. Conversely, there was no difference in the incidence of anemia in the subjects who received iron rather than placebo in spite of the differences in iron levels. In patients who received iron postoperatively, ferritin levels were similar to preoperative measurements, whereas placebo patients had significantly lower postoperative ferritin levels in comparison with preoperative values. There was no difference in the incidence of either vitamin B_{12} or folate levels between the two groups, suggesting that regular menstrual blood loss does not contribute to the development of deficiencies in these levels to the same degree it does for iron levels.

The incidence of folate deficiency after RYGB varies widely in clinical reports, ranging from 0 to 38%.[11–13,22] Foods rich in folate include green leafy vegetables, fruits, meat, and eggs. The minimal daily requirement is 50 μg, which is substantially lower than the RDA of 400 μg per day. Total body stores are estimated at 5000 μg, so depletion can occur with sustained inadequate intake. Reduced dietary intake likely contributes to low folate levels in many RYGB patients. Although folate absorption occurs predominantly in the upper third of the small intestine, there is evidence that absorption can occur in both the mid and distal small bowel.[22] Because folate absorption is also facilitated by HCl in the stomach, low acid production by both the upper pouch and lower position of the stomach in RYGB patients may predispose to development of folate deficiency postoperatively. Russel et al. suggest that increased bacterial synthesis of folate in the upper small bowel may compensate for diminished absorption of dietary folate in achlorhydric patients.[23] This finding suggests that folate absorption may gradually improve over time in patients who have had RYGB.

Changes in the postoperative dietary habits also contribute to the development of nutritional deficiencies following RYGB. Red meat and milk are, respectively, major sources of iron and vitamin B_{12} in the diet. Red meat is generally recognized as the most difficult type of food to eat after gastric restrictive operations.[24,25] Milk product intolerance is common following gastric bypass.[24] Avinoah et al., reported a significantly higher incidence of iron, vitamin B_{12}, and folate deficiency in postoperative RYGB patients who ate red meat less often than once a week in comparison with patients who ate red meat more often than once weekly.[25] These authors concluded that decreased meat consumption is a major factor contributing to both iron and vitamin B_{12} deficiency after gastric bypass.

Updegraffe and Neufeld obtained pre- and postoperative diet histories from 12 patients who had gastric bypass and found that postoperative intake of protein and folate were significantly decreased in comparison with preoperative intake.[26] However, postoperative serum folate levels in their subjects were significantly higher than the preoperative measurements. The investigators attributed the increase in postoperative folate levels to multivitamin supplementation because none of the 12 study patients were taking a multivitamin preoperatively.

In our 1998 report,[10] the incidence of postoperative B_{12} deficiency was significantly greater in the patients who had revision than in those who had primary operations. This finding was surprising because 24 of the 27 patients who had revision procedures had some form of gastroplasty as their initial operation, whereas 3 had revisions of jejunoileal bypass to RYGB. Because there was no difference in serum B_{12} levels between primary and revision patients prior to RYGB, the difference in postoperative levels suggests that B_{12} stores were substantially depleted in the revision group. Reduced dietary intake of vitamin B_{12} after the primary procedure leading to a total body depletion of vitamin B_{12} even before the revision provides a plausible explanation for the significantly lower postoperative B_{12} levels in patients who had revisions. Although the estimated blood loss in revision procedures was usually two to three times greater than in primary operations, the incidence of postoperative iron deficiency and anemia were similar in these two groups.

Patient noncompliance is probably the most important factor contributing to both development and persistence of metabolic deficiencies after RYGB. Only 33% of the patients in our 1998 study were consistently compliant in taking multivitamin supplements throughout the duration of followup.[10] In the same study, we found that only 35% and 54% were compliant in taking prescribed iron and B_{12} supplements, respectively, for treatment of recognized deficiencies, even though the consequences of these deficiencies had been extensively discussed. Compliance was defined as taking vitamin supplements $\geqslant 5$ times per week. Development of severe anemia, defined as HGB $\leqslant 10$ g, was invariably associated with not taking multivitamin and iron supplements and with missing scheduled followup visits. This frequency of noncompliance occurred despite a detailed preoperative discussion regarding the potential for developing metabolic deficiencies after RYGB. The need for vitamin supplements and the risk of metabolic deficiencies are also emphasized at each postoperative visit.

An important unanswered question regarding post RYGB metabolic deficiencies is whether there is steady progression of untreated deficiencies over time. Figure 15–3 shows the changes in the mean HGB, iron, and vitamin B_{12} over time in 85 patients who were followed for at least 5 years. Postoperative changes in hematocrit were virtually the same as the pattern observed for HGB. Moreover, at each successive interval through 5 years postoperatively, HGB and hematocrit were decreased significantly versus the prior interval. After 5 years, both HGB and hematocrit were increased relative to values obtained between 3 and 5 years postoperatively. This finding is not explained, but may relate to the characteristics of the patients who continue to return for followup. Although iron levels declined during the first 12 months postoperatively, there were no significant differences in mean iron levels over time. Vitamin B_{12} levels (Figure 15–3B) were more variable showing an initial decline during the first 24 months postoperatively, with a subsequent increase after 48 months. However, postoperative B_{12} levels were significantly lower than mean preoperative values only at 12 and 24 months postoperatively. Mean postoperative folate levels were significantly greater than preoperative measurements at all time periods. These data weakly suggest that most post-RYGB deficiencies tend to either stabilize or improve between 4 and 5 years postoperatively. However, our experience is muddled by haphazard compliance with treatment regimens and inconsistent long-term followup.

There are no published longitudinal studies of calcium metabolism after conventional RYGB. Crowley et al. evaluated 41 selected patients between 6 and 9 years after RYGB and found that 14 had lost height, 26 had musculoskeletal symptoms, and 1 had developed radiographic evidence of osteoporosis with vertebral compression fractures.[27] Surprisingly, only 1 of these 41 patients had a subnormal calcium level. However, neither parathyroid hormone levels nor bone densitometry were measured in these patients. Our group has performed bone densitometry measurements in more than 30 women at 3 or more years after RYGB. Although there have been no abnormal densitometry studies to date, parathyroid hormone levels have been consistently elevated in these patients. Because milk intolerance is common after RYGB, inadequate calcium intake may contribute to deficiencies in some cases. Clearly, more longitudinal data are needed to evaluate the long-term effects of RYGB on calcium and bone metabolism.

Remarkably, there have been virtually no sophisticated studies of energy expenditure after bariatric operations. Flancbaum et al. measured resting energy expenditure in 60 patients who had RYGB at 6 postoperative intervals ending at 24 months.[28] To their surprise resting energy expenditure was consistently normal based upon Harris-Benedict equation predictions. This "paradoxical" response in resting energy expenditure after RYGB contrasts with the expected reduction in resting energy expenditure associated with fasting, starvation, and low-calorie diets. These normal measurements were recorded as early as 6 weeks postoperatively when dietary intake is generally less than 1000 kcal/d.

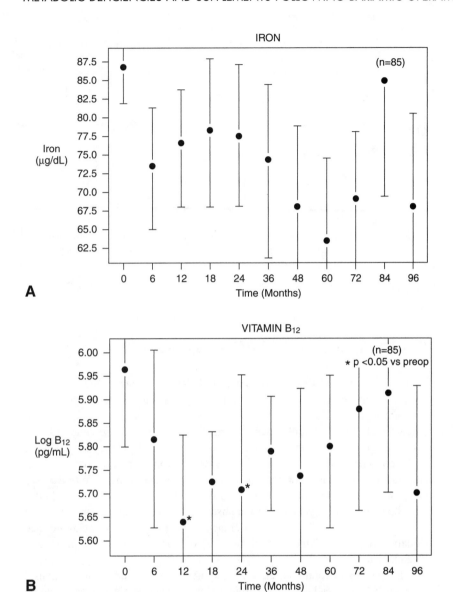

FIGURE 15–3   Data expressed as mean ± SD. * indicates significant difference versus the preoperative measurement (p = 0.05 by analysis of variance with Student-Newman-Keuls test). Log scale E was used to normalize the distribution of the B_{12} values (B). (Reproduced by courtesy of Quality Medical Publishing Co., St. Louis, MO.)

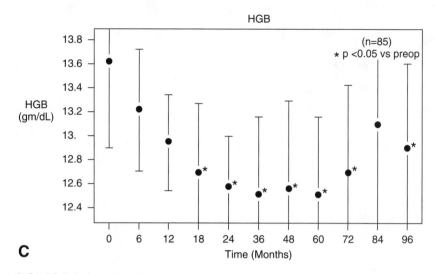

FIGURE 15–3   (Continued)

Clinical Consequences/Symptoms

There is a paucity of longitudinal data on the clinical consequences of metabolic deficiencies after RYGB. Symptoms of B_{12} deficiency include numbness and paresthesias in the extremities and vague gastrointestinal complaints. The tongue can be enlarged and appear inflamed (glossitis). Because vitamin B_{12} is essential for myelin synthesis, clinical presentation of deficiency may include peripheral neuropathy. Symptoms may progress from diminution of vibration and position sense to poor muscular coordination and ataxia. Central nerve symptoms include mental dullness, confusion, memory loss, delusions, hallucinations and overt psychosis. In the absence of replacement, neuropathy can progress to the point of irreversible damage. Severe B_{12} deficiency can produce a qualitative platelet defect that inhibits aggregation and results in a prolonged bleeding time.

Symptoms of folate deficiency are typically subtle and include malaise, diarrhea, and vague dyspepsia. Clinical signs include slightly icteric sclerae and a smooth, atrophic tongue. Although the diagnosis of folate deficiency is based on serum levels, red blood cell folate more accurately reflects tissue stores. Although low B_{12} and folate levels are common after RYGB, I have not recognized symptoms that could be attributed to either deficiency over a 19-year experience.[29] This observation suggests that B_{12} and folate deficiency are rarely clinically important after RYGB. On the basis of these observations, we do not recommend prophylactic supplements of vitamin B_{12} or folate to our RYGB patients. Moreover, because folate deficiency is consistently prevented by taking multivitamin supplements, we no longer routinely measure serum folate either before or after RYGB.

Fatigue and weakness are commonly associated with iron deficiency and anemia in many RYGB patients. Symptoms of iron deficiency include fatigue, lethargy, headache, anorexia, and paresthesias or feeling "cold." Clinical signs include, dry and wrinkled skin, pallor, alopecia, atrophy of the tongue, and, in more severe cases, brittle, flattened, or concave fingernails that fracture easily. A complete blood cell count and measurement of serum iron are sufficient to make an accurate diagnosis of iron deficiency. Microcytic, hypochromic indices suggest iron deficiency as the primary cause of anemia, whereas macrocytic, normochromic indices suggest vitamin B_{12} or folate deficiency as the likely cause. Although serum ferritin is a better estimate of iron stores than serum iron, ferritin need not be routinely measured after RYGB.

Unfortunately, there has been a resurgence of cases of acute thiamin deficiency after RYGB.[30,31] Virtually all of these cases resulted from delayed treatment of protracted vomiting during the first few weeks postoperatively. I believe that the increased number of these cases can be attributed to lack of awareness of this heretofore rare syndrome by inexperienced bariatric surgeons.

Treatment and Prevention

Daily oral multivitamin supplements are recommended for all patients who have RYGB because these patients decrease the quantity of food they consume. In spite of these recommendations, our cumulative experience, with more than 1500 operations performed over 19 years, is that there is no correlation between regularly taking multivitamin supplements and the development of either iron or B_{12} deficiency after RYGB. Both compliant and noncompliant patients develop iron or B_{12} deficiencies. Conversely, there is a significant difference in the incidence of folate deficiency between patients who regularly take multivitamin and noncompliant patients.[10,26,32] Multivitamin supplements, which typically contain 400 μg of folate, consistently correct low folate levels.[10,32] Hence, there is no need to give additional folate supplements for low folate levels after RYGB. The absence of megaloblastic anemia in our 1998 report may be the result of a combination of generally good compliance in taking multivitamins postoperatively and earlier treatment intervention in patients with vitamin B_{12} and folate deficiency.

There is also little published information on the results of treatment of micronutrient deficiencies after RYGB. Low serum levels of iron, B_{12}, and folate should be treated with either multivitamins or supplements of the deficient micronutrient. In our 1998 report, more than 80% of the vitamin B_{12} deficiencies responded to oral B_{12} supplements. Rhode et al. showed that a minimum daily dose of 350 μg of crystalline B_{12} is necessary to maintain normal serum levels after RYGB.[33] Our group has found that 500 μg of oral B_{12} is sufficient to correct the great majority of deficiencies. Intramuscular injections are usually reserved for patients who refuse to take oral B_{12}. Initial injections of 1000 μg are given every 2 to 4 weeks. Maintenance doses of 100 to 500 μg per month should maintain normal serum levels. Fortunately, doses of up to 10,000 times maintenance levels are nontoxic in humans.[34] Nasal sprays and gels also provide effective prophylaxis.

A complete blood cell count and serum levels of iron, total iron-binding capacity, and vitamin B_{12} should be obtained in each patient preoperatively and again postoperatively at 6-month intervals during the first 2 years postoperatively, then annually thereafter. We no longer routinely measure serum folate because multivitamins consistently correct low folate levels in deficient patients. There is considerable controversy regarding the need for prophylactic B_{12} supplements after RYGB. Our group does not recommend prophylactic B_{12} because I have yet to identify clear-cut symptoms of deficiency in any patient. There is also controversy regarding the need for prophylactic calcium supplements after RYGB. Most surgeons neither measure serum calcium nor provide prophylactic supplements to their RYGB patients.[35] However, the risk of developing osteoporosis and/or osteomalacia after RYGB remains undetermined. Prophylactic calcium supplementation is relatively harmless and may be of long-term benefit to some RYGB patients.

In our experience, low serum iron levels do not respond consistently to treatment with multivitamin and oral iron supplements.[13,21] Although there was a significant correlation between taking oral iron supplements and improvement of postoperative iron deficiency in our 1998 report, oral iron supplements corrected iron deficiency in only 43% of cases. Treatment of severe iron-deficiency anemia (HGB $\leqslant 10$ g) is particularly problematic. Patients with severe anemia rarely respond to oral iron supplements alone. However, severely anemic patients may eventually respond to intramuscular iron injections, intravenous iron dextran, erythropoietin (Procrit) given as subcutaneous injections or blood transfusion. Some patients with menorrhagia may require total abdominal hysterectomy to correct anemia. The resistance of iron deficiency to oral iron supplements coupled with the high incidence of iron deficiency anemia in menstruating women have led us to prescribe prophylactic oral iron supplements containing at least 50 mg of elemental iron to premenopausal women who have RYGB.

Anemia is a serious clinical problem after RYGB because of its incidence and the expense that can be incurred for its evaluation, especially if a physician does not understand the patient has had a gastric bypass or that anemia occurs frequently after gastric bypass. If a woman who is menstruating is not symptomatic and has a hemoglobin greater than 8 g/dL, the anemia will usually resolve with menopause. Although iron deficiency is the most common factor predisposing to development of anemia, 50% of low HGB levels in our 1998 report were not associated with iron deficiency. Further studies are needed to elucidate the mechanisms involved in the development of anemia after RYGB in order that more effective strategies for prophylaxis can be developed. This is especially true for younger women who may want to become pregnant because we have little knowledge of how anemia after gastric bypass affects pregnancy outcomes.

MALABSORPTIVE OPERATIONS

Weight loss after the first widely performed bariatric operation, jejunoileal bypass, resulted entirely from malabsorption of ingested nutrients. Malabsorptive operations currently used for treatment of morbid obesity include biliopancreatic diversion (BPD), the duodenal switch (DS) and the distal or very, very long limb Roux-en-Y gastric bypass (D-RYGB). The primary mechanism of malabsorption in these procedures is diversion of biliary and pancreatic secretions from the digestive stream. The current biliopancreatic diversion operations also incorporate a small element of gastric restriction.

Incidence of Deficiencies

Table 15–3 shows an estimated incidence of metabolic deficiencies after the three currently performed biliopancreatic diversion operations. These deficiencies are primarily a consequence of malabsorption rather than of inadequate intake. There is little apparent difference in the incidence of metabolic deficiencies following these three procedures. There is a remarkable paucity of data on B_{12} absorption after the duodenal switch. Serum measurements of vitamins E and K have been rarely reported in the published series of these operations. There are no reports suggesting that vitamin K deficiency is problematic. Coagulopathy secondary to isolated vitamin K deficiency has not been reported after biliopancreatic diversion. I believe that the prevalence of severe nutritional deficiencies following biliopancreatic diversion operations is underreported.

Malabsorption of calcium has been noted in a number of patients following biliopancreatic diversion procedures with an incidence reported in the range of 10 to 35%%.[37–39] Deficiency occurs despite prophylactic oral calcium

TABLE 15–3. INCIDENCE OF METABOLIC DEFICIENCIES FOLLOWING BILIOPANCREATIC DIVERSION			
NUTRIENT	BPB	DUODENOL SWITCH	D-RYGB
Protein/albumin	5–30%	20%	15%
Calcium	20–25%	20–35%	10%
Vitamin A	5–50%	5–10%	10%
Vitamin B_{12}	20–35%	—	8%
Vitamin D	30–60%	25–50%	51%
Vitamin E	30%	—	—
Anemia	20–50%	20–40%	74%
Iron	30–40%	25–30%	49%

Abbreviations: BPB = biliopancreatic bypass; D-RYGB = distal Roux-en-Y gastric bypass.

supplements. Serum alkaline phosphatase is frequently elevated postoperatively suggesting active mobilization of calcium from bone. Serum calcium levels do not reflect bone status. Secondary hyperparathyroidism with increased parathyroid hormone levels suggesting inadequate absorption of calcium is present in a high percentage of patients. Unlike jejunoileal bypass, magnesium deficiency and electrolyte imbalance are apparently uncommon after biliopancreatic diversion.

The incidence of anemia following biliopancreatic diversion procedures ranges from 30 to 74%.[36-38] We recently reported a comparison of a distal malabsorptive RYGB with two types of RYGB performed using shorter, more conventional Roux limb lengths. There was a significantly higher incidence of anemia in patients who had distal RYGB (74%) despite a similar incidence of iron deficiency.[38] Red blood cell indices in the D-RYGB group were typically normochromic, normocytic which are consistent with anemia of chronic disease. Sugerman et al. also noted a preponderance of normochromic, normocytic indices in a group of anemic patients who had a malabsorptive modification of RYGB.[39] Conversely, Skroubei et al. reported a 37% incidence of anemia in a series of 95 patients who had D-RYGB.[40] They also reported significantly lower ferritin levels in D-RYGB versus conventional RYGB patients. Megaloblastic anemia is rare following biliopancreatic diversion.

The reported incidence of protein deficiency has varied widely after biliopancreatic diversion. In 1986, Scopinaro reported that 7.5% of his BPB patients required hospitalization for treatment of protein deficiency.[36] Marceau reported that 20% of their patients developed hypoalbuminemia after the DS, although fewer than 5% required hospitalization.[37] In our experience with D-RYGB, 13% of patients developed low albumin levels with two patients (4.3%) requiring hospitalization to receive TPN.[38] Conversely, other clinical reports do not mention hypoproteinemia following biliopancreatic diversion. I believe that protein deficiency with overt manifestations of malnutrition is a potential risk for patients who have these operations.

Progressive hepatic dysfunction with cirrhosis was the most feared late complication of jejunoileal bypass. Isolated cases of liver failure have been reported after biliopancreatic diversion. However, there is a paucity of objective data on the incidence of progressive liver dysfunction following these operations. We had a late death in a patient with preexisting cirrhosis 9 months after D-RYGB.[38] Sugerman et al. reported two deaths from liver failure among five patients who had D-RYGB with a 50-cm (19.7-inch) common channel.[39] Conversely, Marceau et al. reported improved hepatic histopathology in 11 patients with cirrhosis who underwent the DS.[41] At present, there are insufficient data on the subject of liver dysfunction associated with biliopancreatic diversion. However, it seems reasonable to recommend not performing a malabsorptive operation in a patient with recognized cirrhosis.

Causes of Deficiencies

All of the currently used biliopancreatic diversion operations are designed to produce steatorrhea resulting from incomplete absorption of dietary fat via diversion of bile from the digestive stream. Consequently, all of the fat-soluble vitamins (A, D, E, and K) are not absorbed normally, and patients who have these operations are prone to develop deficiencies in these vitamins. Inadequate intake does not appear to be a major contributory factor to fat-soluble vitamin deficiency following biliopancreatic diversion.

Because protein and carbohydrate are absorbed throughout the length of the small bowel, malabsorption associated with biliopancreatic diversion is theoretically "selective" for fat.[36] Nonetheless, hypoproteinemia has been reported in many patients who have undergone biliopancreatic procedures.[36,37,39] Inadequate intake of protein is thought by many to play a role in such cases,[42] although there are no well-controlled postoperative diet intake studies that support this hypothesis. I have seen several cases of protein-calorie malnutrition after a distal malabsorptive modification of RYGB.[38] Nausea and vomiting that limited oral intake were noted in each case.

The volume of the residual stomach is greater after BPD and the DS in comparison with RYGB. Therefore, it might be expected that the incidence of vitamin B_{12} deficiency would be lower after biliopancreatic diversion. In our experience with D-RYGB, however, which incorporated a 75-cm (29.5-inch) common channel, the incidence of B_{12} deficiency (8%) was significantly lower in comparison with conventional RYGB.[38] The duodenal switch has the theoretical advantage of preserving most of the gastric antrum, which would allow cleavage of food-bound B_{12} in the stomach, thereby improving dietary absorption. Moreover, the common channel of ileum is long enough to permit resorption of B_{12}. It seems likely that the lack of published data on B_{12} deficiency after the DS is a result of the surgeons' comfort in a relatively intact mechanism of B_{12} absorption.[43] This concept requires further study.

Although there are a number of possible causes for anemia after biliopancreatic diversion, there are no careful studies of anemia associated with these procedures. Iron deficiency is likely the most common treatable cause. However, a substantial number of patients have normochromic, normocytic red cell indices consistent with anemia of chronic disease. Although it seems likely that the "chronic disease" in these cases is malnutrition, only a small number of these anemic patients had other clinical stigmata of poor nutrition.

Calcium is absorbed predominately in the duodenum and proximal jejunum, which is excluded from digestive continuity in both the Scopinaro BPD and the duodenal switch. A second mechanism likely contributing to malabsorption of calcium is the fat malabsorption inherent in biliopancreatic diversion. It is well known that unabsorbed fatty acids can interfere with calcium absorption. Sophisticated studies of bone metabolism have been performed by two groups after biliopancreatic diversion.[44,45] Remarkably, both reports showed generally normal bone densitometry measurements despite consistently elevated parathyroid hormone levels. Other indicators, however, showed that manifestations of metabolic bone disease (increased bone turnover, decreased cortical thickness) were present in the majority of patients. Neither hypocalcemia nor vitamin D deficiency correlated with other parameters of bone disease. Marceau et al., however, found that hypoalbuminemia correlated with long-term bone loss.[44] Although symptoms of bone disease (pain, fractures) were noted in 10 to 15% of patients, both groups concluded that bone disease was generally manageable and rarely severe after BPD.

I have observed two cases of symptomatic hypocalcemia after distal RYGB. One patient, who was entirely noncompliant with both multivitamin supplements and follow up after a malabsorptive RYGB, developed pathologic rib fractures as a consequence of severe osteoporosis. Although nephrolithiasis secondary to calcium oxalate stones was common after jejunoileal bypass, calcium oxalate stones appear to be infrequent following the current biliopancreatic diversion procedures.

Clinical Consequences/Symptoms

Patients who have biliopancreatic diversion operations are considerably more prone to nutritional problems than are patients who have gastric-restrictive procedures. In addition to symptoms of anemia, patients may develop symptoms and signs of any of the metabolic sequelae known to follow biliopancreatic diversion that are shown in Table 15–4. Virtually all of these signs and symptoms have been recognized in patients who have undergone biliopan-

TABLE 15–4. METABOLIC DEFICIENCY SYNDROMES ASSOCIATED WITH BILIOPANCREATIC DIVERSION		
DEFICIENCY	SYMPTOMS	SIGNS
Vitamin A	Night blindness, xerophthalmia, photophobia, rash (phyrnoderma)	Dry eyes, papular rash
Vitamin D	Muscle cramps, tetany (rare)	Osteomalacia
Vitamin E	Weakness, phlebitis hypercoagulability	Anemia,
Calcium	Bone pain, irritability, numbness/paresthesias, myalgia, diarrhea, tetany	Bone tenderness, fractures, carpopedal spasm
Protein/albumin	Weakness, peripheral and central swelling, hair loss	Edema, anasarca, muscle wasting, alopecia
Liver	Weakness, jaundice, swelling, bleeding, tremor, coma	Jaundice, edema, bleeding, tremor, coma

Note: These deficiencies have been anecdotally reported and are quite rare. Symptoms associated with iron deficiency and anemia, described previously, are far more common after biliopancreatic diversion.

creatic diversion, but full-blown manifestations of these deficiencies are either rare or underreported. Stigmata of protein-calorie malnutrition are more commonly reported than manifestations of either calcium or fat-soluble vitamin deficiency.

Prevention and Treatment of Deficiencies

There is virtually no information on the efficacy of prophylactic vitamin and mineral supplements after biliopancreatic diversion operations. Effective prophylaxis for potential metabolic deficiencies after malabsorptive procedures would likely include a daily multivitamin supplement and daily oral supplements of iron and calcium. Some surgeons provide prophylactic supplements of vitamin A, vitamin D, vitamin B_{12}, and protein after biliopancreatic diversion.

Patients who have biliopancreatic diversion operations should have a variety of blood tests performed at regular intervals including HGB, iron, protein/albumin, calcium, vitamin A, 25-hydroxyvitamin D, and vitamin B_{12}. These micronutrients should be measured every 6 months for the first 2 years and annually thereafter, if there are no ongoing metabolic problems. Patients with evolving or severe nutritional deficiencies should have appropriate blood tests performed every 3 to 6 months, depending on the severity and refractoriness of the problem.

Recognized metabolic deficiencies after biliopancreatic diversion should be treated with appropriate supplements of the deficient micronutrient. Oral supplements of specific vitamins (A, D, B_{12}) are generally effective in correcting these deficiencies. Likewise, oral iron supplements are used initially to treat postoperative iron deficiency. Treatment of iron-deficiency anemia could include parental iron supplementation, transfusion, or surgical revision. Treatment of protein and/or hepatic deficiency would include TPN given either at home or in an inpatient setting. A 4- to 6-week course of TPN will generally reverse both hypoproteinemia and mild hepatic dysfunction in conjunction with improved oral intake.[38,39] However, if oral intake does not improve over a period of a few weeks, further intervention should be considered. Such intervention could include insertion of an enteral feeding tube, lengthening of the common channel, or reversal (takedown) of the biliopancreatic diversion procedure. Surgical revision (takedown versus lengthening of the common channel) should also be considered if TPN does not restore adequate nutrition. Lengthening of the common channel can be expected to correct protein-calorie malnutrition in most cases.[37,39]

CONCLUSION

In conclusion, biliopancreatic diversion generally results in weight loss and weight loss maintenance that is superior to that provided by RYGB. However, this greater weight loss is associated with an increased risk of a variety of metabolic problems. To date, there are no well-controlled clinical studies that compare the long-term risks and benefits of biliopancreatic diversion to those of RYGB.

REFERENCES

1. Miskowiak J, Monore K, Larsen L, Andersen B. Food intake before and after gastroplasty for morbid obesity. *Scand J Gastroenterol* 1985;20:925–928.
2. Naslund I, Jarnmark I, Anderson H. Dietary intake before and after gastric bypass and gastroplasty for morbid obesity in women. *Int J Obes* 1988;12:503–513.
3. Andersen T, Larsen U. Dietary outcome in obese patients treated with a gastroplasty program. *Am J Clin Nutr* 1989;50:1328–1340.
4. MacLean LD, Rhode, BM, Shizgal HM. Nutrition following gastric operations for morbid obesity. *Ann Surg* 1983;198:347–355.
5. Andersen T. Gastroplasty and very-low-calorie diet in the treatment of morbid obesity. *J Med Dent Pharm Sci* 1990;37:359–370.
6. Raymond JL, Schipke CA, Becker JM, et al. Changes in body composition and dietary intake after gastric partitioning for morbid obesity. *Surgery* 1986;99:15–19.
7. Sugerman HJ, Londrey GL, Kellum JM, et al. Weight loss with vertical banded gastroplasty and Roux-en-Y gastric bypass for morbid obesity with selective vs random assignment. *Am J Surg* 1989;157:93–102.
8. Brolin RE, Robertson LB, Kenler HA, Cody RP. Weight loss and dietary intake after vertical banded gastroplasty and Roux-en-Y gastric bypass. *Ann Surg* 1994;220:782–790.
9. Haid RW, Gutman L, Crosy TW. Wernicke-Korsakoff encephalopathy after gastric plication. *JAMA* 1982;247:2566–2567.
10. Brolin RE, Gorman JH, Gorman RC, et al. Are vitamin B_{12} and folate deficiency clinically important after Roux-en-Y gastric bypass? *J Gastrointest Surg* 1998;2:436–442.
11. Halverson JD, Zuckerman GR, Koehler RE, et al. Gastric bypass for morbid obesity: a medical-surgical assessment. *Ann Surg* 1981;194:152–160.
12. Amaral JF, Thompson WR, Caldwell MD, et al. Prospective hematologic evaluation of gastric exclusion surgery for morbid obesity. *Ann Surg* 1985;201:186–193.
13. Brolin RE, Gorman RC, Milgrim LM, Kenler HA. Multivitamin prophylaxis in prevention of post-gastric bypass vitamin and mineral deficiencies. *Int J Obes* 1991;15:661–668.
14. Dosherholmen A, McMahon J, Ripley D. Impaired absorption of egg vitamin B_{12} in post-gastrectomy and achlorhydric patients. *J Lab Clin Med* 1971;78:839–840.
15. Schade SG, Schilling RF. Effect of pepsin on the absorption of food vitamin B_{12} and iron. *Am J Clin Nutr* 1967;20:636–640.
16. Schilling RF, Hardie GH, Gohdes PN. Low vitamin B_{12} levels are common after gastric bypass for obesity. *Clin Res* 1983;31:759A.

17. Mason EE, Munns JR, Kealy GP, et al. Effect of gastric bypass on gastric acid secretion. *Am J Surg* 1976;131:162–168.
18. Halverson JD. Micronutrient deficiencies after gastric bypass for morbid obesity. *Am Surg* 1986;52:594–598.
19. Behrns KE, Smith CD, Sarr MG. Prospective evaluation of gastric acid secretion and cobalamine absorption following gastric bypass for clinically severe obesity. *Dig Dis Sci* 1994;39:315–320.
20. Rhode BM, Shustik, C, Christon NV, MacLean LD. Iron absorption and therapy after gastric bypass. *Obes Surg* 1999;9:17–21.
21. Brolin RE, Gorman JH, Gorman RC, et al. Prophylactic iron supplementation after Roux-en-Y gastric bypass: a prospective, double-blind randomized study. *Arch Surg* 1998;133:740–744.
22. Rosenburg IH. Intestinal absorption of folates. In: Johnson RR, ed. *Physiology of the Gastrointestinal Tract.* New York: Raven Press; 1981:1221–1230.
23. Russel RM, Dhar J, Dutta SK, et al. Influence of intraluminal pH on folate absorption. *Lab Clin Med* 1979;93:438.
24. Kenler HA, Brolin RE, Cody RP. Changes in eating behavior after horizontal gastroplasty and Roux-en-Y gastric bypass. *Am J Clin Nutri* 1990;52:87–97.
25. Avinoah E, Ovnat A, Charuzi I. Nutritional status seven years after Roux-en-Y gastric bypass surgery. *Surgery* 1992;111:137–142.
26. Updegraffe TA, Neufeld NJ. Protein, iron and folate status of patients prior to and following surgery for morbid obesity. *J Am Diet Assoc* 1981;6:135–139.
27. Crowley LV, Seay J, Mullin G. Late effects of gastric bypass for obesity. *Am J Gastroenterol* 1984;79:850–860.
28. Flancbaum LF, Choban PS, Bradley L, et al. Effect of Roux-en-Y gastric bypass for clinically severe obesity on resting energy expenditure. *Surgery* 1997; 122:943–949.
29. Brolin RE, Gorman JH, Gorman RC, et al. Are vitamin B_{12} and folate deficiency clinically important after Roux-en-Y gastric bypass? *J Gastrointest Surg* 1998; 2:436–442.
30. Chaves LCL, Faintuch J, Kahwage S, Alenear FA. A cluster of polyneuropathy and Wernicke-Korsakoff syndrome in a bariatric unit. *Obes Surg* 2002;12:438–324.
31. Juhasz-Pocsine K, Archer RL, Rudnicki SA, et al. Retrospective review of neurological complications associated with surgical treatment of morbid obesity. *Neurology* 2002;58(Suppl):A247–A248.
32. Mallory GN, Macgregor AMC. Folate status following gastric bypass surgery (the great folate mystery). *Obes Surg* 1991;1:69–72.
33. Rhode BM, Arseneau P, Cooper BA, et al. Vitamin B_{12} deficiency after gastric surgery for obesity. *Am J Clin Nutr* 1996;63:103–109.
34. Grant JP, ed. *Handbook of Total Parenteral Nutrition.* Philadelphia: WB Saunders; 1980:185.
35. Brolin RE, Leung M. Survey of vitamin and mineral supplementation after gastric bypass and biliopancreatic diversion for morbid obesity. *Obes Surg* 1999; 9:150–154.
36. Scopinaro N, Gianetta E, Friedman D, et al. Evolution of biliopancreatic bypass. *Clin Nutr* 1985;5(Suppl):137–146.
37. Marceau P, Biron S, Bourgue RA, et al. Biliopancreatic diversion with a new type of gastrectomy. *Obes Surg* 1993;3:29–35.
38. Brolin RJ, LaMarca LB, Kenler HA, Cody RP. Malabsorptive gastric bypass in patients with superobesity. *J Gastrointest Surg* 2002;6:195–205.
39. Sugerman JH, Kellum JM, DeMaria EJ. Conversion of proximal to distal gastric

bypass for failed gastric bypass for superobesity. *J Gastrointest Surg* 1997; 1:517–525.

40. Skroubei G, Sakellarolpoulos G, Kanstantinos P, et al. Comparison of nutritional deficiencies after Roux-en-Y gastric bypass and after biliopancreatic diversion with Roux-en-Y gastric bypass. *Obes Surg* 2002;12:551–558.

41. Marceau P, Biron S, Hould FS, et al. Liver pathology and the metabolic syndrome X in severe obesity. *J Clin Endocrinol Metab* 1999;84:1513–1517.

42. Gianetta E, Friedman D, Adami GF, et al. Etiological factors of protein malnutrition after biliopancreatic diversion. *Gastroenterol Clin North Am* 1982;16:503–504.

43. Lagace M, Marceau P, Marceau S, et al. Biliopancreatic diversion with a new type of gastrectomy: some previous conclusions revisited. *Obes Surg* 1995;5:411–418.

44. Marceau P, Biron S, Lebel S et al. Does bone change after biliopancreatic diversion? *J Gastrointest Surg* 2002;6:690–698.

45. Compston JE, Vedi S, Gianetta E, et al. Bone histomorphometry and vitamin D status in patients with biliopancreatic bypass. *Gastroenterology* 1984;87:350–356.

REOPERATIVE OBESITY SURGERY

GEORGE COWAN, JR. / M. LLOYD HILER / LOUIS F. MARTIN

EVALUATION

Morbidly obese patients present with many different problems following bariatric surgery. Chapter 14 outlines how most acute postoperative complications present and how they need to be approached. This chapter is devoted to the more long-term set of problems that people sometimes present with to their original surgeons, but probably equally as often to an unfamiliar surgeon because the patient may believe the first surgeon did not provide the success they were initially seeking. A systematic, informed approach to evaluation and appropriate management of the reoperative bariatric surgery patient is essential to try to identify why the patient thinks the initial procedure failed and what the patient expects from revisional surgery. This chapter addresses this need by presenting reoperative bariatric surgical indications, workup, differential diagnosis, operative considerations, procedures, and techniques in a systematic fashion. It draws upon the authors' combined experiences of more than 1000 reoperative bariatric surgeries. Every bariatric surgeon, and many general surgeons with little bariatric surgical experience, will be asked to evaluate patients who present with problems that appear to be associated with prior bariatric surgery. These presentations can, on the surface, appear anywhere from straightforward to frustrating and baffling. To help address these problems, a careful, systematic, workup is needed based on whether the patient is complaining of (1) excessive weight loss, nutritional deficiencies, or inadequate energy; (2) pain; (3) inadequate weight loss; or (4) other symptoms or problems which may be associated with prior bariatric surgery.

Each patient's presentation should be managed as a unique case, employing the experience-derived guidelines, options, precautions, and differential diagnoses presented in this chapter. The evaluation and treatment of unsuccessful bariatric surgery patients is often quite exasperating. The operations to treat their problems have at least double the mortality and morbidity rates of those associated with original bariatric procedures (this is our opinion rather than an evidence-based fact), and it is often very difficult to obtain insurance approval to provide the appropriate procedures and to obtain adequate reimbursement for your time and the added malpractice risk you accept by becoming involved, especially when it was someone else's patient originally.

The patients themselves may have been initially noncompliant or the surgeons may have provided little aftercare or assistance to the patients as they tried to make the behavior modifications necessary for bariatric procedures be successful long term. Some of these patients resist completing another psychosocial evaluation if they underwent even such a brief evaluation before their first procedure. The surgeons who decide to interact with such patients have to have an excellent, experienced multidisciplinary team supporting them to be successful. Generally, bariatric surgeons just starting this specialized type of practice should refer these patients (unless it is your patient) to the most experienced bariatric surgeon in your region. It is also very difficult for general surgeons without extensive experience with bariatric patients, at least during their residency or in prior practice years, to be able to successfully diagnose and treat all but the most straightforward cases of stricture or obstruction. We suggest, for the best outcome for the patient and the piece of mind of the nonbariatric specialist, that these patients be referred, even if the patient is reluctant to travel.

Potential reoperative bariatric surgery candidates are those patients who have had bariatric surgery at least 90 days previously and who experience significant chronic, subacute, or acute problems that appear related to this surgery. Their prior bariatric surgery may consist of a wide variety of restrictive, malabsorptive, restrictive plus malabsorptive, open or laparoscopic procedures. Additional patient variables include prior complications leading to additional procedures, varying body mass indices (BMI = kg/m^2), weight loss/gain/regain, gender, age, race, comorbidities, dietary habits, medications, presenting complaints, national origin, compliance, and psychosocial status.

Even with our experience with more than 1000 reoperative bariatric surgery patients, there are too few individuals with sufficiently matching variables among all these possibilities to establish data-based protocols. The suggestions in this chapter are consensus opinions from ourselves and multiple other senior bariatric patients. We need to develop the apparatus to conduct randomized controlled trials involving 10 to 100 busy bariatric practices so that we can compare different treatments, allowing us or others to produce the data necessary to satisfy the tenets of evidence-based medicine so that this information will be available for everyone. We hope that the recent announcement by the National Institutes of Health requesting applications to establish multiple Centers of Excellence in Bariatric Surgical Research and a unique national database center will provide the leadership to organize and oversee multicenter trials where solutions to these rarer reoperative problems can be proposed and tested. Outcome evaluation for reoperative bariatric problems are often extremely difficult because it is often necessary to "fix" at least two or more apparent problems at one time. For instance, while repairing a gastrogastric fistula, we may additionally perform a ventral, incisional herniorrhaphy, and an extensive enterolysis. Therefore, we cannot claim with any validity which one, if not all, of the different operative procedures solved, worsened, or improved any of the patient's problems.

Presenting Problems and Indications

Reoperative bariatric surgery may be indicated when nonsurgical management of significant problems (Table 16–1) fails to provide adequate relief. This relies upon a sufficiently thorough prior workup to justify and guide possible operative therapies.

WORKUP

A detailed history and physical examination, in conjunction with basic studies (Table 16–2), is essential for documentation and to direct further workup as required. While the basic workups are similar to those of primary bariatric surgery, additional gastrointestinal tract (GI), nutritional, and other evaluations are important. Table 16–3 lists some additional studies that might be undertaken. Also of note, we have found a surprisingly large number of reoperative candidates with positive alcohol–drug screens; we strongly recommend global screening.

When available, prior operative note(s) are valuable. Well-performed upper GI studies provide useful "road maps," augmenting endoscopic study. When referring a bariatric surgery patient to a radiologist or an endoscopist, it is essential to warn them what the altered anatomy should look like and what you expect to be wrong. Ideally, it is helpful to be present for these diagnostic studies.

Differential Diagnostic Considerations

Jumping to immediate diagnostic conclusions from "obvious" presentations can be dangerous. To avoid this error, carefully ponder all differential diagnostic possibilities and follow relevant leads with appropriate, detailed, "detective work." When in doubt, work-it-up further. The following differential diagnostic possibilities and suggestions are offered as a start.

EXCESSIVE WEIGHT LOSS, NUTRITIONAL DEFICIENCIES, OR INADEQUATE ENERGY

The bariatric patients' most dramatic weight loss will occur in their first 3 to 4 postoperative months, especially in the malabsorptive or malabsorptive/re-

TABLE 16-1. PRESENTING PROBLEMS FOLLOWING EARLIER BARIATRIC SURGERY

EXCESSIVE WEIGHT LOSS, NUTRITIONAL DEFICIENCIES, OR INADEQUATE ENERGY

Nausea
Vomiting
Dysphagia
Pain in the abdomen, chest, flank, other location
Hyperesthesia
Hyperactive bowel sounds
Abdominal distention
Shifting dullness
Foam regurgitation
Excessive nasal/sinus drainage
Dumping syndrome
Obstipation
Occult blood positive stool
Hematochezia
Hematemesis
Cirrhosis
Halitosis
Vitamin deficiences
Low protein, albumin, prealbumin, or ferritin levels
Low trace element(s)
Salt(s)
Essential fatty acids
Cheilosis
Red tongue
Pallor
Anemia
Dysosmia
Dysgeusia
Night blindness
Alopecia
Poor healing wound(s)
Lower extremity edema
Significant change in vital signs
Wrong eating habits

INADEQUATE WEIGHT LOSS

Vomiting
Pain in the abdomen, chest, flank, other location
Abdominal distention
Dumping syndrome
Obstipation
Hepatomegaly
Hepatosteatosis
Wrong eating habits

EVALUATION OF PAIN AFTER BARIATRIC PROCEDURES

Nausea
Vomiting
Dysphagia
Pain in the abdomen, chest, flank, other location
Megacolon
Occult blood-positive stool
Hematochezia
Hematemesis
Hepatomegaly
Halitosis
Biliary colic
Wrong eating habits

OTHER SYMPTOMS ASSUMED TO BE SECONDARY TO A PRIOR BARIATRIC OPERATION BY PATIENTS OR PHYSICIANS

Gastrointestinal contents draining through abdominal wall
Jaundice
Biliary colic
Ventral hernia (including giant hernia)
Panniculitis, cellulitis, intertrigo
Excessive flatus and related odors
Significant change in vital signs
Disability
Problems with activities of daily living
Rash(es)
Bone, muscle, or joint pain
Faintness
Seizures
Dizziness with movement
Wrong eating habits
Shortness of breath
Possible psychiatric problems including:
  Weakness
  Tiredness
  Insomnia
  Irritability
  Poor self-esteem
  Inability to cope
  Confusion
  Excessive crying
  Mood swings
  Poor memory
  Poor compliance
  "Fantastic" history

TABLE 16-2. BASIC WORK UP FOR MOST REOPERATIVE BARIATRIC SURGICAL CANDIDATES

Detailed history and physical examination

Psychological screening including a Beck Depression Index and an interview with a psychologist/psychiatrist to look for psychosis, schizophrenia, drug or alcohol addiction, personality disorders (i.e., borderline and/or severe depression)

Nutritional evaluation

Pulmonary function tests if body mass index is greater than 35 kg/m^2 or if symptoms suggest these tests are necessary

Electrocardiogram, echocardiogram, stress test, and cardiologist consultation

Urinalysis

Complete blood cell count

Hemoglobin A$_{1c}$; electrolytes, including Mg, Ca, K, and renal function testing

Fasting lipid profile

Ferritin, prealbumin, total iron-binding capacity

Vitamins A, D, B$_{12}$

Folate

Zinc

Amylase, lipase

Thyroid function tests

Prothrombin time, advance partial thromboplastin time, and possible bleeding time

Posteroanterior and lateral chest radiographers

Drug and alcohol screen witnessed

Pregnancy test (females in fertile years)

Stool occult blood

Possible upper GI endoscopy (gastric and enteric biopsies)

Upper GI barium series with possible small bowel follow through (if this is abnormal, then a computed axial tomographic (CAT) scan of the abdomen and pelvis may be necessary)

Bone densitometry

TABLE 16-3. ADDITIONAL STUDIES THAT MIGHT BE UNDERTAKEN IF NEEDED

Specialist consultations as the basic workup indicates

Radioisotope liquid, solid-phase gastric emptying, and intestinal transit time studies

CAT scan of abdomen and pelvis, with contrast

CAT scan of head

Fistulogram

Fever of unknown origin workup

Culture and antibiotic sensitivities of wound drainage

Stool studies

Clostridium difficile endotoxin assay of stool

Contrast enema

Colonoscopy

Serum cortisol (A.M. and P.M.)

2-Hour oral glucose tolerance test

Parathyroid hormone level

Other studies as indicated by presentation

strictive operations that rearrange the GI tract. These operations rearrange the GI tract, interrupting the natural pacemaker functions of the stomach (see Chapter 13) and the chain of normal peristalsis that propels the food and associated GI tract secretions from the stomach to the duodenum to the jejunum. The older the patients, the longer it takes for their GI tract to adjust to the rerouting that has occurred and the longer they will complain about swallowing difficulties (even if they have just had a band externally wrapped around their stomach or vertical-banded gastroplasty; see Chapter 10), nausea, bloating, difficulty meeting dietary goals for protein intake, and the like. The absolute amount of weight loss after a bariatric procedure is directly related to the patients initial BMI, because the patients with the highest BMIs will lose the most absolute weight in the first 4 postoperative months, but because they are much more obese at baseline, they will lose the least percentage of their excess body weight (%EBW).[1] Therefore, in addition to following absolute weight loss per month, the surgeon also needs to follow the %EBW lost or, if it is easier to calculate, use the percentage of initial body weight lost (%IBWL), the standard suggested by the Institute of Medicine because one does not have to refer to tables that list ideal body weights or subtract a reference weight from actual weight.

People with BMIs greater than 55 or 60 will usually lose 11.3 kg (25 lb) to 13.6 kg (30 lb) the first month and 9.1+ kg (20+ lb) per month for the next 2 to 3 months. Therefore, they may lose 36.3 kg (80 lb) in the first 3 to 4 months and be well above the average weight loss expected for someone with a lower BMI. However, if someone with a BMI between 35 and 40 lost 36.3 kg (80 lb) in 3 to 4 months, this would be excessive.

To help yourself and the patient know what they should be losing, the dietician should meet with the patient at each visit within the first 6 postoperative months and the patients should bring in a 24-hour list of all food and beverages consumed; or the dietician should go through a 24-hour recall of the foods consumed as part of their interaction. Both calories and grams of protein intake should be estimated and recorded. Patients with initial BMIs of less than 50 kg/m^2 can usually maintain muscle mass by consuming 60 to 70 g of protein per day. Patients with BMI >60 to 70 kg/m^2, however, will need more than 100 g of protein per day. Caloric intake should be between 1000 and 1500 kcal.

When patients are unable to consume adequate amounts of protein and calories, they will lose too much weight and will usually lose a disproportionately high amount of their muscle mass, making them feel weak. They will begin to develop nutritional deficiencies (see also Chapter 15). The reasons that patients develop these problems are multifactorial, but need to be addressed aggressively.

If it is not just poor peristalsis as a consequence of age or diabetes, medications that can improve GI tract motility include Reglan (metoclopramide hydrochloride) and erythromycin. Before starting these types of medications, an upper GI series should be completed to document a slow transit time and to eliminate the possibility that the poor intake is the result of a stricture at the gastrojejunostomy, or at the site of a gastric band placement, or a bowel obstruction.

Extensive workup of these symptoms may not result in a definitive diagnosis. During earlier nutritional work, we developed a regimen that worked well for undernourished patients who lacked an appetite, were nauseated, or were intermittently nauseated for no apparent reason. Older patients (older than age 50 years) may not redevelop anything approaching normal peristalsis for 4 to 6 months after bariatric operations that rearrange the intestinal tract. Even swallowing liquids is much harder than it was preoperatively, and occasionally patients become very depressed. They need to be constantly reassured that it will get better within 6 months and that eating will become enjoyable again. An antidepressant may be necessary for 6 months. In addition, these three prescriptions, each given po tid, are often helpful: zinc sulfate 220 mg, vitamin B_6 50 mg, and Periactin (cyproheptadine hydrochloride) 2 mg. Sometimes nausea develops because of intermittent hypoglycemia. Eating frequent meals of small portions instead of three normal-size meals or, in more extreme instances, enteral feeding through a gastrostomy or nasogastric tube often resolves the symptoms without need for chronic antinauseants. Excessive sinusitis secretions can drain into the gastric pouch and cause these symptoms, as can hypersalivation and other throat and nasal disorders. Psychiatric etiology of these problems is a diagnosis of exclusion.

Dumping Syndrome

Dumping occurs in approximately 50% of postoperative primary bariatric surgery patients who have operations that exclude the pylorus from the food limb of malabsorptive procedures. Contrary to earlier belief, the presence or absence of dumping has not been found to correlate with long-term weight loss results.[2] Dumping does cause abdominal pain and cramping, diarrhea, tachycardia (sometimes with palpitations), sweating, headaches, fatigue, and general malaise. Patients who initiate dumping by eating concentrated sweets or fats need to have the cause-and-effect relationship of their behavior pointed out to them. Occasionally, it occurs because they do not read food and medication labels and ingest sauces or soups designed for children that contain sugars or medications that contain fructose or sucrose. It is important to stop these behaviors because the gastrointestinal tract often begins to tolerate higher sugar solutions without dumping as it adjusts. This adjustment will decrease weight loss. Remedial surgery is rarely required if adequate instruction is provided to the patient and there are no psychological barriers to the patient wanting to lose weight. However, on rare occasion, remedial surgery is required.

CONTROLLING DUMPING

Remedial surgery was required on five patients referred to us at Memphis with uncontrollable dumping following gastric bypass Roux-en-Y. In each case, we divided and reanastomosed the two ends of a 90-cm (35.4-inch) segment of the common limb in situ. We also divided the intestinal mesentery down to its root at both intestinal division points. This appeared to effectively interrupt intestinal hyperperistalsis sufficiently to control each patient's dumping.

Stomal Obstructions

Overfilling of an adjustable band, or a nonadjustable band, or a vertical-banded gastroplasty (VBG) that is too tight (usually a stoma opening less than the width of a pencil) will result in poor intake and can even lead to esophageal dilation where peristalsis in the esophagus "gives up" because the esophagus is not strong enough to push food through the restriction (see Chapter 14).[1] Usually at 5 to 8 weeks, the gastrojejunostomies that have been created for gastric bypass or biliopancreatic diversions (or bypasses) have healed and should be between 12 and 15 mm (0.5 and 0.6 inches) in diameter. In patients where healing is too aggressive, the stomach may try to seal itself off and the diameter of the stoma may progressively decrease to 10 mm (0.4 inches) or 8 mm (0.3 inches) or 6 mm (0.2 inches) or even 3 mm (0.1 inches) to 4 mm (0.2 inches) in diameter. An opening of <6 mm (0.2 inches) usually restricts the patient to liquids or soft foods such as yogurt or creamed soups. An opening of less than 4 mm (0.2 inches) will make it hard to even swallow liquids. Usually these strictures can be stretched to the desired stoma diameter of 12 to 15 mm (0.5 to 0.6 inches) endoscopically by using a pyloric channel balloon of 16 or 18 mm (0.6 or 0.7 inches). The balloon should be inflated to a PSI (pounds per square inch) >60 to 65 and held at that for 2 to 3 minutes. If this does not reopen the stoma to 12 to 15 mm (0.5 to 0.6 inches), the balloon dilation can be repeated several times over days or weeks. The goal is to be able to push the endoscope [that usually has a 12- to 13-mm (0.5-inch) diameter] through the stoma into the jejunum or Roux limb. If this cannot be done at the initial endoscopy, the patient should be brought back daily until it can be accomplished. If the patient presents early enough, approximately 50% of patients will need only one dilation. Another 25% will need two to three dilations to maintain this diameter. The other 25% will need more than three dilations, which should usually be done weekly or bimonthly until the stoma remains open. Somewhere around 8 to 12 dilations means that this technique is not working and a revision of the anastomosis, VBG, or nonadjustable band is necessary.

MARGINAL ULCERATION

Marginal ulceration alone, or in conjunction with gastroenteric stomal stenosis, occurred in approximately 10% of our earlier patients at Memphis when gastric pouches for gastric bypasses were approximately 30 mL or larger, because at that size, the pouch always contained acid-secreting cells and the jejunum is not designed to withstand an acid milieu without ulceration. Since reducing gastric pouch size to 15 to 20 mL, marginal ulceration and stenosis now occur in only 1.5 to 2% of patients because the pouches do not contain acid-producing cells. A history of chronically regurgitating "lots of foam" is stomal stenosis until proven otherwise, but pain with eating or vomiting blood or having blood pass per rectum is most often marginal ulceration and can be diagnosed by upper endoscopy or an upper GI barium series.

GASTRIC BAND EROSION

Nonadjustable or adjustable gastric band erosion occurs in 1% or fewer patients. It can be caused by chronic ingestion of nonsteroidal antiinflammatory drugs (NSAIDs), inflammation, ischemia, and other causes that have not yet been identified. The band must be removed, which can occur by spontaneous passage, endoscopic maneuvers, or surgery. At laparotomy, in order to reduce risk of leakage, we prefer to remove eroded bands from inside the gastric pouch via a longitudinal enterotomy and transverse closure just distal to the gastroenterostomy stoma. When nonadjustable bands are made of Marlex mesh, Dacron, or Gore-Tex, removal often requires resection, which can often be performed laparoscopically with the underlying gastric wall, making it easier to reconnect the patient by using a Roux-en-Y gastrojejunostomy than it is to mobilize the stomach to perform a gastrojejunostomy. Noneroded stenotic nonadjustable bands may be divided or replaced as deemed appropriate. Usually, band erosion does not produce peritonitis because the stomach and other overlying tissues surround and cover the band in a tissue capsule so the band erodes internally into the stomach, eliminating its effectiveness but not causing a life-threatening situation.

GASTRIC POUCH BEZOAR

Patients with a gastric pouch bezoar usually present with a history of acute dysphagia and "bringing up white foam." This often results from their having not learned or not been instructed to take small bites, chew all food until it is the consistency of toothpaste, and to eat slowly. It sometimes occurs in edentulous patients or those with poorly fitting dentures. If slow sipping of Adolf's meat tenderizer, 0.5 teaspoon in 1 glass of water, does not dissolve the bezoar, its removal via upper GI endoscopy is required, sometimes together with stomal stenosis dilatation.

GASTRIC BAND ANGULATION

With massive weight loss, the previously enlarged liver may shift craniad, placing traction upon any adhesions between it and an existing nonadjustable or adjustable gastric band. This may result in band angulation or displacement, which causes some degree of pouch obstruction. It is relieved with band removal, replacement, or enterolysis. We prophylactically interpose omentum between the gastric pouch, the band, and the liver at the time of band replacement. This also aids reoperative dissection.

ZENKER-LIKE GASTRIC DIVERTICULUM, SLIPPAGE OF THE BAND, OR POUCH DILATION

The dynamically motile stomach may migrate relative to the gastric band, thereby enlarging the pouch, causing the more distal stomach to herniate up into the band from below, beside the tube of stomach initially compressed by the band, causing a partial or complete stomal obstruction by having too much stomach tissue within the confines of the band and sometimes producing a

Zenker-like diverticulum hanging over the band.[1] Band replacement or removal is necessary, potentially with conversion to a different bariatric procedure.

GASTROENTERIC AXIAL TORSION

Another relatively unusual cause of stenosis is gastric pouch–enteric torsion around its longitudinal axis. Symptoms similar to pouch angulation usually occur soon after surgery. Detorsion often occurs from endoscopic air insufflation allowing the scope to pass through the previously twisted and obstructed site without any apparent resistance. Torsion reoccurs following the exam. It requires surgery with reanastomosis or detorsion plus suturing the untwisted segments securely to surrounding tissue.

SWITCHED INTESTINAL LIMBS

Intractable nausea, vomiting, and dysphagia may also occur following "switched limbs" of the small intestine during a gastric bypass or, more rarely, a biliopancreatic bypass. After dividing the small intestine distal to the ligament of Treitz, the proximal end of the divided intestine may be anastomosed to the gastric pouch instead of being adjoined to the end-to-side enteroenterostomy. This produces a "Roux-en-O" with the esophagus, the proximal pouch, the distal stomach, and the duodenum, with part of the proximal jejunum connected together without any connection to the distal jejunum, ileum, or colon. The remaining distal, intestinal end may then be anastomosed to the proximal jejunum at some point distal to the gastroenterostomy to then allow the Roux-en-O a connection to the distal bowel and anus. The alimentary limb thus formed from the stoma to the enteroenterostomy is a reversed, antiperistaltic limb. Patients will complain of severe nausea, vomiting, and dysphagia. However, when this limb is relatively short, approximately 45.7 cm (18 inches) in length, some patients have been able to ingest some food but characteristically lose excessive weight because of their continuing symptoms. Radiographic studies may show "sluggish" passage of contrast into the distal intestine without any apparent stenosis or other reason for the delay. Radioisotope-tagged liquid- and solid-phase studies document pathologically delayed gastric emptying, suggesting the need for exploration and probable reoperative bariatric surgery where it can be difficult until all adhesions are removed to understand the initial surgeon's error.

Another variety of switched intestinal limbs is the so-called acute Roux-en-O in which the initial mistake is made, but this closed loop obstruction is given no outlet to the distal bowel because the confused surgeon creates a jejunojejunostomy exclusively in the distal jejunum by connecting different parts of it to itself. The closed-loop obstruction of this Roux-en-O is immediately diagnosed by the radiologist on the postoperative films because the contrast all pools in the distal stomach or the patient continuously vomits.

BILIARY REFLUX GASTRITIS

Short alimentary limbs, less than 75-cm- (29.5-inch) long Roux limbs, may permit bile reflux into the gastric pouch or more proximally, causing intractable pain, nausea, vomiting, sometimes bilious, and dysphagia. Gastric or esophageal bile staining may be seen at endoscopy as well as an unusually inflamed, sometimes velvet colored, edematous, pouch and distal esophagus. The diagnosis of biliary reflux gastritis relies upon clinical and endoscopic documentation because there is no definitive histopathologic appearance.

Small intestinal length is notoriously difficult to accurately measure because the bowel may contract one-half of its length with handling. Therefore, we use a 90-cm (35.4-inch) alimentary limb so that, even in the worst-case scenario, the gastroenterostomy stoma remains at least 45 cm (17.7 inches) from the enteroenterostomy. This length is usually sufficient to prevent bile reflux into the gastric pouch.

GASTROGASTRIC FISTULAE

The body's marvelous homeostatic abilities sometimes frustrate gastric division when several staple cartridges are fired to divide the stomach to form a gastric bypass, but the stomach is not physically divided so that permanent scars are formed, allowing disruption in these staple lines to produce gastrogastric fistulae. We have occasionally seen acute staple line disruption heralded by significant gastrointestinal bleeding, but, more usually, the patient reports regaining the ability to "eat anything I want" accompanied by significant weight regain. Some small fistulae, however, may be asymptomatic and discovered during contrast upper gastrointestinal radiography; here, correction may be deferred. When the stomach is not physically divided, any significant wounds, pregnancies, episodes of malnutrition, or cancers can cause reabsorption of protein from the staple line scar leading to disruption.

OTHER FISTULAE

Other fistulae may result from a gastric or intestinal leak, in various combinations. In the superobese [BMI >60 kg/m^2 or weight >226.8 kg (500 lb)] that often require open procedures if a gastric bypass or biliopancreatic diversion (BPD) are the preferred procedure by the surgeon and the patient. Enterocolonic fistula have occurred twice in one author's experience (LFM). These patients had very little free intraabdominal space and the abdominal fascial closure was difficult because it was hard to get the rectus fascia reapproximated. Because postoperative swelling does not peak for 36 to 48 hours, these patients required mechanical ventilation with positive end-expiratory pressure to maintain adequate intraarterial oxygen pressures. On the fourth postoperative day, these patients began leaking liquid stool through their midline wounds. In each case, the sutures used to close the fascia had sawed through a small area [less than 13 mm (0.5 inches) in each case] of the colon. Both were treated by creating a colostomy, resectioning the damaged area of colon, and leaving the blind distal end of the colon attached to the lateral internal oblique fascia marked by multiple metal clips on the colon and fascia, and the insertion of a 35.6-cm × 20.3-cm (14-inch × 8-inch) sheet of polypropylene mesh to increase the size of the abdominal cavity. Both did well, but the woman chose to have the colostomy closed and the mesh removed; the man wanted no additional surgery.

Because of pressure differentials, a gastrocolic fistula cannot be reliably ruled out by upper gastrointestinal contrast radiography; often, it may only be demonstrated with a barium contrast enema. This type of fistula is usually caused by intraoperative injury to both the colon and the stomach leading to inflammation and adhesions, and then a fistula will develop, especially if there is delayed opening of the pylorus, usually because of vagus nerve injury with a tight pylorus that infrequently reflexes. Delay in reoperation is often advisable to allow maturing of adhesions, as well as to compensate massive weight loss by nutritional supplementation including, total parenteral nutrition or enteric feeding, depending on the patient's nutritional status.

Massive, difficult-to-control fistula losses may demand an earlier reoperation. If mucosa is visible at or near the skin level, the fistula should not be expected to close spontaneously. Likewise, foreign materials including bands and excessive suture material, seen on upper GI endoscopy, will prevent or delay fistula closure. Drains that are adjacent to or overlapping the bowel or stomach from which the fistula arises internally can help the formation of a controlled enteral cutaneous fistula that will close as the drain is slowly removed. Occasionally, a hard drain may be a continuing source of injury. Contrast studies, including fistulograms, are often helpful. Persistent fistulae sometimes have closed following smaller diameter drain replacement by interventional radiology, and then drain removal in stages. If a drain is suspected of causing an injury, it should be removed, but this can lead to peritonitis.

THAL-TYPE PATCHES

On occasion, the surgeon may become concerned about the integrity of a gastric pouch, suture or staple line during a gastric bypass where tension on the anastomosis might contribute to the creation of a leak or fistula in the first few postoperative days. To buttress it, we have rotated the native (bypassed) stomach sufficiently to place a tension-free row of interrupted no. 3–0 silk sutures between the seromuscularis of the posterior distal stomach wall and the proximal pouch's wall posterior to the staple or suture line. We then complete encirclement of the site with an anterior row of sutures between the two stomach segments, tying them when completed.

This variation of a Thal patch has also successfully functioned as a buttress over closure of a fistula or acute gastric leak. It is important to avoid tension between the structures and not use the gastrostomy tube for enteral feeding since the distended native stomach may damage the repair.

PROXIMAL JEJUNAL DIVERTICULA RESECTED AND AS REINFORCEMENT PATCHES

The end-to-side anastomosis of gastric pouch to small intestine may leave a stapled end of small intestine protruding laterally. With time, the intestine may enlarge and become dependent, overlapping the gastroenterostomy like a Zenker diverticulum. The patient may fill this blind pouch until they get abdominal pain and then suddenly vomit. This may also be accompanied by intermittent pain, then nausea, without vomiting but with the development of dysphagia. At endoscopy, the scope may advance directly into the diverticulum or blind, dilated end of the proximal part of the Roux limb, rather than pass down the Roux limb after the gastroenterostomy stoma. Upper GI radiography may show the diverticulum filled with contrast material or food that may not readily empty. To minimize this occurrence during primary bariatric surgery, we advance the jejunum craniad to the anastomosis and suture it with three no. 3–0 silks to the lateral distal half of the gastric pouch.

When a jejunal diverticulum at the stoma is present, we have either resected it or tacked it to the lateral aspect of the gastric pouch, sometimes surrounding a stapled and divided gastrogastric fistula as a reinforcement. It is sometimes a convenient alternative to the Thal-type gastric patch.

PROXIMAL JEJUNAL ADVANCEMENT AS A STOMAL PATCH

About 14 years ago, in an attempt to control the gastroenterostomy outlet diameter in a series of our Memphis patients, we advanced the jejunum circumferentially up across the distal gastric pouch over a 34-French bougie, holding the intestine in place with interrupted no. 3–0 silk sutures, as a "jejunal flange." Two years later, there was no significant weight loss difference between these 50 jejunal flange patients and 50 controls.

During this time, however, we experienced a few instances in which sutures tore out of the gastroenterostomy during surgery or our postgenerative GI contract study the next day demonstrated a leak at anastomosis. After repairing the problem sites with no. 3–0 sutures, we found that the jejunal advancement adequately reinforced the closures and there was no subsequent leakage. We then successfully adapted this technique to reoperative patients by advancing a tension-free fold of jejunum over any questionable area and securing it in place with interrupted no. 3–0 silk Lembert or horizontal mattress sutures.

Short-Bowel Syndrome

During the early stages following gastric bypass surgery, the weight-loss curve resembles that of some forms of short-bowel syndrome (SBS) created by vascular disasters or by inflammatory conditions like Crohn disease. When the weight-loss curve from a bariatric surgical patient becomes flat, usually at an acceptable weight of 50 to 75% EBW lost, the SBS is "cured" with the formerly morbidly obese patient able to ingest and absorb sufficient nutrition to sustain the lower weight level.

However, a minority of patients are unable to absorb sufficient nutrients enterally to sustain themselves. In addition to the possibility of excessively short alimentary and/or common limbs (Figure 16–1), this may be due to preexisting, but occult, celiac sprue, sprue-like conditions or lactose intolerance. Correction of nutritional and fluid abnormalities with enteral or parenteral feeding, special dietary regimens to treat lactose intolerance, oral or enteric pancreatic extract to help absorption of fats, atropine, Metamucil, or cholestyramine may be sufficient to allow patients who have lost excessive weight or developed low energy levels to recover.

Also a workup for *Clostridium difficile* or other alimentary tract infection, should be completed. Antimicrobial treatment with oral Flagyl (metronidazole)

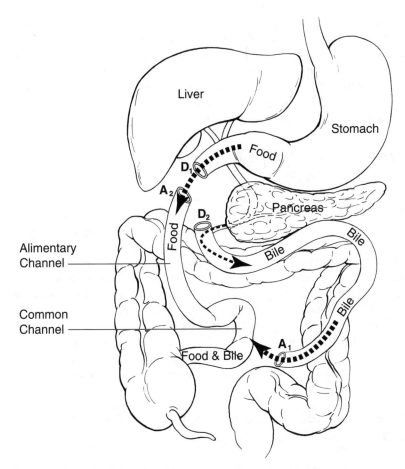

FIGURE 16–1 A malabsorption operation is created by rearranging the small bowel (connecting D_1 to A_2) using the distal segment for food (alimentary or enteral limb), and the proximal segment only as a conduit for bile and pancreatic juice (biliopancreatic limb connecting A_1 to the terminal ileum and closing off the proximal segment D_2 as a "blind" proximal end) to be connected further down for food and bile to mix (common channel). The level at which the division between A_1 and A_2 is made will determine the length of intestine for food absorption, and the site at which the distal end, A_1, will be connected to the terminal ileus will determine the role given to bile in the digestive process.

or vancomycin may be required. We have also seen some severe cases of diarrhea corrected by parenteral correction of vitamin D deficiency. Vitamin A deficiency may also be accompanied by alimentary tract problems. Finally, once all other avenues have been explored, there will be a group of patients who become malnourished with low prealbumin, albumin, and total protein levels; who will usually have anemia and possibly some vitamin deficiencies even though they are following their surgeon's instructions, taking vitamins, and consuming more than 100 g of protein a day; and who develop peripheral edema, lethargy, and symptoms associated with vitamin deficiencies. Usually, these patients have had a distal gastric bypass or one form of the biliopancreatic diversions or duodenal switches, but it can occur even after a gastric bypass. These patients need additional length in their common channel so that they can absorb more food and nutrients. The amount of length that should be added depends on how long the common channel is when the malnutrition occurs. Usually, the addition of 100 to 200 cm (39.4 to 78.7 inches) is sufficient.

EVALUATION OF PAIN AFTER BARIATRIC PROCEDURES

Most evaluations for chronic abdominal pain that occur in bariatric patients at least 3 months after surgery are associated with excessive weight loss and the problems discussed above should be reviewed. There are also acute presentations of abdominal pain after the first 3 months, which are often associated with the development of a small-bowel obstruction, the formation of gallstones, or a late disruption of an anastomosis that might be precipitated by endoscopy with balloon dilation of a stricture at a gastrojejunostomy. Many of these issues are discussed in Chapter 14. Often, unusual forms of small-bowel obstruction can occur that will be missed by a radiologist if insufficient clinical information is provided so that the radiologist does not take a personal interest in watching fluoroscopy as barium transverses bariatric procedures.

Excess, Coiled Alimentary Limb Craniad to Mesocolon

The alimentary limb ordinarily follows a short course from the gastrointestinal stoma of a gastric bypass or a BPD through the opening made in the transverse mesocolon. However, excess alimentary limb may remain coiled craniad to the mesocolon following primary surgery if a retrocolic approach is used. Excessive lengths of the nonanchored limb can also migrate craniad to the mesocolic opening and coil upon itself. Regardless of the mechanism, this condition may cause symptoms of intermittent pain, nausea, vomit and dysphagia. Careful inspection of upper gastrointestinal radiographs will show the misplaced intestine which sometimes is not described in the radiology report. When found, the redundant alimentary limb is reduced distally through the mesocolon and secured with sutures.

Small-Bowel Obstruction (Partial or Total, Recurrent)

Severe, intractable periumbilical, colicky pain, poorly responsive to narcotics, often with nausea and without a recent bowel movement or flatus, is a small-bowel obstruction until proven otherwise. Patients with distal obstruction may not vomit early in the clinical course, but if they have a gastric bypass, they will show excessive air in the small bowel and also the duodenum and distal gastric pouch. A distal gastric pouch massively distended by air or fluid [sometimes only seen on computed axial tomography (CAT) scan] is pathognomonic for a small-bowel obstruction distal to the jejunojejunostomy. Alternatively, if the small-bowel obstruction is proximal to the jejunojejunostomy, there may be no air in the small bowel unless an upper GI endoscopy was recently performed.

We have had a 2% incidence of small-bowel obstruction following bariatric surgery, with 2.5% of these patients developing recurrent obstruction. The majority of obstructions are caused by an obstructing band in the ileum, around which the small intestine may form a volvulus or a severe angulation.

Massive weight loss lengthens and thins out the intestinal mesentery making it capable of twisting around adhesions that shift with massive weight loss. We have seen only 2 cases of intussusception in more than 6000 bariatric surgical patients. Others, however, have reported this complication.[3,4]

During surgery for possible obstruction, it is important to explore for internal herniation, particularly following an initial laparoscopic bariatric procedure.[5] Potential sites include the enteroenterostomy mesenteric junction and the mesocolic opening for retrocolic alimentary limb passage.[6]

Biliopancreatic (Afferent) Limb Obstruction

Biliopancreatic (afferent) limb obstruction or partial obstruction is a potentially lethal condition, particularly because it may be overlooked by the unsuspecting clinician. The biliopancreatic limb represents the bypassed small intestine; consequently, orally ingested contrast material does not reach it. The back pressure of a complete or partial biliopancreatic limb obstruction on the common bile duct, pancreatic duct, native (distal, bypassed) stomach increases with time, which may cause elevations in serum amylase, lipase, and liver function tests, as well as produce tachycardia and hypotension. Antecolic alimentary limb blood supply may be interrupted by marked distention of the native (bypassed) stomach that displaces and overstretches the limb anteriorly. This can result in limb gangrene, perforation of the native (bypassed) stomach, and/or stomal disruption.[7] CAT scan of the abdomen will usually detect a distended C-loop, abnormally enlarged native stomach, and, sometimes, an abnormal alimentary limb.

Colon Pathology

Four of our patients at Memphis developed severe obstipation and pain, with apparent colonic dysmotility and megacolon. Left hemicolectomy resolved their problem, which initially was ascribed to partial small-bowel obstruction.

Colonoscopies have yielded polyps and diverticula among other pathologies. These findings are limited in occurrence as a consequence of the average patient age of 36 years for primary, and 41 years for reoperative, bariatric surgery. When right colon pathology exists, it is desirable, where feasible, to avoid ileocecal valve resection. Such resection may result in increased malabsorption caused by bacterial overgrowth of the distal small intestine.

Massive Ventral Hernia

We have encountered sufficiently massive ventral hernias with loss of domain with the bowel in the subcutaneous fat causing pain and intermittent obstructions for which closure without using a polypropylene patch or patch of other material was not prudent until the bariatric patient lost most of their excess weight. Repair could have resulted in abdominal compartment syndrome, overly long surgery, or unacceptable risk of need for prolonged mechanical ventilator support.

Nongastric or Enteric Intraabdominal Surgical Problems

While intraabdominal pathology following prior bariatric surgery is mostly enteric or gastric related, gall bladder, liver, kidney, gynecologic, pancreatic, and other diseases need to be excluded. Cancer, all forms, has a higher incidence among the obese, and may appear unexpectedly, presenting with pain, rectal hemorrhage, vaginal hemorrhage, jaundice, or abnormal urinanalyis.[7] If pain and other symptoms or laboratory abnormalities are found in the bariatric patient, it must be dealt with initially by the bariatric surgeon to provide the best chance of cure, where cure appears possible, with referral for a diagnosis to the best consultant. Later, a decision can be made whether to modify or reverse the bariatric surgery.

Obstetric/Gynecologic Considerations

Massive weight loss in many women may reverse infertility or produce more normal ebb and flow of monthly hormone levels, causing the return of abdominal pain or cramps in either case. Many obese women are infertile because the estrogen rise produced by follicular stimulating hormone is partially blunted by fat cell storage and then the fat cells release estrogen inappropriately later in the monthly cycle, when serum estrogen levels fall precipitously. The effect is similar to that produced by standard birth control medication. Undetected pregnancy may explain nausea and vomiting complaints in some patients. Testing is advisable in all potentially fertile female patients. Demanding a recent Papanicolaou smear and breast exam is also wise. Two of our Memphis patients developed stomal obstruction during their first trimester of pregnancy. We deferred reoperative surgery with total parenteral nutrition until their middle trimester when fetal loss was less likely. They both delivered healthy infants at term.

INADEQUATE WEIGHT LOSS

Most busy bariatric surgeons will have a certain percentage of their patients return to them because they have not lost at least 50% of their excess weight or they suddenly began to regain weight after successfully having lost weight and keeping it off for several years. Only bariatric surgeons who use a distal gastric bypass or some form of BPD will not have this problem, and they have the opposite problem—some of their patients return with excessive weight loss with nutritional deficiencies.

In the 1970s through the early 1990s, surgeons who primarily performed gastric bypasses saw mostly failure of the staple line that was used to separate the proximal small pouch from the rest of the distal stomach when most surgeons did not cut the stomach to divide it. Subsequently, most surgeons began physically dividing the stomach into two separate pouches, which prevents this type of failure from occurring after the first 90 days. A barium upper GI series in these patients without physical separation of the stomach would show the break in the gastric staple line with some of the barium going into the antrum and down the duodenum. This is corrected by revising the gastric bypass, reducing the proximal pouch to less than 15 to 20 mL and creating a new gastrojejunostomy after performing a partial gastrectomy to remove the excessively large gastric pouches (often 50 to 100 mL) that were created in the 1970s and usually part of the Roux limb at the prior site of the gastrojejunal anastomosis.

Gastric Pouch Remodeling and "Bermuda Triangles"

Enlarged gastric pouches are reduced by stapling off a new pouch above the old one and then removing the portion of the stomach with the broken staple line and prior gastrojejunostomy, removing at least 5 cm (2 inches) of stomach so that no part of the prior staple line is left inside the patient.

This is done because straight gastric staple lines do not always remain straight. Over time, they can become irregular, often S-shaped. During reoperative surgery, firing a straight stapler over an incompletely defined S-shaped staple line can unintentionally entrap one or more gastric segments, appropriately named "Bermuda Triangles." These segments, without distal exit sites to the rest of the GI tract, may become cystic because of gastric mucosal secretion, enlarge further, and disrupt.

To prevent Bermuda Triangles, we carefully mark prior gastric staple lines near to gastric restapling or resection sites, visualize or palpate the staple lines, and mark them with through-and-through no. 3–0 silk sutures 2 to 3 cm (0.8 to 1.2 inches) apart. An intragastric nasogastric tube or bougie may be manipulated against, or through, staple-line defects to identify their location if gaps in the staple line cannot be located by palpation. Occasionally, a gastrotomy is required to determine exact staple-line location. Traction on the preexisting sutures guides precise stapler placement.[8]

Composite Banding

For about 15 years in Memphis, we have been placing a "composite band" around selected reoperative gastric pouches to maintain the pouch diameter long term. It appears to be responsible for an additional 6.8 to 18.1 kg (15 to 40 lb) of weight loss in our series. The band consists of a 1.5-cm × 9-cm (0.6-inch × 3.5-inch) midline fascial strip obtained while opening the abdomen. The central 6.5 cm (2.6 inches) is measured and marked at its extremes with metal clips. Multiple no. 5 Ethibond suture bites are taken in the band along the 6.5-cm (2.6-inch) marked length. The band is placed through a previously channeled posterior gastric pouch track with the no. 5 suture on the outside and sutured to its opposite end at the 6.5-cm (2.6-inch) clip marker level. The suture is tied with a 34-Fr or 36-Fr bougie in place. We have had no recorded erosions of any composite band, an experience that supports the theory that fascial bands (fashioned from the patients' own tissue) buffers the suture from eroding into the gastric pouch.

This "belt-and-suspenders" construction provides the band and sutures to maintain the desired diameter of the pouch in case the fascia weakens. Some surgeons in Europe report using an adjustable gastric band in place of the fascia strip that we use. Our hypothesis needs a prospective randomized trial to establish that the fascia strip improves weight loss, but this can only be accomplished if we can gather forces to complete multicenter trials in patients who need revisions.

Intestinal diverticula may result following functional end-to-side or end-to-end stapled anastomoses. Careful dissection and resection of large enteric diverticula, especially when part of the biliopancreatic limb, may prevent problems with blind loop syndrome.

Perigastric Dissection

When anterior gastric dissection becomes tedious and bloody, pack the area and dissect posteriorly through another approach, such as the lesser sac via the gastrocolic ligament, around the lesser curvature, or over the angle of His. Tracking along the alimentary limb is another option and leads to the gastroenteric stoma. It helps to avoid injuring short gastric or lesser curvature vessels by periodically pausing and reorienting dissection toward the bougie located in the gastric pouch. With prior horizontal gastric stapling, cautiously handle the staple line near the greater curvature, as it often adheres to the splenic hilum.

Vagotomy

Complications secondary to peptic ulcer disease, or chronic gastritis in the distal gastric pouch, may be managed by vagotomy. In such cases, if the anatomy is not too distorted by adhesions and scarring, we may perform a highly selective anterior vagotomy and posterior truncal vagotomy.[9] Where anatomy precludes this approach, we perform bilateral truncal vagotomy.

Other Causes of Insufficient Weight Loss after Gastric Bypass

If after a standard gastric bypass the proximal pouch is intact and the Roux limb and other components appear to be functioning normally, the evaluation on whether or not a revision is needed becomes more complicated and a surgical solution using medical insurance may be precluded if the patient is no longer morbidly obese.

In our patients who present with this problem, we immediately evaluate our prior experience with them to determine how much weight they have lost; how much if any weight has been regained; what our initial evaluation revealed about the patient's psychological stability; the amount of social support being provided the patient; the patient's compliance with our preoperative and postoperative instructions; and the patient's attendance at our support meetings. Superobese patients who have lost more than 20 BMI units, yet are still morbidly obese, may need conversion to a shorter common channel and a longer biliopancreatic limb. Patients who have become disabled and are no longer able to exercise at their previous level, or who develop new diseases that require medications that cause weight gain, are problems that also may require a revision. We still complete a totally new workup on these patients with updates from our dietician and psychologist. Someone who is abusing alcohol or eating high-fat snacks all day needs education, not surgical treatment. Patients with the onset of severe depression, especially after very traumatic events, need psychotherapy rather than surgery. It is usually much easier to diagnose and decide what treatment plan is necessary for patients you have known for years.

It is much more difficult to evaluate patients presenting de novo to your clinic. We treat these patients as new patients and have them complete all medical, psychological, exercise, and dietary evaluations that we perform on our new patients. We like to have them start in our support group at least weekly, where they will often reveal more of themselves in front of their peers and our psychologist than they will to us, especially because they have some idea of why they have failed that they may not be willing to reveal to us until we gain their trust.

Many patients who have bariatric operations by surgeons who are not primarily bariatric surgeons received little preoperative evaluation or postoperative followup. Some welcome our more intensive approach to helping them change their habits, while others think they "know it all" already and initially resent not being able to schedule their surgery within the next week or two. Sometimes we believe that these patients will not benefit from revisional surgery because they do not want to to learn how to use their operations to help themselves lose weight.

When the common channel is shortened and the biliopancreatic limb is lengthened, there is no well-defined formula that lets one calculate these lengths. We measure each limb and will not usually make the common channel shorter than 200 cm (78.7 inches). Surgeons in Canada (see Chapter 12) and Italy often recommend shorter common channels. The socialized health care systems in these countries make it easier to follow patients and check them regularly so that nutritional deficiencies do not develop. Often they need to see a dietician weekly for 2 to 3 months, which can be expensive in our fee-for-service system. Even using common channels of 200 to 250 cm (78.7 to 98.4 inches) in length, we have had several superobese patients who have lost more than 90.7 kg (200 lb), become protein deficient with albumins that drop below 2.0 or even 1.5 mg/dl with leg edema, anemia, hair loss, and other problems. They are happy, however, with their weight loss so they do not want their new operation tampered with. We have found that patients with low levels of social support from their families, even if this is mainly poverty related, or with learning disabilities, are not good candidates for conversion to a distal gastric bypass.

These operations can be difficult and have numerous problems that are not present on initial cases. The portion of the small bowel that has not seen food for years, the biliopancreatic limb, is smaller in caliber, has a much thinner wall, and less peristalsis than does the alimentary limb and the common channel. Rearranging the distances in these limbs can affect the blood supply to them, especially if the surgeon shortens the alimentary limb by dividing the proximal part of the Roux limb from the rest of the jejunum it is in continuity with and then reanastomoses it 200 cm (78.7 inches) from the ileocecal value. Although this works well in more than 90% of cases, in the other 10%, dividing the vascular arcade that runs parallel to the jejunum can cause ischemia in this proximal Roux limb. Also, when the new mesenteric defects are closed that are made to create new limb lengths, stitches can compromise the blood supply anywhere along the small bowel. The biliopancreatic limb mesentery is thinner after disuse, and will often twist acutely, compromising the blood supply. Even if the small bowel is without ischemia at the end of the revisions, remember that when the patient begins to move in bed, roll over, and walk, new twists can occur. The white blood count should be watched closely for at least 4 days and if it starts to rise to levels above the level obtained in the recovery room, then reexploration should be considered early.

In all reoperative cases, the higher rate of complications needs to be emphasized. We suggest giving all such patients a reoperative fact sheet (Table 16–4) to read and sign, and a test (Table 16–5) where wrong answers are reviewed and the patient changes his or her answer and signs it (this is discussed later under "Informed Consent").

Inadequate Weight Loss after Restrictive Operations

As outlined in Chapter 10, several bariatric surgeons have been able to achieve equal weight loss using either VBG or gastric bypass, while others have achieved significantly better results with gastric bypass. This could be tech-

TABLE 16–4. REOPERATIVE OBESITY SURGERY FACT SHEET

Reoperative obesity surgery is done for a variety of different reasons. Because there is no formal, broadly accepted doctrine concerning reoperative obesity surgery, these reasons largely depend on your surgeon's judgment relative to your problems with the results of the earlier obesity surgery. Therefore, your surgeon reserves the right to accept or reject patients for reoperative surgery based upon his or her clinical judgment.

There are many operations available to modify, change, correct, or alter previous obesity surgery. Your surgeon will tell you what is the most likely plan, but you must understand that what the surgeon finds at surgery may change this plan considerably. For example, heavy amounts of scar tissue or unexpected findings can cause the surgeon to change plans from something relatively simple to a very complex procedure or vice versa.

While reoperative obesity surgery usually produces benefits, it is nothing "magic" or guaranteed. *You* may be asked to cooperate and make changes in your lifestyle and in your eating and drinking habits. The surgeon may also require that you be involved in certain behavioral training and exercise programs, usually together with a diet program.

Almost every surgeon who has performed reoperative obesity surgery has complications at some time or another. Every patient has a real risk for one or more complications, There are no guarantees that a serious complication will not occur in any case. The more frequent or serious complications that can occur are:

- Infection in the wound, body cavity (abdomen or chest especially), or lungs (pneumonia, for example) can occur. A lesser problem is collapse of small parts of lung tissue, which is called atelectasis: it is most often a result of difficulty taking deep breaths after surgery. It is a frequent cause of increased body temperature and is treated by breathing treatments or exercises.
- Inflammation or infection of these organs can occur: pancreas (pancreatitis); stomach (gastritis, stomach ulcer); esophagus (esophagitis with chest pain, burning, etc.); liver (hepatitis); gallbladder (cholecystitis, gallstones); kidney (pyelonephritis, kidney failure, nephritis); bladder (cystitis); duodenum (duodenitis, duodenal ulcer).
- The spleen may be injured during surgery and need to be removed. This can seriously increase the risks of infection in the patient's body.
- Organ failure, such as of the heart, kidney, liver, and lungs, has occurred after reoperative obesity surgery.
- Clots in the lower limbs, pelvis, or elsewhere in the body can form and travel to the lungs, causing difficulties with breathing or even death. These clots can also result in temporary or permanent swelling or ulceration, especially in the legs.
- Fluids from the stomach or intestines can leak into the body cavity, other organs, or through the skin. They may continue to drain into a bag for a long time.
- Changes in taste and food preferences often occur. Many patients have difficulties eating certain foods, such as red meats, which they may have liked before surgery. After surgery certain cravings for some foods may occur.
- Food or liquids may not be able to pass through the pouch, lower stomach, or intestines, which may need stretching (dilating) by instruments or endoscopes (which have their own risks). Tubes for nourishing fluids may have to be placed into stomach, intestines, or veins, if the patient is unable to eat or drink enough by mouth. Operation may be necessary.

TABLE 16–4. (CONTINUED)

- Vomiting or diarrhea frequently occurs after this type of surgery and may make it difficult to eat certain types or quantities of food. This can be, in one sense, a benefit of this surgery, because it prevents eating or drinking of certain food(s) for fear of diarrhea or vomiting.
- Bleeding from the stomach or formation of a hernia because of the breakdown of the surgical stitches may require reoperation. Complications of anesthesia and psychiatric problems, such as depression, requiring care and admission to a psychiatric ward, and even resulting in death, are all possible as a result of surgery. Approximately 1 in 200 (0.5 %) of all morbidly obese patients die after open (not laparoscopic "keyhole") gallbladder surgery; the risk is about the same for morbidly obese patients following obesity surgery, with or without the gallbladder being removed.
- Persistent vomiting, nausea, swelling of the abdomen, and heartburn, can occur and may make the patient think seriously about having the operation undone in certain instances.
- The stomach pouch or its outlet may get bigger, or the staple lines may open up, allowing the patient to eat more at a mealtime, or even regain the original, or greater, weight.

Reoperation may be necessary, and no patient should have reoperative obesity surgery performed who is not prepared to accept the need for further reoperation should it be necessary. When this occurs, the risk of surgery is usually somewhat greater than the risk of the original surgery, but it varies with the type of original and reoperative surgery involved. Risk of injury to spleen, bleeding, and need for blood transfusion also increase. Many experienced obesity surgeons order blood transfusions approximately 50% of the time following reoperative obesity surgery. Admission to an intensive care unit may be necessary to observe the patient closely or to treat any of the problems that can arise from surgery.

Over months and years, any type of nutrition problem or infection may occur, including lack of vitamin(s), protein, calories, and mineral(s). Signs of this include weakness, paralysis, confusion, rashes, anemia, hair loss, bone or joint problems, wounds that heal poorly, tongue soreness, night blindness, and numbness. After obesity surgery of any kind, taking vitamins and minerals and follow up by the obesity surgeon, or by a physician well-experienced in this area, is necessary for life. It is the patient's responsibility to make sure that such appointments are regularly made and kept, regardless of whether the patient "feels well" or not. The patient may need to have vitamin B_{12} injections every month for life. Food may get stuck in the stomach pouch and may need to be taken out with a special tube or a scope.

The patient's weight loss goal, no weight loss, or even further weight gain may occur after reoperative obesity surgery.

With weight loss, the skin on the arms, legs, neck, abdomen, face, and elsewhere may become wrinkled, sag, droop, or hang as large folds, and may develop rashes, infections, or odors. It may become quite annoying or embarrassing. As a result, you may feel a need for further surgery.

As soon as any problem arises, proper medical help must be obtained quickly—you have the duty to call for help quickly and without delay.

All of the currently performed types of reoperative surgery for obesity are still relatively new. Therefore, the extremely long-term results of such surgery, including weight loss or possible complications, are unknown at this time.

I have read the above, which has been described to me by my surgeon. I understand this material, the risks, possible complications, other choices, and the possible benefits of obesity surgery, as well as the type of operation that my surgeon recommends for my case.

By signing this statement, I am showing that I have read and accept the above and that I understand it. I have been encouraged to ask all the questions I want; they have been answered well, and I understand the answers.

_____   _____
(Patient Signature)   (Witness)

_____   _____
(Date)   (Time)

Table 16–5. TRUE/FALSE EXAM FOR REOPERATIVE BARIATRIC SURGERY PATIENTS

This examination is given so that your surgeon will know whether you understand the information that has been discussed with you. If you answer any question incorrectly, it will be an alert to review this area with you and to request that you work on it until it appears that you satisfactorily understand the material/concept(s) involved. If you retake the exam using this same sheet, please initial and date your changes beside each answer.

True/False   1. In reoperative surgery patients, the spleen, which may have adhesions to the stomach from previous surgery, has no greater chance of having to be removed than first-time obesity surgery.

True/False   2. Reoperative obesity surgery patients have a higher chance of needing to receive blood than first-time obesity surgery patients.

True/False   3. It is occasionally necessary to not perform part or all of the surgery planned because of unexpected events or findings.

True/False   4. Reoperative obesity surgery absolutely guarantees that additional surgery will not be necessary.

True/False   5. It is definitely guaranteed that all of the problems for which reoperative obesity surgery is performed will be cured.

True/False   6. It is *not* important to take nutritional supplements recommended to me by my surgeon and staff.

True/False   7. Diarrhea, nausea, vomiting, or constipation *never* follow reoperative obesity surgery.

True/False   8. Reoperative obesity surgery has all of the possible problems that can occur with the first-time surgery plus some additional ones.

Date:_____
Signature of the Person Examined_____
Examiner's Signature:_____

nique-related, a result of different levels of postoperative support, a result of the biases of the treatment teams, or a combination of these possibilities. Dr. Paul O'Brien, who has achieved excellent weight-loss results with minimal complications using the Inamed Corporation's LAP-BAND System, a form of adjustable gastric band, converts patients who have had either a VBG or a gastric bypass to an adjustable gastric band with excellent results for these difficult reoperative situations.[10]

Most bariatric surgeons, however, believe that people who have failed a restrictive operation will lose more weight if they are converted to a gastric bypass.[11,12] This is especially true for patients—more often men than women—who had been eating too many nutritionally balanced meals of a size that contains too many calories (big meal eaters) for their level of physical activity (e.g., a former college level offensive lineman who becomes a businessperson but who does not change his eating habits). Alternatively, after a restrictive operation, some big meal eaters begin eating soft, high-calorie foods, the converted "sweet eaters" become grazers, eating small amounts all day to prevent ever achieving a feeling of satiety. This grazing style can also defeat the weight-loss effects of a gastric bypass. For sweet eaters, however, a conversion from a restrictive operation to a gastric bypass will usually prevent eating high-sugar foods because eating them will cause dumping. A gastric bypass also prevents food and GI fluids (acid, pancreatic enzymes, bile) from mixing until the limbs meet in the common channel, so fewer calories are absorbed.

Silicone adjustable gastric banding, nonadjustable gastric banding, and vertical-banded gastroplasty may also result in intolerable side effects. Common reasons for conversion include band erosion, band migration, esophagitis, and staple-line disruption. These can be treated successfully by conversion to Roux-en-Y gastric bypass (RYGB)[11,12] and is clearly justified. In one comparative study, failed VBG conversion to RYGB produced more weight loss and less risk of reoperation for failure than did repeat VBG.[13]

Foreign Body and Enteric Diverticulum Removal

During reoperative surgery, we prefer to remove preexisting foreign bodies, such as Marlex mesh used to form vertical-banded gastroplasty bands, because they may later erode. Also, already-eroded bands are important to remove because of their potential to cause leakage and sepsis. Foreign bodies can lead to episodes of pyelonephritis, hepatic abscess, and peritonitis, all resulting in life-threatening sepsis.

Some key points regarding foreign bodies: (1) physically divided gastric staple lines are less likely to result in gastrogastric fistula than is stapling in situ; (2) avoid crossing prior gastric staple lines, especially to avoid risks of stenosis or leakage; (3) interposition of intestine between gastric pouch and distal stomach may reduce leakage[14]; (4) drain at a "safe" distance from anastomoses and staple lines; (5) where native (bypassed) stomach remains, gastrostomy is wise.

Conversion of Jejunoileal Bypass to Other Weight-Loss Procedures

Jejunoileal bypasses were commonly performed in the 1960s and 1970s but rarely after the mid-1980s because of the discovery that liver failure leading to death occurred in 5 to 10% of patients in the first years after the procedure, and more than 80% of patients who had the procedure developed cirrhosis within 20 years of their procedure (see Chapter 2). In spite of this high morbidity rate, there are still thousands of people with jejunoileal bypasses who are referred to bariatric surgeons by hematologists, gastroenterologists, and other internists and family practitioners who graduated from medical school during the 1970s and early 1980s when this was a well-discussed problem.

Patients who have lost their excess weight and who have maintained a healthy weight may not be convinced that they should be switched to an alternative bariatric procedure, even after a review of the potential morbidity, unless they have a percutaneous liver biopsy that documents early cirrhosis or they have developed symptoms of more advanced cirrhosis. A certain group will not show even mild fibrosis on a liver biopsy and these patients can be safely followed on a regular basis. If cirrhosis is present, however, the patient should have the jejunoileal bypass reversed.

The major problem with reversal is that the long length of mid-jejunum to mid-ileum has not been used for food absorption for approximately 20 years or more and is usually a smaller caliber than a pencil in diameter, and the lumen may not be patent even to that size in places. Also, with no active peristalsis in years, this section of bowel is not ready to function if a one-stage operation is tried to reinsert this section back into its place in the GI tract, or to use it to anastomose its proximal end to a small divided gastric pouch to form a gastric bypass. The surgeon and the hospital should understand that if a one-stage operation is used, they will be supporting an inpatient for 3 to 8 weeks of total parenteral nutrition and small amounts of oral intake as that unused section of bowel is rehabilitated to part of its prior functional level, allowing the patient to survive on the oral intake the deconditioned bowel can accommodate.

To avoid this long and expensive hospitalization, at the Louisiana State University in New Orleans, we approach these reversals as a two-stage procedure. First, we dissect out the bypassed section of small bowel and bring out its proximal end as an ostomy on the abdominal wall, or at least attach it to the abdominal wall fascia with a pediatric feeding tube (12 or 14 French) inserted through the skin and subcutaneous fat and then into the bowel for at least 10.2 cm (4 inches). If we do not think the bowel will accommodate this initially we insert a 14- to 20-gauge angiocatheter into the closed proximal end and slowly distend it for these 10.2 cm (4 inches) by inserting normal saline into it through a three-way stopcock until we are sure we have the first 10.2 cm (4 inches) of bowel patent. The patient and its family will then have to spend 2 to 6 months flushing saline into this disused bowel until at least 200 mL of fluid can be flushed into it easily. A barium study will then usually show that the intestine has dilated and opened back into its drainage point in the terminal ileum, cecum, or other part of the colon.

The proximal end of the bypassed intestine can then be anastomosed to the gastric pouch just as in primary gastric bypass procedures. Gastrostomy tube insertion is important for possible enteral feeding or decompression. The nonbypassed hypertrophic jejunal segment is then anastomosed end-to-side to the bypassed intestine, 90 cm (35.4 inches) or more from the gastroenterostomy and becomes the biliopancreatic limb. In some instances, we have interposed a segment of previously bypassed intestine between the hypertrophic jejunum and the enteroenterostomy in order to improve projected weight loss following surgery by decreasing backflow of nutrients into this superabsorptive section of bowel. Alternatively, the previously excluded bowel could be reinserted into its position in the intestine and a restrictive bariatric operation performed. We, and others, have noted that jejunoileal bypass patients have more problems, and less weight control, following conversion to a purely restrictive procedure than to a gastric bypass procedure because of the hypertrophied proximal jejunum and distal ileum.[15] Consequently, we avoid jejunoileal bypass conversion to gastroplasty. When the patient has significant cirrhosis, however, a bariatric procedure is not necessary and reanastomosis of the bypassed section after rehabilitation is probably the safest procedure.

Intestinal Measurement

It is wise to document small-bowel limb lengths, particularly when altering them. We use a known length of umbilical tape along the well-stretched antimesenteric border, moving the tape proximally from the ileocecal valve. Despite known inaccuracies in limb length measurements, they do provide "ballpark" figures and are superior to no figures at all.

Gastrostomy Tube

Postoperative native stomach decompression, as well as possible postoperative gastrostomy feedings and medications, are indications for tube placement, where a residual, bypassed stomach exists.

To permit access to the bypassed stomach even years postoperatively or by an interventional radiologist, we suture an approximately 5-cm × 7-cm (2-inch × 2.8-inch) gastric rectangle to the parietal peritoneum with interrupted no. 2–0 silk. This rectangle is centered around the gastrostomy tube during its insertion, which can be performed by using either the Wetzel or Stamm technique. The 7-cm (2.8-inch) sides run anteroposteriorly. Each corner is marked by two large, radiologically opaque hemoclips. In Memphis, we have successfully used this access for enteral feeding, endoscopy, including endoscopic retrograde cholangiopancreatography, medications, and biliopancreatic limb decompression, even years following the procedure.

Drains

Postoperative leakage rarely occurs but, when it does, early warning is important. A drain can serve this function and can also channel any fistulous drainage externally as a "controlled leak." Our preferred drain for a case in which we think a leak is highly likely, is a large triple-lumen surrounded on either side with a wide Penrose or large Blake drain that buffers the intermittent low Gomco drainage suction from adjacent tissues. We suture these drains, as well as the Gomco collar, to the skin with no. 0 silk or no. 2–0 nylon and also place a suture through the collar edge and one of the Gomco sump channels to prevent drain travel. Otherwise, one or two 19-Fr Blake drains are used in reoperative surgery. Any questionable drainage can be sent to the lab for an amylase analysis, which, if elevated, indicates probable leakage. We insist on using a drain in all primary and reoperative patients too heavy to fit into our CAT scanner [158.8 kg (350 lb)] and in all reoperative patients regardless of weight.

Laparoscopic versus Open Approach

Because of minimal adhesions following most laparoscopic bariatric surgeries, reoperative surgery via the laparoscopic route is feasible and, perhaps, preferred. Further studies are necessary to determine the balance of one approach vis-à-vis the other.

Bowel Preparation and Quadruple Antibiotics

Reoperative bariatric surgery may involve different procedures than were planned preoperatively. Dense adhesions may also result in inadvertent spillage of gastric or intestinal content. Prophylactic antibiotics are known to reduce risk of postoperative infection. The contents of the bypassed stomach have about a 67% chance of containing microorganisms.[16] Consequently, we regularly use propylene glycol bowel preparation and triple antibiotics, usually fluconazole, ciprofloxacin, and metronidazole.

Psychosocial Pathology

Considerable psychosocial pathology exists in the bariatric surgical population.[18] Much of it is secondary to the patients' conditions. For example, 89% of patients presenting to our Memphis clinic as primary bariatric surgery candidates tested positive for depression. This appeared largely centered around their inability to achieve a sustained weight loss.[19] This presentation is often exacerbated in patients presenting with significant problems following earlier bariatric surgery. In many, their abdominal pain and other symptoms were considerably magnified by depression. We have documented several cases of Munchausen syndrome associated with incredible histories and clinical courses.

Substance Abuse

Many reoperative candidates receive chronic narcotic prescriptions for headaches, low back pain, abdominal pain and other complaints. A few others test positive for alcohol, marihuana, and nonprescribed medications. It is important to know one's patient sufficiently in order to balance reoperative risks where surgically remediable problems exist in a known addict, substance abuser, or chronic pain patient. When we have performed surgery on these patients, they soon taught us the wisdom of deferring substance abuse treatment until full postoperative recovery.

Psychological Screening

Functional illiteracy can cause patients to misunderstand postoperative instructions, and misread prescription bottles. This results in poor postoperative compliance. Patients who abuse alcohol will not lose much weight or will begin to regain weight after bariatric surgery. Anorexia-bulimia occurs in approximately 5% of primary bariatric surgery patients; some may continue with postbariatric surgery symptoms of pain from overeating and then hematemesis from excessive vomiting. Psychological screening for these and other relevant conditions is very important before considering any revisional bariatric procedures, as mentioned briefly in "Evaluation" above.

Cardiopulmonary Problems

Malnutrition may cause occult myocardial damage that may clinically manifest with complaints of shortness of breath with exertion, lower extremity edema, tiredness, and right-upper-quadrant abdominal tenderness caused by the stretching of the Glisson capsule. Many morbidly obese patients have used phentermine and fenfluramine to lose weight in the past. A small percentage of these patients developed heart valve damage and/or pulmonary hypertension. We advise screening most reoperative patients who used these medications with an echocardiogram and, as indicated, further evaluation by a cardiologist.

Hematology Considerations

We recommend insertion of a inferior vena caval umbrella in patients with a coagulopathy, prior deep venous thrombosis or pulmonary embolism, severe obstructive sleep apnea, or severe obesity-hypoventilation syndrome, and in those who remain supermorbidly obese. Hematology consultation in certain patients is also wise preoperatively. Anemia may occur following gastric bypass or BPD as a consequence of reduced iron absorption; however, it is wise to confirm the absence of occult blood losses prior to reoperative bariatric surgery.

Certain patients lose little blood at reoperative surgery and have no apparent postoperative gastrointestinal bleeding but inexplicably develop significantly lower postoperative hematocrits. Daily postoperative complete blood cell count monitoring is wise.

Liver Pathology

Nonalcoholic steatohepatitis is common in the morbidly obese, but regresses in most patients with massive weight loss following bariatric surgery. Often unaccountably, other pathology may be present.[21] Because the presence of pathology may not be grossly or biochemically apparent, histology is necessary to demonstrate otherwise overlooked fibrosis, cirrhosis, hemochromatosis, and other findings. In some, the liver pathology may not regress and can be associated with problems following reoperative bariatric surgery. We perform an intraoperative wedge liver biopsy in all of our patients as a baseline of record and a diagnostic modality.

Medication Side Effects

Narcotics, NSAIDs, aspirin, antidepressants, and many other medications may be responsible for nausea, vomiting, dysphagia, constipation, diarrhea, and other complaints in bariatric surgery patients. A careful medications history, prescribed and over-the-counter, may lead to problem resolution. Postoperatively, we have seen two patients with refractory hypotension that did not remit until discontinuation of intravenous morphine. Also postoperatively, patients may develop depression, tachycardia, or hypertension as a result of withdrawal from prior medication that was not covered postoperatively.

Postoperatively administered narcotic tablets and other potentially vasoconstrictive oral medications can cause gastric erosions, perforations, and other problems. We insist that all oral medications be administered in a liquid or liquified form for at least the first 5 postoperative weeks.

Other Possible Causes of Weight-Loss Failure

Certain medications adversely affect weight loss following bariatric surgery.[22] Some of these include certain antidepressants, antihypertensives, hypoglycemic agents, and steroids. If a patient is taking such medication and the patient's chief complaint is weight regain or inadequate weight loss, a trial of alternative medication(s) might be worthwhile before committing to reoperative surgery.

Sweets Cravings

Some patients develop a sweets craving 1.5 years or more following bariatric surgery, which may cause weight increase. About two-thirds of our Memphis patients have responded well to 5-hydroxytryptamine over-the-counter medication. An alternative is ingesting a high-protein diet that may dampen or abort the cravings. "Stuffing the pouch" with snacks of low-calorie foods such as celery, raw cauliflower, cantaloupe, cottage cheese, or carrots, is an ancillary strategy that can induce satiety.

REVERSAL

Rarely does bariatric surgery require complete reversal. The surgeon who is inexperienced with bariatric procedures may think that a reversal is easier than understanding and correcting the problems the bariatric surgery patient has developed. The surgeon becomes the "hero" who has "fixed" the problems created by the bariatric surgery. In time, however, this surgeon will be found to have done little favor for the patient who regains all prior weight, and reassumes the burden of their prior comorbidities plus other new ones. The general surgeon lacking extensive, current bariatric surgery experience is wise to avoid reoperative bariatric surgery and to refer these patients to experienced bariatric surgery colleagues.

INFORMED CONSENT

Informed consent is a process. It is usually concluded by the patient signing a document certifying, among other things, that he or she is adequately informed about the proposed operative procedure(s). This process is meant to assure that the patient understands the procedure(s) and alternative options, as well as the risks, benefits, possible complications, and implications of the surgery to be performed by the named surgeon(s). Most bariatric surgeons do an excellent job of informed consent for primary bariatric surgery. However, reoperative bariatric surgery is less frequent, encompasses more variables, and lacks readily available informed consent models when compared with the primary surgery. Our informed consent reoperative fact sheet (see Table 16–4) and true/false examination (see Table 16–5) are reasonably time-tested models, as are our earlier primary bariatric surgical ones, and are recommended for use with this surgery. From a risk-management perspective, it would seem extremely difficult for a patient to claim not to have understood the informed consent material when the patient has signed the consent form and has had his or her signature witnessed, and has correctly answered questions concerning the surgery.

As part of the informed consent counseling, we ask each patient whether at least a 50% improvement of their problems would be satisfactory. They almost invariably agree with this realistic goal, which is usually surpassable.

CONCLUSION

Reoperative bariatric surgery involves complexities best addressed by the well-informed and experienced bariatric surgeon. The surgeon requires knowledge of options to detect and handle different, unique or unexpected situations, many of which have been addressed in this chapter. Another source of current medical opinions from bariatric surgeons is the web site of the American Society of Bariatric Surgeons (www.asbs.org). The Society maintains a privileged section on its web site that only bariatric surgeons can enter. Surgeons can ask a question and obtain many opinionated answers. Although reoperative obesity surgery is not a lucrative part of any bariatric surgeon's practice, it keeps life interesting and often produces tremendous benefits to the treated patients.

REFERENCES

1. Martin LF, Smits G, Greenstein R. Laparoscopic adjustable gastric banding to treat morbid obesity: three-year efficacy and six-year safety data from the US Multicenter Trials. (submitted).
2. Mallory GN, MacGregor AM, Rand CS. The influence of dumping on weight loss after gastric restrictive surgery for morbid obesity. *Obes Surg* 1996;6:474–478.
3. Duane TM, Wohlgemuth S, Ruffin K. Intussusception after Roux-en-Y gastric bypass. *Am Surg* 2000;66:82–84.
4. Norton KS, Brown WA, Johnson LW. Roux-en-Y limb intussusception: two case reports and a review of the literature. *J La State Med Soc* 2003;155:57–58.
5. Schweitzer MA, DeMaria EJ, Broderick TJ, et al. Laparoscopic closure of mesenteric defects after Roux-en Y gastric bypass. *J Laparoendosc Adv Surg Tech* 2000; 10:173–175.
6. Serra C, Baltazar A, Bou R, et al. Internal hernias and gastric perforation after a laparoscopic gastric bypass. *Obes Surg* 1999;9:546–549.
7. Keysser EJ, Ahmed NA, Mott BD, Tchervenhov J. Double closed loop obstruction and perforation in a previous Roux-en-Y gastric bypass. *Obes Surg* 1998;8:475–479.
8. MacGregor AM, Rand CS. Revision of staple line failure following Roux-en-Y gastric bypass for obesity: a follow-up of weight loss. *Obes Surg* 1991;1:151–154.
9. Torress JC. Gastric bypass distal Roux-en-Y jejunal interposition with selective proximal vagotomy and posterior truncal vagotomy. *Obes Surg* 1994;4:279–284.
10. O'Brien P, Brown W, Dixon J. Revisional Surgery for morbid obesity—conversion to the LAP-BAND system. *Obes Surg* 2000;10:557–563.
11. Westling A, Öhrvall M, Gustavsson S. Roux-en-Y gastric bypass after previous unsuccessful gastric restrictive surgery. *J Gastrointest Surg* 2002;6:2:206–211.
12. Balsiger BM, Murr MM, Mai J, Sarr MG. Gastroesophageal reflux after intact vertical banded gastroplasty: correction of Roux-en-Y gastric bypass. *J Gastrointest Surg* 2000;4:276–281.
13. Van Gement WG, Van Wersch MM, Greve JW, Soetes PB. Revisional surgery af-

ter failed vertical banded gastroplasty: restoration of vertical banded gastroplasty or conversion to gastric bypass. *Obes Surg* 1998;8:21–28.

14. Capella JF, Capella RF. Staple disruption and marginal ulceration in gastric bypass procedures for weight reduction. *Obes Surg* 1996;6:44–49.

15. Behrns KE, Smith CD, Kelly KA, Sarr MG. Reoperative bariatric surgery. Lessons learned to improve patient selection and results. *Ann Surg* 1993;218:646–653.

16. Uramatsu S, Cowan GSM Jr, Hiler ML, et al. Infectious potential of the bypassed stomach in gastric bypass patients [abstract]. *Obes Surg* 1996;6:307.

17. Sweet WA. Linitis plastica presenting as pouch outlet stenosis 13 years after vertical banded gastroplasty. *Obes Surg* 1996;6:66–70.

18. Martin LF. The biopsychological characteristic of people seeking treatment for obesity. *Obes Surg* 1999;9:235–243.

19. Cowan GSM III, Buffington CK, Vicjerstaff S, et al. Psychological status of the morbidly obese. *Obes Surg* 1996;6:107–109.

20. Cowan GSM Jr, Battle AO, Buffington C, et al. Munchausen's syndrome in postbariatric surgical patients. *Obes Surg* 1997;7:98–99.

21. Gholain PM, Kotler DP, Flancbaum LJ. Liver pathology in morbidly obese patients undergoing Roux-en-Y gastric bypass surgery. *Obes Surg* 2002;12:49–51.

22. Aronne LJ, Bray GA, Pi-Sunyer X, et al. *Management of Drug-Induced Weight Gain. A Continuing Education Monograph for Physicians.* Madison, WI: University of Wisconsin Medical School's Department of Continuous Medical Education; 2002.

OBESITY IN CHILDHOOD AND ADOLESCENCE

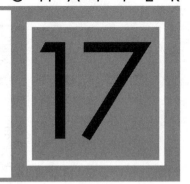

JOHN N. UDALL, JR. / MELINDA S. SOTHERN

DEFINITION AND PREVALENCE

Obesity is the excess storage of energy in the form of fat. There has been a significant increase in the prevalence of obesity in all age groups in the United States, particularly since the early 1980s. In the pediatric age groups between 1973 and 1994, the mean body weight of 5- to 14-year-old children in the Bogalusa Heart Study increased by 3.4 kg (7.5 lb), and the mean weight of 15- to 17-year-olds increased by 5.7 kg (12.6 lb).[1]

Data from the 1988 to 1991 National Health and Nutrition Examination Survey (NHANES) III cohort suggest that approximately 14% of US children are overweight (defined in "Treatment" below). More recent data suggest that overweight is more common among specific population subgroups. The prevalence of overweight in the Practice Partner Research Network, a network of primary care practices across the country, was 18 to 20%, while the prevalence of "at-risk" children was 34 to 36%. Similarly, among third- and sixth-grade children in New York City, 15 to 22% were overweight.[2]

MEASURES OF ADIPOSITY

Measurement of the individual compartments of body mass (i.e., muscle, fat, bone, etc.) is extremely challenging because no direct method exists other than in vivo neutron activation analysis (very limited availability) or chemical analysis of the cadaver (useful for animal studies only).

Some of the more frequently used body composition tests in children include anthropometry and skin-fold-thickness measurements, densitometry, dual-energy absorptiometry, bioelectrical impedance analysis, and the use of

335

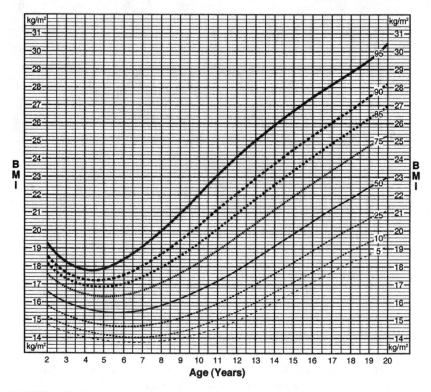

FIGURE 17–1   Body mass index for boys.

radiographic imaging techniques, such as computed tomography and magnetic resonance spectrometry.

Body mass index (BMI) is the standard test in assessing obesity. BMI is defined as body weight in kilograms divided by height in meters^2 (kg/m^2). In 2000, the Centers for Disease Control and Prevention (CDC) introduced BMI charts for boys and girls, ages 2 to 20 years (Figures 17–1 and 17–2). BMI is the most commonly used approach to determine if adults are overweight or obese. An adult with a BMI of <18.5 is considered underweight. A BMI from 18.5 to 24.9 is normal, and a value from 25.0 to 29.9 is considered overweight. Obesity is graded as mild (30.0 to 34.9), moderate (35 to 39.9), or morbid or severe (>40.0). The BMI is also the recommended measure to determine if a child is overweight. The new BMI growth charts can be used clinically beginning at 2 years of age, when an accurate stature can be obtained (Figures 17–1 and 17–2).

COMORBIDITIES

Obesity is widely recognized as contributing to various conditions such as hypertension, hypercholesterolemia, and diabetes, and to an increased incidence

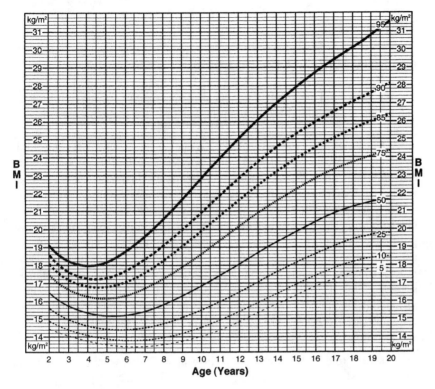

FIGURE 17–2   Body mass index for girls.

of musculoskeletal injuries. Obesity may also be associated with poor self-image and discrimination.[3]

PATHOPHYSIOLOGY

Like many other preventable adverse health states, childhood overweight reflects the convergence of many biological, economic, and social factors. Overweight arises from multiple causes, some as intimate as the family dinner table, others as seductive as television or the latest children's video game. Provision of high-fat meals and snacks in school settings is both a powerful temptation and a clear signal of accepted nutritional norms. Innovative strategies have been evaluated to address each of these concerns.[2] No one intervention, by itself, is likely to produce large reductions in the prevalence of obese or overweight children. Like adolescent smoking, teen pregnancy, and youth violence, childhood obesity is prevalent because it arises from deeply rooted behaviors and from social practices that are hardly confined to children. Given the profound consequences of childhood inactivity, poor nutrition, and overweight throughout the life span, urgency is warranted in responding to this epidemic. Treatment should be based on dietary changes, behavior modification, and increased physical activity.[2]

TREATMENT

Multidisciplinary Program

The recommended and clinical treatment of adolescent obesity includes individual and group multidisciplinary programs using dietary intervention, behavior modification, and exercise.[4]

Over the past 15 years, the authors have published results of treating childhood and adolescent obesity using an integrated, four-level team approach in a weekly outpatient clinical setting.[5–11] Program Methods Committed to Kids is a medical, psychosocial, nutrition, and exercise intervention for overweight adolescents along with their families and is conducted in a weekly outpatient clinical setting. The program is unique because of its integrated, four-level approach that encourages short-term (12 weeks) goal setting, quarterly feedback, and motivational techniques to improve health behaviors. During the 1-year program, adolescents and their families attend weekly, 2-hour, comprehensive sessions (Table 17–1). During these sessions, patients receive medical supervision, nutrition instruction, fitness counseling, exercise, and behavior modification. Program materials are color-coded according to the initial level of obesity as follows:

Level 1 (red): severe obesity defined as >97th percentile age-adjusted body mass index (BMI [US Centers for Disease Control and Prevention])[12] and >200% ideal body weight (IBW)[13]

Level 2 (yellow): moderate obesity defined as >95th percentile BMI and 150 to 200% IBW

Level 3 (green): overweight or mild obesity defined as 85th to 95th percentile BMI and 121 to 149% IBW

The color-coding of the educational materials is used to individualize exercise and diet prescriptions; it is also used as positive reinforcement as subjects reduce weight and achieve a lower level of obesity. In addition, the program workbooks follow the four phases of the 1-year program:

TABLE 17–1. SAMPLE WEEKLY CLINIC SCHEDULE FOR PARTICIPANTS OF COMMITTED TO KIDS

TIME	ACTIVITY
4:30 to 5 P.M.	Weigh-in and medical monitoring
5:00 to 5:15 P.M.	Group session: accomplishments
5:15 to 6:30 P.M.	Group activity session on nutrition, behavior, and/or exercise

Phase I: Beginner (weeks 1 through 12)
Phase II: Intermediate (weeks 13 through 25)
Phase III: Advanced (weeks 26 through 38)
Phase IV: Expert (weeks 39 through 52)

At the end of the expert phase, adolescents are awarded a free membership in the Total Exercise and Weight Maintenance (TEAM) Kids Club. TEAM Kids Club members are encouraged to attend quarterly special events and evaluations free of charge until their 18th birthday. They are also allowed to attend future classes, as needed, to assist with relapse prevention at no additional charge.

MEDICAL SUPERVISION AND GUIDANCE

The medical therapy consists of a complete medical/family history, a physical examination, body composition by dual-energy x-ray absorptiometry (DEXA), exercise tolerance (VO_2max [maximum oxygen consumption] using indirect calorimetry), and a baseline laboratory evaluation. Weight, blood pressure, resting heart rate, symptoms, and complaints are monitored weekly. Quarterly evaluations include height; weight; BMI; %IBW; waist and hip circumference; bioelectrical impedance and skin folds (triceps and subscapular);[14] physical activity rating;[15] and self-esteem, depression, and self-efficacy ratings.[16]

Medical Nutrition Therapy

The medical nutrition therapy consists of a diet history, intake visit, and laboratory assessment of growth, and current weight status. During the intake visit, the dietician establishes an initial 12-week weight loss goal based on the participant's %IBW and BMI. Energy restriction is used if patients are unsuccessful initially in losing weight while on a diet of reduced fat/healthful food choices. The diet prescription for overweight adolescents in the level 3 category includes a balanced hypocaloric diet (BHD) ranging from 1200 to 2000 kcal per day. The focus of the diet is to "reteach" normal portion sizes to patients and parents instead of focusing on a specific energy level. The diet prescription for the moderate and severely obese adolescents (in levels 1 and 2) includes a protein-modified fast diet (Table 17–2) as follows:

High protein: 2.0 to 2.5 g/kg IBW (average 90 to 140 g/d)
Reduced carbohydrate: 50 to 75 g/d
Reduced fat: 30 to 45 g/d
Total energy: 1000 kcal/d (depending on the protein prescription)

The maintenance diet begins once a patient has lost approximately 20% of entrance body weight or is ≤95th percentile BMI. At this point, they are

TABLE 17–2. Protein-Modified Fast Diet for Participants of Committed to Kids
Food composition
Lean meat and substitutes (13 to 20 oz/d)
Vegetables (reduced carbohydrate)
Bread/starch/fruit/milk: 2 to 3 exchanges per day combined
Selected free foods
Fluid
64 to 96 oz (minimum)/d
Supplements
Daily multivitamin with minerals
Elemental calcium: 1200 to 1400 mg/d
Additional potassium, if necessary
Duration
10 to 20 weeks

switched to a balanced hypocaloric diet to maintain steady weight loss or until they reach ≤85th percentile BMI or 120% IBW.

NUTRITIONAL EDUCATION NUTRITION

Education is conducted in group sessions with patients, parents, siblings, extended family, and friends in attendance (see Table 17–1). Patient participation is encouraged during cooking demonstrations, energy-counting, and food-measuring activities. At the end of the 1-year program, families should be able to adequately identify, select, and prepare foods that are appropriate to continued weight maintenance and good health (Table 17–3). Nutrition education sessions include identifying the food groups/nutrients in food laboratories; cooking demonstrations, which are referred to as "Fun in the kitchen," label reading/grocery shopping, and dining out/fast food/menu tips (Table 17–3).

EXERCISE PROTOCOL AND PHYSICAL ACTIVITY EDUCATION

The physical activity education includes the Moderate Intensity Progressive Exercise Program, an educational, curriculum-based intervention designed using social cognitive theory.[5,17,18] The approach includes guidelines for exercise frequency, duration, and intensity, as well as a series of 52 weekly, dynamic, interactive group sessions that promote increased physical activity and improved body-movement awareness.[5] The program also includes specific recommendations for type or modality of exercise based on the individual overweight level and physiologic function of the adolescent (Table 17–4).[18–20] Exercise instruction is conducted at each visit by a clinical exercise physiologist and includes fitness counseling. The exercise activities correspond with the group's physiologic condition of obesity and ability to comprehend, synthesize, and apply health and fitness information to daily life situations. The mus-

WEEK	TOPIC	ACTIVITY DESCRIPTION	TIME (P.M.)
		TABLE 17–3. SAMPLE WEEKLY CLINIC INTERVENTION SCHEDULE FOR PARTICIPANTS OF COMMITTED TO KIDS	
1	Nutrition	Diet instruction	5:00–6:00
	Behavior	Goal setting and self-monitoring	6:00–6:20
	Exercise	Safety and exercise/MPEP step	6:20–6:30
2	Nutrition	Questions and answers	5:00–5:15
	Behavior	Commitment rating	5:15–5:30
	Exercise	The metabolic systems of the body: aerobic vs. anaerobic metabolism, low impact aerobics to music	5:30–6:30
3	Nutrition	Fun in the kitchen—oven-fried chicken	5:00–5:30
	Behavior	Benefits and sacrifices: limit setting and rules for eating	5:30–5:50
	Exercise	Aerobic field sports	5:50–6:30
4	Nutrition	Fun in the kitchen—low-calorie pizza	5:00–5:30
	Behavior	Habit formation: ABCs of behavior, behavior chain	5:30–6:00
	Exercise	MPEP/strength training	6:00–6:30
5	Nutrition	Restaurant choices	5:00–5:30
	Behavior	Eating patterns: practical solutions; goal check	5:30–6:00
	Exercise	The flex test—stretch and flex series	6:00–6:30

Abbreviation: MPEP = moderate intensity progressive exercise program.

cular strength, endurance, and flexibility exercises are illustrated in detail in the workbooks and demonstrated in the exercise videos.[5,18–21]

BEHAVIOR-MODIFICATION PROTOCOL

Weekly sessions begin with group discussion highlighting the patients' accomplishments for the week (see Table 17–1). Positive reinforcement is given for trying new vegetables, turning down high-energy snacks, or participating in physical activity. Behavior-modification skills are introduced by using discussion, modeling, role playing, and guided problem solving.[16,21] Topics such as self-monitoring, commitment, setting limits, habit formation, goal setting, and action plans, decision-making skills, attitudes, relapse prevention, and assertiveness training, are discussed. Patients with psychological problems are referred to a therapist for additional individual counseling while continuing in the program. Award certificates, inexpensive sports equipment, and other incentive items are given quarterly as positive reinforcement for achieving short-term goals (Table 17–5). Special events, such as roller skating parties, park/field

TABLE 17–4.   INITIAL EXERCISE GUIDELINES* FOR PARTICIPANTS OF COMMITTED TO KIDS

Overweight adolescents

- <150% IBW, 85th to 95th percentile BMI
- Recommended aerobic activities: weight-bearing activities such as brisk walking, treadmill, stair-climbing, field sports, rollerblading, hiking, racquetball, tennis, martial arts, skiing, jump rope, indoor gym sports, and swimming

Obese adolescents

- 150 to 200% IBW; >95th to 97th percentile BMI
- Recommended aerobic activities; primarily non–weight-bearing activities such as swimming, cycling, strength/aerobic circuit training, arm-specific aerobic dancing, arm ergometer (crank), recumbent bike, and interval walking†

Severely obese adolescents

- >200% IBW; >97th percentile BMI
- Weekly supervision by trained exercise professional
- Recommended aerobic activities: non–weight-bearing activities only, such as swimming, recumbent bike, arm ergometer, seated (chair) aerobics, and seated or lying circuit training

Abbreviations: IBW = ideal body weight.
BMI = body mass index.
*Guidelines should be readjusted every 10 to 15 weeks based on evaluation results.
†Walking with frequent rests as necessary. Gradually work up to longer walking periods and fewer rest stops.
Source: Used with permission from Sothern M, et al.[4]

TABLE 17–5.   QUARTERLY AWARDS FOR PARTICIPANTS OF COMMITTED TO KIDS

New target weight
New 10-week weight-loss goal
Attendance award
Graduation certificate
Exercise award for most minutes of exercise
Nutrition award for trying new vegetables
Evaluation report form and new education materials

days, and holiday parties, are organized during the 1-year program to encourage continued participation.

OUTCOME DATA

For a 1-year period, 93 adolescents (age 13.1 to 17.7 years) were enrolled in the program. At the end of the year, 56 patients (22 boys, 34 girls; 44 whites and 12 African Americans) participated in evaluations (60.7%). Subjects reduced BMI from 32.3 ± 1.3 at baseline to 29.35 ± 1.9 at 10 weeks and further reduced BMI to 28.2 ± 1.2 at 1 year; %IBW was reduced from 177

$\pm$ 34.0 at baseline to 156.2 $\pm$ 23.7 at 10 weeks and further reduced to 141.9 $\pm$ 20.1 at 1 year (P <.001).

Surgery

Bariatric surgery has been used by some surgeons to treat obesity in children and adolescents. It may induce long-lasting (>1 year) effects on body weight in severely obese adolescents.

Randolph et al. was one of the first groups to report surgical treatment of morbid obesity.[22] The group performed jejunoileal bypass for morbid obesity in four children ages 11, 15, 15, and 16 years. Children were followed for 1 year following surgery. The authors concluded that "adolescents and preadolescents can deal with the operation and postoperative problems of massive intestinal bypass." They noted that linear and skeletal growth was not impaired and that "adolescents and younger children who are markedly overweight and who are incapable of effective dietary therapy should be considered for jejunoileal bypass."[22] Silber et al. described 11 morbidly obese adolescents who underwent jejunoileal bypass.[23] Ten years later, they had maintained a weight loss ranging from 45 to 90 kg (99.2 to 198.4 lb). Unfortunately, each adolescent had at least one complication of the procedure, including encephalopathy, cholelithiasis, nephrolithiasis, renal cortical nephropathy, hypoproteinemia, and other nutritional deficiencies. Several adolescents had complications that required reversal of the surgery.

Because of the severity of the complications of jejunoileal surgery, this procedure is rarely performed now.[24] Instead, the Roux-en-Y gastric bypass (RYGB) is the most commonly performed bariatric surgery in children. Vertical-banded gastroplasty has also been performed in adolescents.[24,25]

In one study of RYGB and vertical-banded gastroplasty, 34 adolescents aged 11 to 19 years at the time of gastric surgery for obesity were interviewed an average of 6 years postoperatively.[25] Patients' preoperative BMI averaged 47; at follow-up, their BMI averaged 32. Two thirds of the patients weighed within 9 kg (19.8 lb) of their lowest postsurgical weight at the time of follow-up; three had had additional obesity surgery. Patients reported excellent psychosocial adjustment, including improved self-esteem, social relationships, and appearance. No patient was unemployed, which is significant considering the degree of discrimination young adults who are severely obese face when entering the workforce. Patients reported poor compliance with exercise and dietary instructions. More seriously, only four patients reported taking vitamin B_{12}, multivitamin supplements, and calcium as directed,[25] illustrating the problems often associated with delivering complicated, high-risk therapies to adolescents and young adults who feel immortal and do not want to be reminded that supplemental medications are necessary for good health after gastrointestinal surgery.

The risks and benefits of intensive weight-management therapies, including bariatric surgery should be weighed carefully before they are used with pediatric patients. Until further controlled trials become available, intensive therapies for pediatric obesity should be considered only for children who have not responded to conventional weight-management programs but have significant complications of their obesity[24] or under trial-like settings where an Institutional Review Board is helping to supervise the risks that the adolescents are being exposed to when surgical therapy is offered. Pediatric patients who demonstrate compliance in nonsurgical weight-loss programs, even if they do not lose weight, are better surgical candidates than ones who have never demonstrated compliance.

REFERENCES

1. Slyper AH. Childhood obesity, adipose tissue distribution, and the pediatric practitioner. *Pediatrics* 1998;102(1):4.
2. Strauss RS, Pollack HA. Epidemic increase in childhood overweight, 1986–1998. *JAMA* 2001;286:2845–2848.
3. Dietz WH. Health consequences of obesity in youth: childhood predictors of adult disease. Pediatrics 1998;101(Suppl):518–525.
4. Sothern MS, Schumacher H, von Almen TK, Carlisle LK, Udall JN. Committed to Kids: an integrated, 4-level, team approach to weight management in adolescents. *J Am Diet Assoc* 2002;102(Suppl):381–385.
5. Sothern M, Hunter S, Suskind R, Brown R, Udall J, Blecker U. Motivating the obese child to move. The role of structured exercise in pediatric weight management. *South Med J* 1999;92:577–584.
6. Sothern M, Loftin M, Suskind R, Udall J. The impact of significant weight loss on resting energy expenditure in obese youth. *J Invest Med* 1999;47:222–226.
7. Sothern M, Despeney B, Brown R, Suskind R, Udall J, Blecker U. Lipid profiles of obese children and adolescents before and after significant weight loss: differences according to sex. *South Med J* 2000;93:278–282.
8. Brown R, Sothern M, Suskind R, Udall J, Blecker U. Racial differences in lipid profiles of obese youth before and after significant weight loss. *Clin Pediatr* 2000;39:427–431.
9. Sothern M, Blecker U, Suskind R, et al. Weight loss and growth velocity in obese children after very-low-calorie diet, exercise, and behavior modification. *Acta Paediatr* 2000;89(9):1036–1043.
10. Suskind R, Blecker U, Udall J, et al. Recent advances in the treatment of childhood obesity. *Pediatr Diabetes* 2000;1:23–33.
11. Sothern M, Loftin M, Suskind R, Udall J, Blecker U. The Impact of Significant Weight Loss on maximum oxygen uptake in obese children and adolescents. *J Invest Med* 2000;48(6):411–416.
12. Rosner B, Prineas R, Loggie J, Daniels S. Percentiles for body mass index in US children 5 to 17 years of age. *J Pediatr* 1998;132:211–222.
13. Hamill P, Drizd R, Johnson C, Reed R, Poche A, Moore W. Physical growth: National Center for Health Statistics Percentiles. *Am J Clin Nutr* 1979;32:607–629.
14. Sothern M, Loftin J, Tuuri G, Udall J. A comparison of skinfold analysis and dual-energy x-ray absorptiometry (DEXA) in female youth with increasing levels of obesity. *Med Sci Sports Exerc* 2000;32(5):2338.
15. Godin G, Shephard R. A simple method to assess exercise behavior in the community. *Can J Appl Sport Sci* 1985;10:141–147.
16. von Almen T, Figueroa-Colon R, Suskind R. Psychosocial considerations in the

treatment of childhood obesity. In: Giorgi P, Suskind R, Catassi C, eds. *The Obese Child (Pediatric Adolescent Medicine)*. Basel, Switzerland: Karger; 1992:162–171.

17. Bandura A. *Social Foundations of Thought and Action*. Englewood Cliffs, NJ: Prentice-Hall; 1986.

18. Sothern M, Loftin M, Udall J, et al. Safety, feasibility and efficacy of a resistance training program in preadolescent obese children. *Am J Med Sci* 2000;319:370–375.

19. Sothern M, Loftin M, Blecker U, Suskind R, Udall J. Physiologic function and childhood obesity. *Int J Pediatr* 1999;14:135–139.

20. Sothern M, Loftin M, Ewing T, Tang S, Suskind R, Blecker U. The inclusion of resistance exercise in a multi-disciplinary obesity treatment program for preadolescent children. *South Med J* 1999;92:585–592.

21. Sothern M, Schumacher H, von Almen TK. *Trim Kids: The Proven 12-Week Plan That Has Helped Thousands of Children Achieve a Healthier Weight*. New York: HarperCollins; 2001.

22. Randolph JG, Weintraub WH, Rigg A. Jejunoileal bypass for morbid obesity in adolescents. *J Pediatr Surg* 1974;9(3):341–345.

23. Silber T, Randolph J, Robbins S. Long-term morbidity and mortality in morbidly obese adolescents after jejunoileal bypass. *J Pediatr* 1986;108:318–322.

24. Yanosky JA. Intensive therapies for pediatric obesity. *Pediatr Clin North Am* 2000;48(4):1041–1053.

25. Rand CSW, Macgregor AMC. Adolescents having obesity surgery: a 6-year follow-up. *South Med J* 1994;87(12):1208–1213.

RESOLUTION OF THE COMORBID DISEASES OF MORBID OBESITY AFTER BARIATRIC SURGERY

WILLIAM J. RAUM / LOUIS F. MARTIN

In addition to the obvious problems related to size and weight, morbidly obese patients have multiple associated diseases (comorbidities) that have detrimental effects on many organ systems. It is important to identify these problems preoperatively (see Chapter 5) because these diseases need to be controlled or stabilized to reduce their impact on perioperative surgical risk. During hospitalization, potential rapid exacerbation or destabilization of chronic medical conditions should be anticipated so that they may be addressed promptly (see Chapter 7). Resolution of these chronic and debilitating diseases in the postoperative period helps to justify surgery as an appropriate treatment option. Lastly, recurrence of comorbid disease without weight gain must be identified, which can occur with dietary changes, development of new stressful conditions, or the ongoing effects of aging.

If comorbid disease is not recognized and managed properly other even more serious problems could occur. For example, orthostatic hypotension can be produced if antihypertensives are not reduced or discontinued postoperatively, which may result in stroke, myocardial infarct, or severe trauma from a fall caused by dizziness. Diuretics may cause renal insufficiency or renal stone formation. Hypoglycemic agents may cause prolonged hypoglycemia, neuroglucopenia, coma, stroke, and death. Unrecognized and untreated obstructive sleep apnea may become more severe because of different sleeping positions necessitated by postoperative pain and the use of certain postoperative sedatives and analgesics, resulting in sudden death.

Many chronic comorbid diseases are cured by bariatric procedures in a majority of the patients.[1,2] The likelihood of cure is dependent on the length and severity of the disease, the amount of weight loss achieved and the level of contribution of obesity to the severity of the disease. For example, many primary hyperlipidemias may be exacerbated by obesity but will not be cured by weight loss. On the other hand, more than 80% of type 2 diabetes is cured, depending on the procedure used and duration of the diabetes.[1–3] Blood pressure in hypertensives is normalized within a few days to a few months of the procedure.[1] However, hypertension may return in many patients within 4 to 8 years after the procedure, even without any significant weight regain[4] over the lowest weight achieved after surgery.

The different types of surgical procedures—gastric banding,[5,6] gastric bypass,[7] or biliopancreatic diversions[8]—each have their different impacts on comorbid diseases. Some of their effects depend on the degree of weight loss achieved, some on the changes in hormones and some on the degree of malabsorption induced. Many of these characteristics are just now being reported.[9]

Recognizing the types and changes in comorbid disease that occur in the morbidly obese is essential to reducing the risk of surgical treatment and reducing the number of potential short- and long-term consequences of permanent weight loss. Every entity—the press; insurance companies; local, state and federal government; medical societies; physicians; nurses; dietitians; and all health care providers involved in facilitating or hindering the treatment of the morbidly obese—should be aware of the good and bad consequences of their actions and pronouncements on the disease burden that these people carry.[10] The only effective treatment for morbid obesity and its comorbid conditions is bariatric surgery. There are no drugs, psychotherapy, lifestyle changes, acupuncture, hypnosis, or nutrition programs that remotely approach the capacity of bariatric surgery to reduce or eliminate the diseases caused or exacerbated by morbid obesity.

The comorbid diseases of morbid obesity overlap and interact extensively. For example, feeling tired all the time may be a result of the increased work load of carrying an extra 45.4 kg (100 lb) or more everywhere they go, to the metabolic consequences of diabetes, to hypoxia and hypercarbia from pickwickian syndrome, or to the lack of sleep from obstructive sleep apnea. However, to aid in the discussion of the problems caused by morbid obesity they have been divided into organ systems. Some, but not all of the potential interactions are discussed. Nor is this a complete list of all the potential problems, as new associations are being reported every month. We have attempted to present those problems that cause the most disability and impact on the quality of life to the greatest degree.

PULMONARY

Sleep Apnea

Obstructive sleep apnea (OSA) is a relatively newly recognized disease.[11] The technology and reliable testing, labeled polysomnography or sleep study, became clinically available only about 20 years ago and then was provided mostly in large medical centers with active research programs. Now there are reliable, certified, private testing centers throughout the country in urban and rural areas. The test is conducted during the evening in a sleep center equipped with comfortable rooms, modeled after hotels rather than hospitals, that are monitored by video. Sensors are placed on the patient that measure respirations, snoring, brain electric potentials (electroencephalograph), heart electric potentials (electrocardiogram), and blood oxygen levels (pulse oxygen device). The severity of the disease is measured by an index named the respiratory distress index (RDI). Its value is derived from the number of breathing related events, apneas and hypopneas that occur during the test. The normal RDI is 5. Values from 5 to 14 may require treatment if associated with other problems, such as coronary artery disease or hypertension. An RDI above 14 is considered moderate disease, and should be treated. Severe sleep apnea (an RDI greater than 30) is usually associated with severe deficiency in blood oxygen levels (pulse oximetry), especially during the deepest sleep stage, rapid eye movement (REM) sleep. Normal oxygen saturation levels should be greater than 95%. Levels below 70% are common with severe OSA and may decrease to 45%. Oxygen levels this low commonly lead to cardiac arrhythmias, cortical nerve damage, and severe morning headaches. Depending on other cardiopulmonary pathology, OSA is probably the most common cause of sudden death in morbid obesity. Some laboratories also calculate an RDI separately during rapid eye movement sleep (a REM RDI), when the most severe obstructive events occur.

The treatment for OSA in morbid obesity is weight loss. The cure rate is nearly 100%.[12,13] A drastic intermediate treatment is to have removal of tissue from the oropharynx, tonsils, adenoids, and uvula. While this may provide temporary relief, the soft tissue and fat deposition in the upper airway will regenerate and again cause obstruction. A small portable device that delivers continuous positive airway pressure (CPAP) to the upper airway may be used to prevent apneas by preventing the lax soft tissue from closing off during inspirations. A second sleep study is performed, usually the following night, to titrate or adjust the setting on the CPAP device to abolish the apneas. Alternatively, many sleep laboratories offer "split" studies where a patient identified with 30 apneas or more in the first half of the night, confirming a diagnosis of apnea, is fitted with CPAP for the second half of the night and a titration completed. This saves the patient time and the insurance company money when the patient's sleep apnea is severe enough to reach diagnostic criteria in <4 hours. Settings for CPAP device range from approximately 4 to 20 cm of water. Several fittings and accessories can be supplied to increase compliance and comfort of the treatment. A swivel connection to allow more movement in bed, a humidifier, nasal mask, and facemask or nasal pillows are among some of the variations. Some patients may require a gradual ramp of increasing pressure to reach treatment levels, or supplemental oxygen delivered through the CPAP, or two levels of pressure treatment, called BiPAP. The sleep laboratory should test these fittings to see which is most comfortable and appropriate for the patient before the system is ordered.

Probably 80% of patients with morbid obesity have sleep apnea with 60% being moderate to severe. There is no close correlation of BMI to the incidence of sleep apnea although the most common characteristics for people who have sleep apnea are obese hypertensive males who snore. Even patients with a body mass index (BMI) of less than 35 can have severe OSA. Neck circumference may be a better correlation, where 17 inches in men and 16 inches in women is a good predictor of the risk of OSA.[11] However, weight loss through bariatric surgery is near universal cure where both BMI and neck circumferences are drastically reduced. Medically induced weight loss will also eliminate OSA. However, more than 98% of patients regain their weight and their OSA. Therefore, it is the permanent weight loss associated with bariatric surgery that cures sleep apnea, not the procedure used.

We routinely test all our patients with a quiz (Figure 18–1) to determine the likelihood of the presence of OSA. Those who score above a certain threshold are given a sleep study. More than 90% of patients who scored above 30 on this quiz had sleep apnea. So far, only one patient who scored less than 30 demonstrated moderate sleep apnea during hospitalization.

Pickwickian Syndrome

Severe obesity leads to decreased ventilation from abdominal fat impeding the movement of the diaphragm and adipose tissue in and around the thorax reducing thoracic expansion. Hypoventilation leads to hypercarbia that leads to daytime somnolence.[14] Collapse or atelectasis of the lower lobes of the lungs leads to shunting or lack of oxygenization. Untreated, this syndrome can lead to prolonged intubation and mechanical ventilation after surgery. Prolonged hospitalization and complications secondary to extended intubation and mechanical ventilation can occur including pneumothorax, adult respiratory distress syndrome, wound dehiscence, anastomotic leaks, and pneumonia to name a few.

We perform full pulmonary function tests before and after bronchodilation, and arterial blood gases. Patients with pickwickian syndrome are given incentive spirometry, other breathing exercises, bronchodilators (if indicated), and put on a low-calorie weight-loss program to reduce weight by 20 to 50 pounds or more until pulmonary function tests and blood gases show a substantial improvement. Most patients reach normal blood gases with this treatment (pCO_2 of less than 45 mmHg and pO_2 of greater than 80 mmHg).

Pickwickian syndrome is cured by substantial weight loss, regardless of the procedure used.[14,15]

Asthma, Dyspnea on Exertion

Small airways disease, whether caused by seasonal allergens, unidentified triggers, smoking, or other toxins, appear to be much less symptomatic after weight loss.[16] Dyspnea on exertion and most other forms of respiratory symptoms are diminished or totally cured. If patients are identified with chronic asthma by history and demonstrate improvement after bronchodilation during pulmonary function testing, their bronchodilator treatment is optimized or intensified. If inhaled steroids were not being used, they are added in a moderate dose range (Flovent 110 µg, 2 puffs b.i.d.), and incentive spirometry is used for several

▌ St. Charles
▌ General Hospital
Tenet Louisiana HealthSystem

NAME _____

M.R.# _____

WEIGHT MANAGEMENT

Restful, restorative sleep is essential to your well-being. In fact, most of us spend nearly one third of our lives asleep. The quality of that sleep can directly affect your life.

Nearly 17 million people have sleep apnea, a breathing disorder that disrupts sleep and makes waking hours miserable. This daytime suffering is needless. Once diagnosed nearly every patient with sleep apnea can be helped. Many are unaware that this problem even exists. Sleep apnea is frequently the cause of sudden death in people with morbid obesity. Please answer the questions below. The quiz is designed to alert you to any problems resulting from poor sleep. If you have had any of the symptoms in the past year, mark the box, fill in the number in ( ) on the blank line and add up the total.

☐ _____ 1. I have been told that I snore or I know that I snore. (20)

☐ _____ 2. I definitely do not snore. (-50: subtract 50 points)

☐ _____ 3. I do not know if I snore (0)

☐ _____ 4. I have been told that I stop breathing when I sleep (10)

☐ _____ 5. I wake up choking (10)

☐ _____ 6. I sweat excessively at night (5)

☐ _____ 7. (If female and above is true) I have hot flashes related to my cycle (-5)

☐ _____ 8. I am tired and sleepy during the day even after 8 hours of sleep (2)

☐ _____ 9. I wake up tired and unrested (2)

☐ _____ 10. I suddenly wake up unable to breath (10)

☐ _____ 11. I have fallen asleep while driving (5)

☐ _____ 12. I am a restless sleeper (toss and turn a lot) (5)

☐ _____ 13. My neck circumference is more than 17 inches (20)

(Ask nurse to measure if unknown)

☐ _____ 14. I frequently have morning headaches (5)

_____ TOTAL (more than 30 points suggests that you have SLEEP APNEA.

Please share this with your doctor so that a sleep test can be ordered. Sleep apnea is a life threatening sleep disorder that causes you to stop breathing. It can happen hundreds of times per night while you sleep and you may not be aware of it.

2-7281-11

FIGURE 18.1   Sample sleep study quiz. (Courtesy of St. Charles General Hospital, New Orleans, Louisiana.)

weeks prior to surgery. Both treatments are rarely needed for more than 1 month postoperatively.

The resolution of small airways disease may be the result of a decrease exposure to certain food allergens that are no longer in the patient's diet. Alternatively, the decrease in adipose tissue in all organs including the lungs and thorax may reduce the intensity of symptoms.

Dyspnea on exertion most certainly improves simply from the reduction of weight that is being carried. With increased activity, and increased pulmonary function there is an increase in overall cardiopulmonary fitness after weight loss.[17]

CARDIOVASCULAR DISEASE

Generalized Atherosclerosis

Many of the comorbid diseases associated with obesity, as well as obesity it-self, are risk factors for the development of atherosclerosis of the major arteries. These risks factors include elevated lipid levels, diabetes, and hypertension. Two studies have shown that atherosclerotic plaque either reverses or progresses less rapidly in morbidly obese persons who have had bypass procedures that lower lipid levels. Buchwald et al. showed that a terminal ileal bypass reversed plaque in coronary angiograms (see Chapter 2) and have combined this with gastric restrictive surgery to also induce weight loss.[18] Karason et al.[19] demonstrated that plaques in carotid arteries of morbidly obese patients did not progress in thickness after gastric bypass, reverting to thickness levels of normal weight patients over several years time.

Coronary Artery Disease

Obesity has been identified by the American College of Cardiology as an independent risk factor for coronary artery disease (CAD).[20,21] Like hypertension, hypercholesterolemia, and smoking, obesity may lead to a myocardial infarction. Resolution of this risk factor through weight loss eliminates this risk factor. For patients with previously diagnosed CAD, we seek clearance from the patient's cardiologist to ensure that treatment is maximized and that there are no reversible ischemic changes on cardiac stress tests that should be treated. For patients with stable CAD, protective drugs, such a beta-blockers, nitrates, or calcium channel blockers, are maintained, as the blood pressure will allow. If symptoms or a screening electrocardiogram suggests the presence of undiagnosed CAD, we obtain a cardiology consult for stress testing, advice on preoperative treatment, and clearance for surgery.

Congestive Heart Failure

We have performed gastric bypass on patients with left ventricular ejection fractions as low as 25%. With weight loss, all cardiovascular drugs were discontinued and the ejection fractions rose to greater than 55%. Patients with milder degrees have returned to normal function. A dilated cardiomyopathy in a normal weight patient will probably never improve significantly. However, a dilated cardiomyopathy in a patient more than 45.4 kg (100 lb) overweight has room for considerable improvement.[22] The heart in a morbidly obese patient has considerable reserve that will become apparent with weight loss. The essential step to be able to attain sufficient weight loss is proper preparation for surgery. These high-risk patients must be highly motivated to change their lifestyle before bariatric surgery. They must reduce salt intake, lose weight, and increase activity and cardiovascular fitness. Other associated diseases must be maximally treated including hypertension, sleep apnea, and diabetes. Some patients may require 3 or more months of intensive therapy before they are ready to undergo bariatric surgery. With this preparation, risks are markedly reduced and a good outcome is expected.

Karason and colleagues[23] have shown that after bariatric surgery morbidly obese patients decrease the thickness of their left ventricular wall and overall ventricular mass as they lose weight. Morbidly obese patients who do not have surgery and do not lose weight continue to increase left ventricular mass over time.

Dependent Edema, Venous Insufficiency, Cellulitis

Venous return from the lower extremities of morbidly obese individuals is reduced from the pressure exerted by abdominal and pelvic fat on top the femoral veins as they transverse the pelvic bone leading to varying degrees of venostasis, lymph edema, and increases the risk of deep venous thrombosis as a consequence of stasis. This may, and usually does, occur in the absence of right heart failure. When the edema becomes chronic, it can lead to changes in the skin that allow for the development of cellulitis, venous stasis skin ulcers, especially as small veins permanently clot, and varicose veins.[23] Recurrent cellulites can result in life-threatening systemic infections and other complications from antibiotic therapy including renal failure.

As long as the deep venous system remains relatively intact, weight loss can cause complete resolution of even the most severe forms of venous stasis with brawny edema, stasis ulcers, and recurrent cellulitis. Varicose veins usually require other therapy.

Deep Venous Thrombosis, Pulmonary Emboli

The risks of these diseases are actually significantly increased by bariatric surgery before they are decreased.[24,25] Abdominal surgery adds an additional impediment to venous return by increasing intraabdominal pressure, and the supine and feet-down positions used for bariatric surgery increases the risk of venous stasis and deep venous thrombosis. The release of these clots may cause fatal pulmonary infarction. To avoid this complication, women are advised to stop taking all estrogens and progestogens at least 30 days before surgery and to not restart until 60 days after surgery. Patients with a prior history of deep venous thrombosis or pulmonary emboli are implanted with a Greenfield filter prior to bariatric surgery. All patients are treated with a prophylactic heparin preparation. We usually use Lovenox given as the patient's BMI in milligrams, 6 hours before surgery and every 12 hours after surgery until discharge. Plexi-Pulse or other devices to enhance venous flow are applied immediately after surgery and maintained until the patient is fully ambulatory.

METABOLIC DISEASES

Entire books have been written about the metabolic consequences of obesity, especially diabetes. Only an overview of these diseases can be presented here, along with some information on the effect of the different procedures on these diseases.

Diabetes Mellitus Type 2

Diabetes mellitus type 2 is caused by even mild obesity and can be very severe in the morbidly obese. Treatment of diabetes with insulin and some oral hypoglycemics in the attempt to control blood sugar actually increases fat deposition, increases resistance to treatment (insulin) and stimulates appetite to cause more obesity. Diabetics are especially resistant to medical weight loss treatment[26] because of this hormonal drive to gain more fat. Successful weight loss, regardless of the method of treatment (medical or surgical), results in a marked decrease in insulin requirements to maintain blood sugar because of a marked reduction in insulin resistance. The reason for this reduction of insulin resistance is unclear.[27] Insulin levels decrease far more rapidly than the decrease in weight or even fat mass. The reduction in calories that pass through the gut are thought to reduce some gut hormone secretion that leads to insulin resistance. A more extensive discussion of the hormones involved in weight regulation is given in Chapter 3. The reduction in insulin resistance is reason for the improvement in diabetes control.

Less than 1% of morbidly obese diabetics are able to maintain diet-induced weight loss for more than a year, and diabetes returns rapidly as they regain their weight. Surgery, especially gastric bypass and biliopancreatic bypass, is the cure of diabetes.[28] Food is permanently rerouted from the stomach, and duodenum, which may affect the secretion of ghrelin,[29] reduce appetite and enteroglucagon, and reduce insulin resistance. Gastric restrictive procedures are not as effective in reducing weight in general and have no effect on gut hormones related to the control of diabetes,[26] but do reverse diabetes in patients who lose at least 40% of their excess weight.

For other than mild diabetes (glycated hemoglobin less than 7 to 8) we highly recommend that gastric bypass or biliopancreatic bypass be used to treat morbid obesity. Most diabetes will be cured by these procedures. Those who have had diabetes for more than 20 years and who are on multiple medications may not be cured but will require much less intense treatment to maintain normal blood sugars.

Be prepared for the marked decrease in the number and types of drugs needed to control blood sugar after surgery. In most cases, no treatment other than the gastric bypass diet is need after discharge to maintain blood sugars of less than 180. Usually by 1 month postoperatively blood sugar levels are normal or even low if patients are having difficulty maintaining adequate calorie intake on a regular basis. For this reason, it is better to provide only loose control of blood sugar during this time. Tight control may result in prolonged hypoglycemia that may result in trauma from falling or central nervous system damage from neuroglucopenia.

If treatment is required for several months to keep blood sugars below 180, we recommend that agents that are less likely to cause hypoglycemia be used, including Glucophage or the glitazones. Sulfonylureas or insulin should be avoided. Just as blood sugar is controlled, most of the complications, depending on their severity, are cured, including proliferative diabetic retinopathy, nephropathy, and neuropathy (peripheral and autonomic).

The economic impact on society and the patient of a diabetes cure is tremendous. The costs for drugs, supplies for sugar testing, trips to the physician, and hospital admissions are eliminated. Diabetes can be very debilitating and resolution of this disease can release patients from disability to become productive members of society.

Irregular Menses and Polycystic Ovarian Syndrome

Menstrual irregularities abound in morbidly obese women. The most detrimental is excessive menstrual flow leading to severe anemia. Weight loss can occasionally reduce anemia secondary to these menstrual irregularities, but many times the cause is uterine fibroids or some other malady that could be relieved by a hysterectomy, but cannot be performed because of the risk associated with surgery in morbid obesity. Many gynecologists will require morbidly obese patients to lose 22.7 kg (50 lb), or 45.4 kg (100 lb), or more before they will attempt pelvic surgery because of the increase risk of complications which has been documented in their literature.

Polycystic ovarian syndrome (PCO) is, indeed, a syndrome and not a single disease entity. Some forms of the syndrome are caused by abnormal hormonal profiles during fetal development induced by the environment or genetic anomalies. Some of these cause obesity and are therefore resistant to treatment except by weight loss.[30,31]

If the PCO is not caused by a fetal anomaly or a genetic abnormality, weight loss will cure this syndrome. Insulin levels drop, fat mass decreases, and cycles return. Hirsutism may linger because once the hair follicles are stimulated they are slow to recede. The amount of hair growth will decrease and gradually the number of hair follicles will decrease. Patients who have been morbidly obese since childhood need to be warned that their menstrual cramps may increase dramatically as their menstrual cycles normalize with the return of peaks of estrogen and progesterone in each cycle.

Hyperlipidemia

Lipid metabolism may be a primary genetic defect and completely unresponsive to weight loss. There are many normal-weight people with very severe forms of hypercholesterolemia. For some, only one or two of the multiple gene abnormalities are present and if weight and fat intake were low or normal, there would be no lipid abnormalities. For many, hyperlipidemia is secondary and only a result of excessive fat intake and or secondary to diabetes.

Secondary forms of hypercholesterolemia and mixed hyperlipidemia are cured by weight loss and the change in diet and lifestyles imposed by bariatric surgery. Even gastric restrictive procedures may be effective.[32] More severe forms of hyperlipidemia and those secondary to diabetes are cured by gastric bypass. For those with severe primary hyperlipidemia or milder primary disease exacerbated by obesity, biliopancreatic diversion, long-limb gastric bypass, or a gastric restrictive procedure with a partial ileal bypass may be required to control the lipid abnormalities.[18] The latter two procedures cause some malabsorption of fats to reduce the enterocolic circulation and reabsorption of cholesterol.

If the correct procedure is selected, hyperlipidemias can be cured, or at least better controlled, by bariatric surgery.

Hyperuricemia and Gout

Gout is an inherited disease of abnormal excretion or production of uric acid. Morbid obesity can exacerbate this condition by affecting uric acid metabolism. Foods rich in purines, red meat, organs (liver, sweetbreads), will result increased uric acid production. However, it is more likely that gout is exacerbated more by the treatment of other problems than by diet. Diuretics are the most common offenders; thiazide and loop diuretics impede the excretion of uric acid. In patients with gout, acute arthritic attacks can occur with rapid changes in uric acid levels, especially with intermittent use of diuretics for dependent edema. Hyperuricemia induced by diuretics may result in the development of uric acid renal stones or even uric acid nephropathy. The morbidly obese are more prone to these problems because of intermittent dieting that results in ketosis. Ketones prevent the excretion of uric acid further increasing levels.

Allopurinol may be used to decrease the production of uric acid. If patients truly require a diuretic, indapamide (Lozol) may be used, because it does not increase uric acid levels.

The number and severity of gout attacks will be reduced by weight loss,[33] however, weight loss itself can induce attacks because of the increased production of uric acid from the breakdown of endogenous muscle and the production of ketones from the metabolism of fat. Careful management of gout is needed in the perioperative period to reduce the number and severity of attacks.

Hyperuricemia and uric acid stones can be prevented by eliminating the use of loop or thiazide diuretics, maintaining adequate urine output, minimizing the loss of lean body mass with mild exercise, the intake of low purine protein, and the judicious use of allopurinol.[34]

Dysmetabolic Syndrome

This is a new diagnosis code (277.7), designed to reflect the association of metabolic diseases with morbid obesity. The diagnosis may be used for a patient with morbid obesity who has any combination of metabolic disorders such as hyperlipidemia, diabetes, hyperuricemia, or PCO.[35] The designation is a major step in recognizing that obesity is a metabolic disease and not simply a voluntary lifestyle choice.

MUSCULOSKELETAL

Joint Disease

Morbid obesity has a major impact on the development of pain in the weight-bearing joints, hips, knees, ankles, and feet.[36] Pain that reduces mobility and activity leads to more obesity. The range of disease extends from joints that cause pain after some significant activity, to pain with any activity, to pain at rest. Pain involved with activity is probably more related to tendonitis, fascitis, and injury to cartilage or synovial membranes. This type of pain and disability is remarkably reversed by weight loss, regardless of the method used.[36] Pain with any activity or at rest is usually not reversed by weight loss, and may require surgical intervention with joint replacement or repair. However, weight loss does make these orthopedic procedures easier to perform and the results more durable.

Lack of activity is one of the primary causes of obesity and for its resistance to treatment. It is also one of the most common causes for granting disability payments. Pain medications, use of ambulatory devices, and trips to physicians, physical therapists, and chiropractors place a heavy burden on society and the individual. The economic impact and emotional impact on patients relieved of this disability is tremendous.

Low Back Disease

Like joint disease, low back disease, or back pain, comes in a variety of presentations and reversibility. Back pain that is musculoskeletal, or involves the sacroiliac joints responds remarkably well to weight loss. Degenerative disk disease, osteoarthritis of the facets, or bone spurs are much less responsive. Again, like joint disease, where orthopedic surgery is indicated, patients respond far better after weight loss and have a more durable outcome. Back disease has a much greater prevalence in the obese and is much more disabling than joint disease.

Neuropathy

Neuropathic pain has numerous causes. Sciatica occurs from the pressure on the sciatic nerve from weight or arthritis involving the sciatic notch. Various type of nerve impingement can occur in the back from bone spurs in the nerve canals, disk disease that presses on the spinal cord or nerve roots. Nerves can also be compressed by synovial cysts in the wrist (carpal tunnel syndrome) or even the feet (tarsal tunnel syndrome). Weight and the effect of gravity could exacerbate any of the neuropathies involving the back. The tunnel syndromes are less likely to be related to weight and more likely to be related to certain activities or posture.

GASTROINTESTINAL

Gastroesophageal reflux disease, hiatal hernia, heartburn, and esophagitis are all caused by or exacerbated by morbid obesity. Increased intraabdominal pressure can render the gastroesophageal sphincter incompetent, allowing acidic gastric juices to bathe the esophagus. The discomfort from heartburn, loss of sleep, and the use of multiple drugs—proton pump inhibitors, H_2 blockers, and antacids—can be disabling and expensive. The development of Barrett esophagitis and cancer of the esophagus may be lethal.

Bariatric surgery resolves these problems regardless of the procedure used, but the gastric bypass is most effective.[37] Any procedure or even medical treatment that reduces abdominal girth and the volume of food being consumed will reduce or eliminate heartburn. The gastric bypass has the additional advantage that the acid-producing cells of the mid and distal stomach can no longer reach the esophagus through the divided stomach. Smaller, sliding hiatal hernias require no further intervention to prevent reflux. Because restrictive procedures can still potentially reflux acid into the pouch, and because the sleeve gastrectomy of the biliopancreatic diversion still contains acid-secreting cells, these procedures are less well-suited to the treatment of the more severe forms of reflux disease.

Steatosis of the Liver

Fatty liver or steatosis is a common consequence of morbid obesity[38] that is further exacerbated by hyperlipidemia. For the most part, it is a rather benign condition.[39] Fat is lost rapidly from the liver with weight loss by any means. However, steatosis can become severe and cause cirrhosis, and eventually liver failure, if left unchecked, or if an additional chemical insult, such as alcohol, is encountered.

An enlarged liver masquerading as steatosis may actually be a more silent cirrhosis with portal hypertension. Cirrhosis is a relative contradiction and cirrhosis with portal hypertension is an absolute contraindication to bariatric surgery.

Cholelithiasis

The incidence of cholelithiasis in morbidly obese patients is approximately 25 to 30%.[40,41] The solubility of bile salts is reduced when overweight, gaining weight, or reducing weight, leading to sludge and eventual stone formation. Defective gall bladders, even if asymptomatic should be removed if bariatric surgery is being performed. The risk of acute cholecystitis after bariatric surgery is high. The treatment, a second intraabdominal surgery during the early postoperative recovery phase, causes higher risks to the patient than having a single procedure. The consequences of gallstone-induced pancreatitis during this period could result in very prolonged hospitalization and even death.

If the gall bladder is normal, it is not routinely removed, but the incidence of developing gallstones is approximately 30% when losing weight following gastric bypass surgery. Actigall given at 300 mg q.i.d. reduces the risk of developing cholelithiasis to approximately 1 to 2%. Actigall should be taking throughout the time that the patient is losing a significant amount of weight (2.3 kg [5 lb] per month or more).[40]

Hemorrhoids

Morbid obesity and other causes of increased abdominal pressure, such as pregnancy, increase the incidence of hemorrhoids. If thrombosis has not occurred in the vein, weight loss may reduce the pressure enough to avoid the need for surgical resection.

PSYCHOLOGICAL

There are numerous issues intertwined with psychological problems and morbid obesity. Sexual, physical, and mental abuse as a child can lead to the development of morbid obesity. Depression can cause obesity secondary to using food to cope with certain problems. Depression can result from the development of obesity and its medical and social complications and lack of self-esteem. Addictive behaviors may use food to satisfy certain cravings. Personality disorders, bipolar psychosis,[42] and schizophrenia can occur in the morbidly obese without any cause or effect.

Depression caused by obesity is cured by weight loss.[43] None of the other disorders is necessarily improved by weight loss and some may be contraindications to bariatric surgery. For surgery to be successful patients must be able to follow treatment protocols. Most patients with psychoses such as schizophrenia, and many with severe personality disorder, are unlikely to be able to meet that criterion. Patients with severe addictive behaviors may have substituted food for alcohol or drugs. If food is removed, they may revert to these old habits. Although not an absolute contraindication, these patients should be in therapy and assurance provided by their therapist that they are under control and that the therapist will provide continued treatment if exacerbated by weight loss.

In addition to interviews by a clinical psychologist and medical social worker, testing is performed to assess the patient's psychosocial status. This is vital to avoid doing more harm to some patients, or recognizing those that should undergo more psychological therapy or drug treatment to enhance their ability to cope with the many changes that occur following bariatric surgery.

CONCLUSIONS

There are many comorbid diseases and conditions related to morbid obesity. Some of the most prominent comorbid conditions and the improvements seen after surgery have been presented but others, such as psoriasis, pseudotumor cerebri, renal insufficiency,[44] and glaucoma, have also shown improvement in small series. Clearly, obesity and its comorbid diseases have a profound and increasing effect on the individuals affected and the society to which they belong. Medical treatment of obesity has an extremely low success rate, whereas bariatric surgery has a very high success rate.[45] Better access to surgical treatment for adults and children is essential to control the obesity epidemic.

REFERENCES

1. Sjostrom CD, Lissner L, Wedel H, Sjostrom L. Reduction in the incidence of diabetes, hypertension, and lipid disturbances after intentional weight reduction by bariatric surgery: the SOS intervention study. *Obes Res* 1999;7:477–484.
2. Torgerson JS. The Swedish Obese Subjects (SOS) study. What does weight loss really accomplish? *Fortschr Med* 2002:144(40):24–26.
3. Rubino F, Gagner M. Potential of surgery for curing type 2 diabetes mellitus. *Ann Surg* 2002;236(5):554–559.
4. Sjostrom CD, Peltonen M, Wedel H, Sjostrom L. Differentiated long-term effects of intentional weight loss on diabetes and hypertension. *Hypertension* 2000;36:20–25.
5. Pontiroli AE, Pizzocri P, Librenti MC, et al. Laparoscopic adjustable gastric banding for the treatment of morbid (grade 3) obesity and its medical complications: a three years study. *J Clin Endocrinol Metab* 2002;87(8):3555–3561.
6. Arribas del Amo D, Elia Guedea MN, Aguilella Diago V, Martinez Diez M. Effect of vertical banded gastroplasty on hypertension, diabetes, and dyslipidemia. *Obes Surg* 2002;12(3):319–323.
7. Stubbs RS, Wickremesekera SK. Insulin resistance in the severely obese and links with, metabolic comorbidities. *Obes Surg* 2002;12(3):343–348.
8. Scopinaro N, Gianetta E, Civalleri D. Biliopancreatic bypass for obesity: I. Initial experiences in man. *Br J Surg* 1979;66:618–620.
9. Scheen AJ. Results of obesity treatment. *Ann Endocrinol (Paris)* 2002;63(2 pt 1):163–170.
10. Martin LF, Raum WJ. What will society's response be to the obesity epidemic? *Prog Obes Res* 2003;9:591–595.

11. Olejniczak PW, Fisch BJ. Sleep disorders. *Med Clin North Am* 2003;87:803–833.

12. Dhabuwala A, Cannan RJ, Stubbs RS. Improvement in comorbidities following weight loss from gastric bypass surgery. *Obes Surg* 2000;10(5):428–435.

13. Rasheid S, Banasiak M, Gallagher SF, Lipska A, et al. Gastric bypass is an effective treatment for obstructive sleep apnea in patients with clinically significant obesity. *Obes Surg* 2003;13(1):58–61.

14. Kessler R, Chaoutat A, Schinkewitch P, et al. The obesity-hypoventilation syndrome revisited: a prospective study of 34 consecutive cases. *Chest* 2001;120(2):369–376.

15. Sugerman HJ, Fairman RP, Sood RK, Engle K, Wolfe L, Kellum JM. Long-term effects of gastric surgery for treating respiratory insufficiency of obesity. *Am J Clin Nutr* 1992;55(2 suppl):597S–601S.

16. Dixon JB, Chapman L, O'Brien P. Marked improvement in asthma after Lap-Band surgery for morbid obesity. *Obes Surg* 1999;9(4):385–389.

17. Karason K, Lindroos AK, Stenlof K, Sjostrom L. Relief of cardiorespiratory symptoms and increased physical activity after surgically induced weight loss: results from the Swedish Subjects study. *Arch Intern Med* 2000;160(12):1797–1802.

18. Buchwald H, Schone JL. Gastric obesity surgery combined with partial ileal bypass for hypercholesterolemia. *Obes Surg* 1997;7:313–316.

19. Karason K, Wikstrand J, Sjostrom L, Wendelhag I. Weight loss and progression of early atherosclerosis in the carotid artery: a four-year controlled study of obese subjects. *Int J Obes* 1999;23:948–955.

20. Alexander JH, Greenbaum AB, Hudson MP, et al. Session highlighted from the American College of Cardiology Scientific Sessions: March 29 to April 1, 1998. *Am Heart J* 1998;136(1):176–179.

21. Rashid MN, Fuentes F, Touchon RC, Wehner PS. Obesity and the risk for cardiovascular disease. *Prev Cardiol* 2003;6(1):42–47.

22. Alpert MA. Management of obesity cardiomyopathy. *Am J Med Sci* 2001;321(4);237–241.

23. Karason K, Wallentin I, Larsson B, Sjostrom L. Effects of obesity and weight loss on left ventricular mass and wall thickness: survey and intervention study. *BMJ* 1997;315:912–916.

24. Wu EC, Barba CA. Current practices in the prophylaxis if venous thromboembolis in bariatric surgery. *Obes Surg* 2000;10(1):7–13, discussion 14.

25. Scholten DJ, Hoedema RM, Scholten SE. A comparison of two different prophylactic dose regimens of low-molecular-weight heparin in bariatric surgery. *Obes Surg* 2002;12(1):19–24.

26. Greenway SE, Greenway FL 3rd, Klein S. Effects of obesity surgery on non–insulin-dependent diabetes mellitus. *Arch Surg* 2002;137(10):1109–1117.

27. Pories WJ, Albrecht RJ. Etiology of type II diabetes mellitus: role of the foregut. *World J Surg* 2001;25(4):527–531.

28. Sugerman HJ. Bariatric surgery for severe obesity. *J Assoc Acad Minor Phys* 2001;12(3):129–136.

29. Cummings DE, Weigle DS, Frayo RS, et al. Plasma ghrelin levels after diet-induced weight loss or gastric bypass surgery. *N Engl J Med* 2002;346:1623–1630.

30. Hoeger K. Obesity and weight loss in polycystic ovary syndrome. *Obstet Gynecol Clin North Am* 2001;28(1):85–97, vi–vii.

31. Pasquali R, Gambineri A, Biscotti D, et al. Effect of long-term treatment with metformin added to hypocaloric diet on body composition, fat distribution, and androgen and insulin levels in abdominally obese women with and without the polycystic ovary syndrome. *J Clin Endocrinol Metab* 2000;85(8):2767–2774.

32. Bacci V, Basso MS, Greco F, et al. Modifications of metabolic and cardiovascu-

lar risk factors after weight loss induced by laparoscopic gastric banding. *Obes Surg* 2002;12(1):77–82.

33. Pi-Sunyer FX. A review of long-term studies evaluating the efficiency of weight loss in ameliorating disorders associated with obesity. *Clin Ther* 1996;18(6): 1006–1035, discussion 1005.

34. Emmerson BT. The management of gout. *N Engl J Med* 1996;15;334(7):445–451.

35. Adami GF, Ravera GM, Marinari GM, Camerini G, Scopinaro N. Metabolic syndrome in severely obese patients. *Obes Surg* 2001;11(5):543–545.

36. McGoey BV, Deitel M, Saplys RJ, Kliman ME. Effect of weight loss on musculoskeletal pain in the morbidly obese. *J Bone Joint Surg Br* 1990;72:322–323.

37. Jones KB Jr, Allen TV, Manas KJ, et al. Roux-en-Y gastric bypass: an effective anti-reflux procedure. *Obes Surg* 1991;1(3):295–298.

38. Dixon JB, Bhathal PS, O'Brien PE. Nonalcoholic fatty liver disease: predictors of nonalcoholic steatohepatitis and liver fibrosis in the severely obese. *Gastroenterology* 2001;121(1):91–100.

39. Ramsey-Stewart G. Hepatic steatosis and morbid obesity. *Obes Surg* 1993; 3(2):157–159.

40. Sugerman HJ, Brewer WH, Shiffman ML, Brolin RE, et al. A multicenter, placebo-controlled, randomized, double-blind, prospective trial of prophylactic ursodiol for the prevention of gallstone formation following gastric-bypass-induced rapid weight loss. *Am J Surg* 1995;169(1):91–96, discussion 96–97.

41. Abu Abeid S, Szold A, Gavert N, et al. Apolipoprotein-E genotype and the risk of developing cholelithiasis following bariatric surgery: a clue to prevention of routine prophylactic cholecystectomy. *Obes Surg* 2002;12(3):354–357.

42. McElroy SL, Frye MA, Suppes T, et al. Correlates of overweight and obesity in 644 patients with bipolar disorder. *J Clin Psychiatry* 2002;63(3):207–213.

43. Holzarth R, Huber D, Majkrzak A, Tareen B. Outcome of gastric bypass patients. *Obes Surg* 2002;12(2):261–264.

44. Cohen AH. Pathology of renal complications in obesity. *Curr Hypertens Rep* 1999;1(2):137–139.

45. Barrow CJ. Roux-en-Y gastric bypass for morbid obesity. *AORN J* 2002; 76(4):590, 593–604.

Page numbers followed by *f* or *t* denote figures or tables, respectively.